Group Work Reaching Out: People, Places and Power

The *Social Work with Groups* series

• *Group Work Reaching Out: People, Places and Power,* James
  A. Garland, Guest Editor

For information on previous issues of the *Social Work with Groups* series, edited by Catherine P. Papell and Beulah Rothman, please contact: The Haworth Press, Inc., 10 Alice Street, Binghamton, NY 13904

Group Work Reaching Out: People, Places and Power

James A. Garland
Editor

The Haworth Press, Inc.
New York • London • Norwood (Australia)

Group Work Reaching Out: People, Places and Power has also been published as *Social Work with Groups,* Volume 15, Numbers 2/3 1992.

The Haworth Press, Inc., 10 Alice Street, Binghamton, NY 13904-1580, USA

Library of Congress Cataloging-in-Publication Data

Group work reaching out : people, places and power / James A. Garland, editor.
p. cm.
Also published as : Social work with groups, v. 15, nos. 2/3 1992.
Papers presented at the Ninth Symposium, Group Work Reaching Out.
Includes bibliographical references and index.
ISBN 1-56024-304-X (acid free paper)
1. Social group work–Congresses. 2. Social group work–United States–Congresses. I. Garland, James A.
HV45.G7315 1992
361.4–dc20
92-20870
CIP

Group Work Reaching Out:
People, Places and Power

CONTENTS

POWER

ABOUT THE EDITOR

James A. Garland, MSSS, is Professor at the Boston University School of Social Work, Boston, Massachusetts, where he has chaired the Group Work and Human Behavior Sequences. He is consultant to a variety of public and voluntary agencies on the practice of social and clinical group work, program development and organizational development. He is known for his writing and teaching on group developmental theory. Mr. Garland is engaged in the independent practice of group work. He is President of the Association for the Advancement of Social Work with Groups, an international professional organization, and currently serves on the Clinical Commission of the National Association of Social Workers.

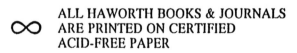

Group Work Reaching Out: People, Places and Power

Introduction

The theme of the Ninth Symposium, Group Work Reaching Out, grew out of concerns expressed in several previous symposia and in the human service field in general that, in the decade of the 1980s, neither the quantity nor the quality of professionally directed group services were sufficient to meet the emerging social conditions and crises facing large segments of populations in North America and worldwide. In a positive light, there is agreement that group work has experienced increased, albeit often sporadic, interest on the part of a variety of caregivers for responding to an array of problems in the clinical, educational and rehabilitative sectors. Groups are viewed in many cases to be the treatment of choice for victims and perpetrators of abuse and for those enslaved by addictions to chemicals or to pathological relationships. They are used in both educational and corrective settings as tools for controlling disruptive and anti-social behavior. They are mobilized, often in "warehousing" fashion, to provide care for a whole range of deinstitutionalized, chronic clients in an era of shrinking financial resources. And they are purported to be taught in professional training programs, social work prominent among them, as part of a "multimethod" or "generic" preparation for practice.

Yet, as the Planning Committee consulted together, questions such as the following proliferated:

- Are our models for practice sufficiently articulated to relate to emergent needs, and are we teaching them to our students?
- Have group workers become unable or unwilling to move out of their offices to encounter and work with clients in their "natural" ground?
- Are we making group work accessible to alienated, isolated, ethnically diverse, poor and stigmatized people?
- Have we deserted neighborhoods, both as places in which to give help and as fragmented small societies in need of reconstruction?
- Have we deserted institutional living milieus as arenas for scientific analysis and professional intervention in favor of only selected, boundaried "talking therapy" groups?
- Are we open to and knowledgeable about radically different power relationships between citizens and governments and between ourselves and our citizen-clients?

1

The Committee, therefore, cast a broad net as it proposed criteria for submission of papers and workshop proposals related to the theme and to the questions. The response was large and impressive (one hundred seventy-five) and resulted in one hundred presentations, out of which fifty-six were gleaned as written, relevant and offered for publication. Selecting twenty of them for inclusion in this volume was not an easy or painless task. All were thoroughly reviewed for quality, relevance to the central themes and representativeness in terms of populations, settings, geographic locales, problem entities, program innovations, conceptual frameworks and the like. Attention was paid as well to authors: new and well-known; geographic, cultural, ethnic, and gender distribution; practitioners and teachers, etc. Many of those not chosen were deemed fully deserving of publication and, in fact, several will have been so recognized both in regular editions of *Social Work with Groups* and in other professional journals by the time that this collection has come into print (an aspect of the vagaries of succeeding Symposium committees lining up to wait their turn, once they activated their own, local "amateur" teams).

All who worked on the Ninth Symposium Committee, whether they ensured the excellence of the program event, oversaw the amenities of the weekend, or, through refereeing, advising and editing, participated in the process that produced this book, are to be commended. Cathie Rocheleau is especially to be thanked for handling the myriad administrative and secretarial functions, indispensable to Symposium and book, with intelligence and skill. They, as did the authors, kept faith with the intent of the Symposium. It is our hope and belief that the following twenty papers, two serving as *overview* and introduction, six focused on *people*, six on *places* and six on *power*, will reflect that commitment and will be of use to planners and practitioners as social group work moves into the decade of the nineties.

The *Overview* introduction of the Symposium and of this collection, presented by Judith Lee, is a stirring call to social workers to value their own classical and emergent theoretical perspectives and practice forms and to honor their activist history. She offers group work values and methods as an antidote to the current slide into alienation, reawakened class and racial/ethnic strife and anti-democratic sentiments and actions. Papell focuses on the knowledge-building side of the equation with specific application to "new" populations, both those who are literally newly arrived in our culture (e.g., Southeast Asians, etc.), and those who are newly identified, such as the homeless, AIDS patients, or incest survivors. She reviews the value of empirical research and of a "world view" that looks at the nature of knowledge and allows for speculation and intuitive investigation as being essential to creative outreach.

The section of the book devoted to *People* was most difficult to cull because of the number of articles submitted that often pitted one population group against another. How does one choose among Vietnamese high school girls, Israeli prison inmates and Bedouin of the Negev desert? Nevertheless, we did. Blitstein leads off this section with a conceptually solid and methodologically dramatic account of the process of empowering mentally retarded and developmentally disabled adults in a residential (intermediate care) group residence. His account of the evolution "from narcissism to team spirit" at Hull House, starting with self-absorbed, dependent, adult "kids" who were challenged to grow through phases into grown up responsible group members speaks both to individual and collective psychology. Chau's discussion of the culture-based elements of needs assessment for people of color as related to group work referral and practice is an intricate and complex formulation. Each major life issue (e.g., role-status changes) is related theoretically and through case example to individual, intragroup, intergroup and systems levels. Employing a task centered, time limited (twice a week for six weeks), goal oriented group approach with chronically mentally ill adults, Garvin employs some familiar "fun" activities (i.e., board games) to reach concrete interpersonal ends. Of particular value in an era of accountability and search for more accurate measures of practice is his employment of empirical measures, explained in clear language, to evaluate every step in the process. Kacen, Anson, Nir and Livneh report on group work with Bedouin young men and young women about to finish high school. Using both a group dynamic and anthropologic analysis in the context of rapidly changing social, political and economic conditions in Israel, they illustrate ethnically sensitive practice as they help these young people to integrate the dramatically different frames of reference and value systems of which they are a part. The case might be said to verge on the exotic; the lessons to be learned are universal. Lovell, Reid and Richey describe a twelve-week, educationally based support group for low-income abusive mothers. Unlike many *parenting* groups, this model focuses on the interpersonal relationships of the individual members themselves (i.e., vs. the increasing use of even shorter groups to pump in "skills of parenting" without regard for the women as persons). Enjoyable metaphorical games are employed to illustrate friendship stages. Although the groups happen in the context of very adequate support programs at the agency, the authors conclude, as do most workers who become knowledgeable in this area, that longer term support groups concurrent with and subsequent to the time limited programs, should be offered.

Louis Lowy, a dynamic leader in the field of gerontology and in group work, died before the publication of this book. His article, a *tour de force* on intergenerational relationships in group work with the elderly may serve as a posthumous testament to a lifetime that began with surviving the Nazi death camps in Europe and moved on to the achievement of a brilliant career on two continents, of writing, teaching and advocacy for excellence in practice and sanctification of human dignity. His chapter serves as well as a passionate finale to the section devoted to people.

The beginning paper in the third of the collection devoted to *Places* is about reaching inner city children in public middle school. True to Bilides' extensive practice background, it offers rich detail on the process of group work, a realistic appraisal of the difficult realities of the setting and a lucid description and conceptual structure for a multi-faceted group program suited to the various needs, capacities and interests of the youngsters for whom and by whom it was designed. A true group work *connector*, Bilides gives credit to everyone else who helped him. Goldberg and Lamont's study of whether and how an MSW graduate's interest and skill fare after she/he has experienced an integrated practice curriculum is the third in a series of empirical investigations on the subject. It speaks to the previously cited question of whether "new" social workers are being adequately prepared to work with groups. Although final judgements on the matter must be made by the reader, the evidence amassed by the practitioner/researchers suggests that the integrated curriculum may not be doing what it was intended to do. Kolodny's retrospective analysis on intensive, long term neighborhood-based group work with socially isolated children is at once an almost poetic memoir and an insightful reminder. It speaks to the efficacy of the use of real life experiences as a powerful therapeutic tool. It also speaks to a reality that is rediscovered about every five or ten years: that even clinically based treatment is feasible in a natural street corner setting. A real contrast to the street corner is Moore and Starkes' conceptual study of the group in the residential institution. This analysis, the latest in Moore's series of investigations into the subject, is systemic, based on values of client self-determination and, in the editor's mind, represents a definitive statement on a paradigm for understanding the individual, the group and the institution. Highlighting the setting typical of those wherein the social group held sway for many decades and where it evolved its identity, its philosophy and much of its technology, Ramey addresses the current plight of group work in neighborhood centers, using an exploratory and qualitative method to gather data on the subject. In an era when community-based, skillfully conceived group approaches might be crucial to treatment, growth, support and activism, Ramey surveys both the lack of professional group work involvement and the potential still inherent in this crucially situated "place." One of the few to focus on group work in the industrial workplace, Wegener's paper offers a comprehensive review of the needs of working people at work, the potential functions that may be played by group work and the ethical, logistical, clinical and political issues that are involved in conceiving, initiating and carrying out a group work program. In addition to reviewing developmental, treatment and work-related stress foci, Wegener introduces the possibility of groups influencing the setting itself — a possibility distressingly absent from most employer-financed programs.

Opening the papers focussing on *Power* is Behroozi's generic model for defining the nature of involuntary participation in groups. His investigation into the ethical, strategic, technical and theoretical considerations of the issue is comprehensive and aimed eventually at helping the involuntary applicant, wherever feasible, "to transform to clienthood, (i.e.,) voluntary membership." It is an exceptionally clear conceptual statement. Berman-Rossi's study of empowerment of groups is applied in the context of evolution in group systems. She analyzes several models of group development as well as the role of authority and power in groups in general. Her articulate and detailed treatment of the phenomenon and implications for worker activity elaborates and adds significantly to work previously done on the topic. Addressing directly the rights of the poor and oppressed to hold power and to exert it in the community, Breton presents a radical position on the function of the social worker. She rejects the concept of a social work dominion or of benevolent protection, therapy or tutoring. Rather, drawing on analysis of liberation theology, she sees reaching out as acknowledging the political and psychological reality of oppression and focussing on "re-enfranchising" the poor as they reclaim their rights to participate in their communities. Group workers are urged to eschew traditional reciprocal and social action models, and to adopt a political action model to truly challenge the power structure. Lewis presents a detailed review of the ways in which knowledge and values coming out of feminist studies and practice can benefit social group work practice in general and vulnerable populations in particular. She notes that the historic qualities of social group work were related to "equality, participation and self and societal fulfillment." The case made in the paper is powerful, compassionate and extremely well-reasoned. Many of the general concepts and principles of empowerment elucidated in the general papers are made explicit and concrete in Mandell and Postel's account of how a group of black mothers confronted a group-worker and a child treatment agency as they moved to achieve "consumer control." It also provides an intimate view of the personal reactions of the African-American, male worker, hired especially to work with these mothers, and how he grew, with the assistance of a Caucasian female graduate student, to work cooperatively with the mothers as they "took on" the agency on behalf of themselves and their children. The vibrancy of this case makes us aware of how few practice papers like this we managed to generate for the Symposium and for this publication. The final offering in the collection raises the investigation to a nationwide level as Wilson describes how a social service system was created to serve a revolutionary, socialist system in Nicaragua. Sweeping away a prerevolutionary, clinical orientation, the new social system approach, as implemented in the national school of social work and in the government bureaucracy, focused on the transformation of the structure and practices of society. Its mission stressed equality, the shaping of society by the people ("workers and peasants") and struggles against imperialist principles, a reference to historic domination by outside political entities and their collaborators. Western liberals might raise questions about the place of the individual in all of this and the role of help with personal problems. Wilson notes that social workers are allowed to provide help to individuals, families, small groups, institutions and communities. Research is also supported. The reader is invited to view the details and ponder on how many of our desires to effect social change might correspond to this mode. While some might be reluctant to enter into such a marriage, honest study of a continuum of possibilities compels us to become familiar with models such as the one related by Wilson.

James A. Garland

OVERVIEWS

Jane Addams in Boston:
Intersecting Time and Space

Judith A. B. Lee

My charge is to address "The State of the World and the State of Social Work with Groups." I will do this from the point of view where we are and where we have been, hence my retitling. The Association For the Advancement of Social Work with Groups exists because social workers who know what social group work is want to make sure it has vitality in these times, that it is not lost, or bastardized or changed beyond recognition. And, most of all, that it regains the momentum and force to have an impact in our world.

We as social workers with groups possess more than a bundle of technologies. The knowledge of group dynamics, group processes, group psychology, and group skills are an important part of our technological equipment, but they also belong to anybody. Gisela Konopka in her comments on Nazi Germany has well pointed out that groups can be used for good or evil. Ruth Middleman has described the use of the small group in the business world in Japan (Middleman, 1983; Marks, 1986). Recently my

Judith A. B. Lee, PhD, is Professor at the University of Connecticut School of Social Work, West Hartford, CT.

young neighbor who is employed by an insurance company gave me an astonishing treatise on groups used for the ultimate purposes of productivity.

Further, the inappropriate and poor use of individual psychology applied to groups, and racial, gender, and class biases in some of the literature on groups is astounding! For example, a group therapy book, (Gibbard, Hartman and Mann, 1976) describes the "group leader as oedipal father" (regardless of gender) and the group members as "the mothers" or the "ever waiting potentially symbiotic mother" (regardless of gender, group purpose, composition, differential individual and group development and a host of other factors). This group worker (well versed in psychoanalytic theory and its offshoots) will never be taken for a father, oedipal or otherwise, and will never see her group members, different individuals after all, as a symbiotic undifferentiated maternal mass. Theorizing about groups requires a new pair of lenses — an appreciation for the "groupness" before us.

It is ridiculous to analyze a group without awareness of person, environment transactions and social context, as done in a later chapter by an author who saw group members' requests of the worker for intervention with the welfare department as "dependent feelings (that) also reflected exaggerated feelings of helplessness" (Gibbard et al., 1976). (Did the author ever try to negotiate the welfare system?) He also saw the scapegoating of one of the two "Negro patients in the group" (his words) as an expression of acting out toward the therapist "in symbolic terms." And, he noted that in the male therapist's planned absence "the two female patients who showed up were dressed in slacks," (another astounding observation!). The theme of the meeting was around the powerful role of mothers as compared to the inadequacy of fathers and of their preference for the female group leader. This was seen as a manifestation of the ambivalence felt toward the male therapist, who was "the dominant leader" of the two therapists.

Giving such a "definitive" explanation for such complex behavior displays, at best, a sense of therapeutic and theoretical egocentricity. There is more to the world than the "here and now" of the therapy group and its "dominant therapist." Clients' lives are more than transference and the real concerns of living *are* grist for the mill in social work practice and critically important. First year students quickly learn to keep "one eye on the content and one eye on the process." Experienced workers see the connection between the two, but hold on to both.

Much group therapy theory (Yalom, 1970) focuses on the group's "here and now" to the exclusion of the content and context of people's lives. Many of us were appalled as we listened to Yalom speak at the NASW Clinical Conference in San Francisco, Sept. 1986 as hundreds of social workers, eager for some knowledge of group work, listened to this approach. The group, in the examples, was only a backdrop. In one example, a battered married woman was trying to tell a specific recent abusive incident and was asked to respond only to what was going on with her and the therapist "here and now." Such group therapists have a lot to learn from social workers who work with groups and are anchored in the mandate of this profession to maintain "dual simultaneous concern with people and environments." We must challenge the use of the group for manipulative means and ends, be they desired by coercive elements of society, by the business community, or by therapists and a range of well-intentioned helpers.

THE TRENDS

The societal and world trends that I will address are: the effects of our super-industrial era on human relatedness; the persistence of oppression based on social class and difference; the increased loss of power to the working person; and the ever present threat of nuclear disaster, an eminent attraction for the here and now mentality. Our heritage, methods, and skills equip us to deal with this level of complexity.

OUR HERITAGE – PEACE, BREAD AND POWER

We are a proud people, the children and legacy of Jane Addams, of her sisters, and brothers, and thereby the inheritors of the settlement movement, the women's movement and the peace movement, of a passion for social equality, social justice and social reform, of a respect for difference and the richness of diverse cultures, and of world consciousness and responsibility (Addams, 1922, 1930). We are the great-great-grandchildren of a woman who never had children, who lived with a woman, among the poor, in a house full of women, and some men, who gave their lives to working with oppressed groups so that reciprocity and a fair share of resources might flow between the classes here and throughout the world (Addams, 1910).

We are the legacy of a woman who came to Boston in September 1914 as President of the "Woman's Peace Party" to help organize women (2500 were present in Boston), to address issues of "Peace and Bread In

Time of War." She saw peace and the meeting of basic human needs as inseparably connected. She tapped into women's sense of relatedness and believed in the power women could have to "make public opinion both for reasonable peace terms and for a possible shortening of the war" (Addams, 1922). She said, "We revolted not only against the cruelty and barbarity of war but even more against the reversal of human relationships which was implied. . . . We were . . . certain that if war prevailed, all social efforts would be cast into an earlier and coarser mold" (Addams, 1922). This peace movement was started "early in the Fall of 1914 when a small group of social workers held a meeting at the Henry Street Settlement in New York, trying to formulate the reaction to war on the part of those who . . . had devoted their energies to the reduction of devastating poverty" (Addams, 1922). From these meetings the Women's International League For Peace and Freedom developed with Jane Addams at its head. She was awarded the Nobel Peace Prize and was the first woman and the first American to be so awarded.

The threats of nuclear extinction with which we live are more frightening and global than Jane Addams could ever have envisioned. We are a finger away from annihilation as we are at War in the Persian Gulf and in Central America and as we prepare for "Star Wars." Our social inequities are so great that we may be on the verge of another Great Depression (Batra, 1987). Addams' connection between the military industrial mentality and basic human needs is equally astute now.

Yet we must note that a difference in Addams and the social workers of today is that she occupied the power position of the "well born wealthy." We, with our clients, need to gain access to that power. Many of us are the children of the immigrant groups she served, the children of the poor who experienced settlement houses and Ys and Camps as consumers of the service. We are a profession of people who know oppression firsthand — the oppressions of religion and race, of caste and of class, the oppressions of gender and of difference. We can not forget what it's like to be left out; to be freezing cold in the winter and unable to escape heat in the summer; to be without in a land of plenty for some and none for others; to live, as a young friend of mine says, "in the ghetto, where you get none, till you get out and you get some." (If you're lucky.) The emphasis we have on groups, says, "we can do it together."

We are not your ordinary social workers, we are your rebels who insist on blending cause and function, (Schwartz, 1959; Germain and Gitterman, 1980); your superb clinicians who abhor the I-It relationship implied in the words therapist, patient, and treatment, and prefer words like guest or member or neighbor, when even the word client conveys immeasurable social distance (Tropp, 1967). We are your holistic thinkers in a fragmented age (Schwartz, 1974), your die hards who will not let go of the poor and who still believe we will all rise up together, or not at all (Lee, 1988).

Among us are those George Getzel called the "righteous gentiles of the new Holocaust," which means that we give priority to practice with oppressed groups. George Getzel is one such "righteous gentile" in the struggle against AIDS. We, in the gay community, embrace him and his work with groups as a brother. Yet, we are here in Boston where recent legislative decisions mean that Jane Addams, and a host of other past and present social work leaders could have never cared for a foster child, where at least one-tenth of the population who are gay would be denied the privilege of parenting while children go waiting and where "Boston marriages" are now open. We are in New England, where the Connecticut Legislature failed once again to pass the "Gay Rights" bill. We are in America where doctors still refuse to treat patients with AIDS, and where the infant mortality rates among minority groups rival that of so called undeveloped countries. This age of misguided moralism is like that of the progressive era that called forth the outraged leadership of Jane Addams and her kin. This is also an era in which invisible minorities have become visible and can now be discriminated against openly. I guess that's progress! Other newly visible groups are the families of alcoholics, including "ACOAs" and the survivors of incest including "AMACs" and the mentally ill and their families in self-help networks.

VIOLENCE – DIFFERENCE AND OPPRESSION

We are here in Boston where Mary Follett lived and worked at the Roxbury Neighborhood House, and campaigned for legislation for Boston After School Centers (Brandwein, 1987), later developing a significant group work theory base. The well known Boston University Model flows from these Settlement House roots, as well as from their famous youth workers and stage development theoreticians, Garland, Kolodny and Jones, and their grandmaster, Saul Bernstein. Yet Roxbury is known as a code word for a poor black community even as South Boston is known as a working class Irish stronghold. "South Boston High" was a symbol of Northern racism for years though more recently harmony has been won by kids whose parents were, earlier, against bussing. Boston is a symbolic microcosm of the ever strong existing tensions between people of difference, and of the need for oppressed groups to come together in unity. The Irish history of oppression persists until this day in Northern Ireland, though assimilating is now possible for most Irish Americans. As we remember how oppression feels, we are moved to compassion, not competition or disdain of other oppressed groups. This same kind of racial tension burst into open conflict in New York City this summer where a black man was killed when his car ran out of gas in the all white Howard Beach, Queens. The signs on the placards of the protests that followed this were the same as we saw in Mississippi in the early 1960s. Racial struggle hasn't gone anywhere but underground. It has to emerge again.

THE GRAVEST SITUATION

Group work has historically been active in the struggles for racial justice and in promoting intergroup communication. The Ys, the Settlement and Neighborhood Houses, and Jewish Community Centers have led in this struggle. Some of our legacy in this area has come down to us through the early writings of group work leaders, like Helen Northen's work with the YWCA (Northen, 1968); and Wilson and Ryland's focus on dealing with "Interracial Relations" through group work (1949). Ivor Echols, Ruby Pernell, Larry Davis, Ken Chau and others continue to instruct us on outreach, on the racial composition of groups, and other ethnic sensitive group practices (Davis, 1980). Danielle Nisivoccia notes that in her Job Preparation groups in a New York Settlement House, a predominant theme of the Black and Hispanic young adults she worked with was "dealing with racism in a white world," and "dealing with the white man on the job." The mutual aid process, the role play, the give and take created an opportunity for dialogue and problem solving that is denied most low income minority youth and most workers. Jewelle Taylor Gibbs (1984) has noted that black youth are an "endangered species." The lack of employment opportunities and the lack of hope is strongly related to this. Jane Addams knew a great deal about youth in general and poor youth in particular. She describes cocaine addicted youth, physically and emotionally abused young women, and alienated young factory workers. Hull House posed alternatives for such youth, much as Edd Lee's Seneca Center does in New York. As Addams noted, "We may either smother the divine fire of youth or we may feed it" (Addams, 1912).

Jane Addams was dedicated to racial justice established in dialogue with the Black community. In their article "A Profile of Black Female

Social Welfare leaders During the 1920s," Robenia and Lawrence Gary documented the social welfare leadership of fifty-six Black women. Noting that the "Black church, mutual aid and fraternal organizations were the major social welfare institutions of the Black community," they emphasize that Black women played important roles in these organizations. They also documented that Black women's clubs worked cooperatively with white women, including Jane Addams. "White and Black women worked together to find jobs and decent homes for Black immigrants, open playgrounds for Black children, breakdown the color barriers in employment, improve health and to protect Black domestics from exploitation of employment agencies" (Gary and Gary, 1975).

One of the important areas of dialogue at Hull House was "Race Relations." Addams recognized the role of economic oppression: ". . . We cannot truthfully say, however much we should like to say, that . . . Worthy will be worthily received. To make even the existing degree of recognition more general requires first of all a modicum of leisure and freedom from grueling poverty." Addams went on to describe an investigation made in 1929 which gives an analysis of Black women in industry from studies made in fifteen states. Like today, their earnings were found to be far below the earnings of most White women. (It does not speak of White men.) She goes on, "Because we are no longer stirred . . . to remove fetters, to prevent cruelty . . . we have allowed ourselves to become indifferent to the *gravest situation in American life*" (Addams, 1930). (I underscore her emphasis.)

Incidents like the killing in Howard Beach happen as the economically oppressed turn against the racially and economically oppressed in the competition for increasingly scarce resources like jobs and housing. Youth from these communities also may indulge in a sport called "gay bashing" where they seek out gay people to attack violently, another growing national shame.

The work with the homeless and hungry, of Margo Breton in Canada and of many others state-side, attests to another violence, to the widespread oppression of the poorest of the poor, particularly in the area of affordable housing and provision for basic human needs (Lee, 1988). There is no doubt that this reflects basic structural flaws to which we must attend (Batra, 1987; Ryan, 1971). William Ryan's story of cholera and the pump describes well the frustration we feel working at the bottom. The sick and dying come floating downstream and we pull them out and attempt to help, but the water from the pump is polluted. How can we get water for a new pump? (Ryan, 1971) I am hopeful that, while we can not do it alone, we can make an impact with our clients/neighbors/friends.

GROUP WORK AND LABOR

Jane Addams' leadership in the social reform issues of her day including those relating to the vote for women, to child and female labor, unemployment and unfair employment is well known. She saw the alliance of settlement houses with labor unions as natural. She said in 1910 "Settlement is drawn into the labor issues of its city . . . as the present industrial system thwarts our ethical demands, not only for social righteousness but for social order . . . That in this effort it should be drawn into fellowships with the local efforts of trades-unions is obvious" (Addams, 1930). In reading her description of residents and neighbors debating on matters such as the Stockyard Strike one is heartened to see people grapple with "the close connection of their own difficulties with national and even international movements" (1930, 168). This societal and world consciousness and connection of social group work with the world of work was picked up by such group work leaders as Grace Coyle and Clara Kaiser, Margaret Berry and Hy Weiner, all prominent group work theoreticians and educators whose theories were grounded in practice in labor and industrial settings. For Hy Weiner, there was no separation of social action and other forms of group work (Weiner, 1961). He was clear that social work had a place in industry but not as a tool of management. He saw group work as facilitating the strengths of unions in serving their own (Weiner, 1967.) He was as much at home with a group of labor organizers or shop stewards as he was in a group of children or concerned parents. He saw no dichotomy of function.

What I learned from Hy Weiner and Bill Schwartz and other Columbia giants of the 1960s (Mitch Ginsberg, Irv Miller and others) was to pull things together, to integrate seemingly diverse elements into a professional whole represented by a common social work method, and not the number in the relational system, to find the unity in the one and the many: the public trouble in the private issue, and the professional function addressed holistically (Schwartz, 1986). Schwartz drew together the streams of influence that became group work's identification with social work as a profession. "The roots of group work were in the activities of the agencies reflecting concern with social conditions and their effects on people. Its origins lay in the general movement for social amelioration and social protest. Even as its workers drew inspiration from educational theory, psychiatric learnings and small-group research, these developments were seen by many as instruments to be used in achieving social objectives. The ensuing efforts to build a scientific base and a unique methodology were undertaken, *not to replace the sense of mission but to implement it"* (Schwartz, 1959) (The emphasis is mine).

Schwartz characterized the 1950s as an "age of anxiety" "fraught with doubts, pessimism and the fear of imminent catastrophe." We can easily relate to this 1955 description of the American scene: "Uncertainty, doubt, confusion and fear are the order of the day, intensified by an ever threatening international situation, the insecurities resulting from a structureless (and) contradictory climate add to the mental health problems of the nation. The reactionary political climate which is accompanying this period of change has brought an attack on our humanistic philosophy . . ." (Schwartz, 1959). The current time has been called the age of narcissism—the "me generation" (Lasch, 1978). The group work of our era also strongly reflects society's pull toward individual growth more than social goals, social gain or social responsibility. We must lead the profession in the re-establishment of these priorities.

THE OPPRESSIONS OF TECHNOLOGY

Alvin Toffler conceptualizes our present time as one of "future shock." We are speeding into a "super-industrial" era so fast that the knowns of our culture, our methods of adaptation, are fast slipping away. "We must invent super-industrialism, not import it . . . We must anticipate not a single wave of change but a series of terrible heaves and shudders . . . There is no whole pattern for us to adopt. More important, the transience level has risen so high, the pace is now so forced, that a historically unprecedented situation has been thrust upon us. We are asked to adapt to a blinding succession of new temporary cultures. This is why we may be approaching the upper limits of the adaptive range. No previous generation has ever faced this test" (Toffler, 1970). We have staggering new tasks of adaptation and many tasks of earlier ages to accomplish while we stand on moving ground trying to grow as individuals. This is an impossible position. Yet it is where we are and why I turn to the origins of our history to illuminate our strengths and tasks. Industrialism was still new in Addams' era, economic slumps were severe, and life moved fast. The needs of the poor remain astonishingly and sadly similar. We were diverted from Addams' method (Settlement Houses, dialogue, and Deweyan style discussion groups were methods) with our need for professional identity, a search for skill and method and a scientific base. While these were valid pursuits we were side-tracked from the kind of vision and methods that could address our concerns even as we face the turn of the 21st century.

Often it is glibly said that we need a "new technology for helping" as we reach a new age. But what is this new technology? I propose that, short of massive structural changes, which groups can also work toward, what we already know in group work might be all that is relevant in our brave new world and that a "new technology" might be the last thing we need. In a world of transience and fear, we need human connection to hold on to, and to empower ourselves to action. As Toffler notes "To create an environment in which change enlivens and enriches the individual, but does not overwhelm him, we must employ not merely personal tactics but social strategies." If we are to carry people through the accelerative period, we must begin now to build "future shock absorbers" into the very fabric of the oppressiveness of our super-industrial society (Toffler, 1970; Frière, 1973).

FUTURE SHOCK ABSORBERS

Toffler suggests the following measures as "future shock absorbers": (1) that we regulate the level of stimulation in our lives so that we don't overload our capacities; (2) that we attempt to hold on to the things, people and experiences that mean something to us and limit the amount of "throw-away" situations we get into; (3) that we create 'stability zones' — certain enduring relationships that are maintained; (4) that we provide temporary organizations — 'situational groupings' — for people who happen to be passing through similar life transitions: That "group members be given the opportunity to pool their personal experiences and ideas before the moment of change is upon them." He notes that such groups not be "devoted to hashing over the past or to soul-searching self-revelation" but to "planning practical strategies for future use in the new life situation," and that "we honeycomb the society with such coping classrooms." (5) that person-to-person crisis counseling be done by "deputizing a large number of non-professional people in the community." That "social service come to be a reciprocal 'love network' — an integrative system based on the system of 'I need you as much as you need me.' (6) that there be "halfway houses" for people facing massive change as a means of gradualizing changes like the retirement process; (7) that we preserve "enclaves of the past;" places where things are slower, "like they used to be," (8) that we pre-adapt people to "enclaves of the future," to future changes through education of what life will be like in another place or time; (9) that we preserve ritual and establish new global rituals and celebrations — e.g., like a global Martin Luther King, Jr. day and (10) that we educate people to cope with the future, including grounding students in "certain common skills needed for human communication and social integration," and "how to think" and "how to learn" (Toffler, 1970).

SOCIAL WORK WITH GROUPS MEETS THE NEED

Group work has been addressing itself to all of these needs. Toffler's suggestions can be divided into the use of informal groups or natural helping networks and the use of formal groups and creating networks at points of transition and crisis. (See Germain and Gitterman, 1980.) His over-arching theme is to stimulate connection and learning in mutual aid groups. Every street worker, gang or club worker knew principles related to mobilizing informal natural helping systems for the social good rather than for destructive aims. Carol Swenson has done very fine qualitative research into natural helping networks (Swenson, 1979). There is a rediscovering of our territory. Groups, whether informal or formed, can be the place to focus on coping, and new role attainment; can be centered on life transitions; can be the place to form, maintain and preserve relationships as well as rituals; can be enclaves of the past and preparatory for the future and can educate for novelty, diversity and newness. They always have. Future shock absorbers are exactly what Settlement Houses were. Groups can also empower for economic, social and political change (Hartford, 1971; Garvin, 1981; Northen, 1988; Addams, 1930; Wilson and Ryland, 1949; Schwartz and Zalba, 1971; Gitterman and Shulman, 1986; Lee, 1988). We are doing all that Toffler suggests and perhaps only need to sharpen our conceptualizations as we approach the 21st Century.

Schwartz's definition of group work and social work function is as relevant today as it was in 1959: ". . . The history of social group work lends itself strongly to a conception of function in which the group worker assumes the task of searching out and clarifying the vital connection between . . . the group members and the external requirements of his social situation. This connection becomes increasingly obscure as a society grows more complex. It is only through social survival that the individual survives . . ." (Schwartz, 1959). We are now talking about survival, and about the relief of oppression, and I believe the definition applies as do the roles and skills that follows in Schwartz's "mediation function" (Schwartz, 1959 and Schwartz, 1974).

Schwartz recognized that we live in an unfair, structurally flawed society. His words ring true today: "There can be no 'choice' or even a division of labor between serving individual needs and dealing with social problems if we understand that a private trouble is simply a specific example of a public issue, and that a public issue is made up of many private troubles" (Schwartz, 1974). (See also Middleman and Goldberg, 1974.) The elements of both aspects of function are inherent in every group with which we work.

SUBVERSIVE ACTS

Paulo Frière in his *Pedagogy of the Oppressed* (*1973*) suggested that real education is a subversive act. The same is true of real social work. Frière believes "every human being is capable of looking critically at his world in a dialogical encounter with others. In this process, the old, paternalistic teacher/student relationship is overcome. A peasant can facilitate this process for his neighbor more effectively than a 'teacher' brought in from the outside." Yet the worker/teacher/student (for we learn reciprocally in this model) has certain separate tasks. One is to promote consciousness, or "conscientization." By this, Frière means learning to perceive social political and economic contradictions, and to take action against oppressive elements of reality. I believe this is the same skill as uncovering and confronting the obstacles between people and systems that Schwartz described. And, I believe that it is part of "lending a vision" of hope. This dialogue to include consciousness would, for example, in the therapy group described earlier (Gibbard et al., 1976) include a discussion of racism when one of the two Black members of the group is scapegoated. It would include a discussion on being poor and class structure with the members wanting help with the welfare department. It would include a discussion of women's status and sexism in the excerpt of the women wearing slacks. And the young adult pre-employment group might include work on how things might be changed in terms of the power dynamics they already discussed so well.

Frière warns against a "banking concept of education," i.e., that we deposit "wisdom" in others. He suggests instead that we encourage what is there to emerge. By being ready for work on the oppressive elements of our society, we will use our skills to encourage members' views to emerge. The other key method of Frière's approach is dialogue. If the worker takes the role of wanting to understand (rather than being the expert) and of being vulnerable rather than master, real dialogue can occur — real talk on real subjects which leads to empowerment. Frière stresses that the worker should be a problem-poser rather than a problem-solver. This means that we work with our group members on the art of critical thinking about the total person-environment context.

The group members in dialogue with the worker and each other can relate to any problem they face on a personal and wider political level. Once there is better awareness of the nature of problems, group members no longer blame themselves for the troubles they face, despair, and become apathetic and ego centered. They learn that they can take the present and the future in hand and challenge the structural arrangements that exist which produce such dysfunction.

PEOPLE HAVE THE POWER

Social work with groups has to be the technology of the future, if there is to be a future. We do know how to work with groups. We do not need new group technologies. We need to teach and practice what we know. Lindemann said "groups are the building blocks of democracy." If we are ever to actualize real democracy then we want people struggling with problems in living to see those problems as bigger than themselves as individuals, yet not so big that they are beyond the power that people can find together. Barbara Solomon cautions that "the worst approach to helping would be to do it in ways that power remains in other than black hands—even when those hands are tender and caring" (Solomon, 1976). To paraphrase her regarding everyone's feelings of helplessness as we speed toward the 21st Century, "The worst approach to helping would be to do it in ways that the power is seen as out of our hands." We do have the power, group members do have the power. This society and this world is ours. We also have the responsibility to move beyond our self-centeredness—and all therapies and helping situations which keep us focussed only on self to a focus on self's connection to the good of the many, the good of our world. *Every* group meeting and helping encounter can bring us closer to assuming the responsibility and power to act as "causal forces capable of exerting influence . . ." (Solomon, 1976) on every level of being. Let us be honest as problem posers. Let us help group members to work on complex person-environment transactions in the economic, social and political context in which they exist. Let us learn to trust the group, and to believe in people, to know that through the process of dialogue and mutual aid, we can find the way to do what needs to be done. It *is* not ours to know answers or to teach or manipulate, or to lead in reform or revolution. It is ours to provide opportunities for people to come together in dialogic communication. If we become "critical co-investigators" with our group members we can work on the solutions to the problems posed here (Frière, 1973).

When Jane Addams was in Boston on that September day in 1914, she drew a parallel between war and human sacrifice. We have spoken of violence, of the oppressions of class, race and difference. We have spoken of transience, alienation and cognitive dissonance in a world moving so fast that we need "future enclaves" to even envision tomorrow. We have spoken of the nearness of war and nuclear destruction. We are speaking of human sacrifice, of the waste of the lives we have nurtured. Addams continued, "It took the human race thousands of years to rid itself of human sacrifice; during many centuries it relapsed again and again in periods of national despair. So have we fallen back to warfare, and perhaps will fall back again and again, until in self-pity, in self-defense, in self-assertion of the right of life, not as hitherto a few, but the whole people of the world, will brook this thing no longer" (Addams, 1930). I urge you to find with your groups the power to "brook this thing no longer."

REFERENCES

Addams, J. *Twenty Years At Hull House*. New York: The Macmillan Company, 1910. Signet Classics, 1961, 60-64.

Addams, J. *The Spirit of Youth and the City Streets*. New York: The Macmillan Company, 1912, 161.

Addams, J. *Peace and Bread In Time of War*. New York: The Macmillan Company, 1922. First NASW Classics, Edition, 1983, 2-10.

Addams, J. *The Second Twenty Years At Hull House*. New York: The Macmillan Company, 1930, 120; 380-413; 400; 121.

Batra, R. *The Great Depression of 1990*. New York: Dell Books, 1987.

Brandwein, R. "Women and Community Organization." In *The Woman Client*, D. Burden and No. Gottleib (Eds.). New York: Tavistock Publications, 1987, 111-125.

Davis, L. Ed., *Ethnicity In Social Group Work Practice*. New York: The Haworth Press, Inc. 1980.

Frière, P. *Pedagogy of the Oppressed*. New York: The Seabury Press, 1973.

Garvin, C. *Contemporary Group Work*. New Jersey: Prentice-Hall, 1981, 47-55.

Gary, L. and Gary R., "Profile of Black Female Social Welfare Leaders During the 1920's." National Institute of Mental Health Study (Grant No. MH 25551-02), 1975.

Germain, C. and Gitterman, A. *The Life Model of Social Work Practice*. New York: Columbia University Press, 1980.

Gibbard, G.; Hartman, J. and Mann, R., Eds. *Analysis of Groups*. San Francisco: Jossey Bass, 1976, 88-93.

Gibbs, J. T. "Black Adolescents and Youth: An Endangered Species." *American Journal of Orthopsychiatry*, 54 (1), January 1984, 6-21.

Gitterman, A. and Shulman, L. *Mutual Aid Groups and the Life Cycle*. Illinois: The Peacock Press, 1986.

Hartford, M. *Groups In Social Work*. New York: Columbia University Press, 1971, 31-61.

Kaplan, S. "Therapy Groups and Training Groups: Similarities and Differences." In *Analysis of Groups*, G. Gibbard, J. Hartman and R. Mann (Eds.). San Francisco: Jossey Bass, 1976, 94-104.

Lee, J. A. B., Ed. *Return To Our Roots; Group Work With the Poor and Oppressed*. New York: The Haworth Press, Fall, 1988.

Marks, M. L., "The Question of Quality Circles." *Psychology Today*, March 1986, 36-38, 42-46.

Middleman, R. M., "Quality Circles." 1983.

Middleman R. and Goldberg, G. *Social Service Delivery: A Structural Approach*. New York: Columbia University, 1974.

Northen, H. *Social Work With Groups*. New York: Columbia University Press, 1969, 212.

Northen, H., *Social Work With Groups*, Second Edition. New York: Columbia University Press, 1988.

Ryan W. *Blaming the Victim*. New York: Vintage Books, 1971.

Schwartz, W. "Group Work and the Social Scene." In *Issues In American Social Work*, A. Kahn (Ed.). New York: Columbia University Press, 1959, 122, 133-135.

Schwartz, W. "The Social Worker In the Group." In *The Practice of Social Work*, R. Klenk and R. Ryan (Eds.). Belmont, CA: The Wadsworth Publishing Co., 1974, 217-227.

Schwartz, W. "Private Troubles and Public Issues: One Social Work Job or Two?" In *The Practice of Social Work*, R. Klenk and R. Ryan (Eds.)., 75.

Schwartz, W. "The Group Work Tradition and Social Work Practice." *Social Work With Groups*. Vol. 8, No. 4, Winter 1985/86, 7-27.

Solomon, B. *Black Empowerment: Social Work In Oppressed Communities*. New York: Columbia University Press, 1976, 5, 26.

Swenson, C. R. "Social Networks, Mutual Aid, and the Life Model of Practice." In *Social Work Practice: People and Environments*. C. B. Germain (Ed.). New York: Columbia University Press, 1979, 213-238.

Toffler, A. *Future Shock*. New York: Random House, Bantam Edition, 1971, 371-427.

Tropp, E. "Three Problematic Concepts: Client, Help, Worker." *Social Casework*, 55(1) 1974, 19-29.

Weiner, H. J. "Toward Techniques for Social Change." *Social Work*, VI, NO. 2, 1961, 26-35.

Weiner, H. J., "A Group Approach to Link Community Mental Health With Labor." *Social Work Practice*. New York: Columbia University Press, 1967, 178-188.

Wilson, G. and Ryland, G. *Social Group Work Practice*. Cambridge, MA: Houghton Mifflin Company, 1949, 121-132; 465-471.

Yalom, I. *The Theory and Practice of Groups Psychotherapy*. New York: Basic Books, Inc. 1970, 30, 109-121, 142-153.

Group Work with New Populations: Knowledge and Knowing

Catherine P. Papell

I was asked by the Symposium Committee to address the subject of "Group Work with New Populations." At first blush one would undoubtedly expect that a "new population" is an immigrant group, a group of persons who are newcomers to the august "land of the free." Of course we must discuss knowledge of specific culture. We must discuss ethnicity, and ethnic differences as these appear in groups of Afghans, Asians from Japan, Taiwan, Korea, Vietnam—perhaps Hmong people, as well as East Indians, el Salvadorans, Haitians, Chicanos, and of course Black, Puerto Rican, and Native Americans. We could discuss working with people who do not know our language. We could compare cultural attitudes towards women, or the roles of men, etc., etc.

But, pause a moment, perhaps a "new population" today refers to a group of persons who are experiencing new, or newly appearing, social problems with whom group workers are now using their skills. For example would a new population be a group of AIDS patients or a group with an AIDS patient in it? Or a group of incest victims or survivors? Or a group of homeless persons in a public shelter? Or a group of high school students whose use of alcohol is at least *abuse* and who are now "playing around" with crack? If these are the new populations we are to address, then as group workers we must search out some very specific knowledge and we must certainly talk about outreach, prevention, education, empowerment as well as treatment. For example, we must acquire knowledge about adolescent alcohol/drug abuse and the bio-psycho-social consequences of chemical dependence in individual and interactional systems. The demands on group workers to know enough in relation to the new populations that appear in our practice today are compelling indeed.

I shall not use this time to consider any one of these or other "new

---

Catherine P. Papell, DSW, is Professor Emerita, Adelphi University School of Social Work, Garden City, NY.

23

populations" in relation to specific knowledge that is needed by the group worker, or whether it is or is not available. I refer the reader to the excellent practice papers that are now present in the group work literature or that are prepared for the Group Work Symposia, and to the widening resources in social work and related professional literature. I also suggest the public knowledge in the media, the press and even the magazines in the local supermarket. To be noted also is the significance of knowledge that is available through the various self-help movements.

KNOWLEDGE AND THE PROCESS OF KNOWING

Instead of specific knowledge about new populations this paper will consider knowledge in general in the contemporary world that is overwhelming us with the newly printed word. I would like to talk about searching for knowledge, using knowledge and about knowing as we pursue the business of helping people as social group workers. A large data bank of information itself is not enough. The quantity of knowing does not determine the effectiveness of a social group worker with a "new population." Rather the question is *how* to know and how to know *what* knowledge is and how to *use* knowledge in a group work context, and flowing from such questions is a crucial one: how to *educate* for today's practice with groups requiring so much special knowledge.

Let us remind ourselves that as group workers we often do not have the luxury of *knowing* before we start. We begin with people in their life space and learn the specialness of their life situations as we engage with them. That is the heritage of group work in the social work profession and its contribution to practice skill, since our practice *creates* life space rather then *isolates* from it. Reviewing something about *knowledge and knowing* can perhaps modify the frantic scramble for information. It can sustain us as we search for the knowledge that is needed and it can free us in sorting out data in relation to social group work practice purposes.

KNOWLEDGE AND FACT

Let us consider that word of elusive meaning, knowledge. Is knowledge "fact"? Bertrand Russell wrote about "fact" as follows:

> "Fact" as I intend the term, can only be defined ostensively. Everything that there is in the world I call a "fact." The sun is a fact; Caesar's crossing of the Rubicon was a fact; if I have a toothache, toothache is a fact. If I make a statement, my making it is a fact, and

if it is true there is further fact in virtue of which it is true, *but not* if it is false. The butcher says, "I am sold out, and that's a fact"; immediately afterward a favored customer arrives and gets a nice piece of lamb from under the counter. So the butcher told two lies, one in saying he was sold out and the other in saying that his being sold out was a fact. Facts are what make statements true or false. (1948)

For us as social group workers, fact is the unadorned reality about existence and the world, that which is real without qualification by my mental processes or yours, without dialectical activity on the part of the knower. I will pick up a stone and put it on a scale; you too may take your turn at putting the stone on the same scale. The weight will be the same regardless of my fascination with the form, color and texture of the stone, or your fascination with the evidences of many minerals in it.

And what of a human group? The facts are simple: seven members, all male, ages 12-14, all Vietnamese school children in a local Junior High School in the inner city, meeting for the first time on invitation of the school social worker. We are all aware that the process of the group will be very different, though possibly equally as meaningful to the group, depending on who is the worker. Each potential worker with this group will perceive the group and its needs differently, filtering perceptions through his/her own mind. Each will make decisions about how to start and what to do as the group worker, based on his/her *unique* mental complex of knowledge, values and skills as well as those that are held as the common property of social work. Fact is not enough to explain "knowledge" or its use. Facts must be organized in the mind of each of us and processed according to what the specific mind knows, what it values, and what it can do.

KNOWLEDGE AND INFORMATION

Let us talk *now* about "information." Information is the key word in computer technology today. Information is the data that is put into the machine and brought out in remarkable combinations for problem-solving if you and I push the buttons correctly. In a world that has this marvelous electronic toy that can produce and exchange data with mind-boggling speed and range, we may need to be wary of elevating "information" as transmitted by the computer to a superordinate position in the knowledge base of the profession, even as we try to use it to its fullest.

As an aside, perhaps you read Russell Baker's column on "Computer

Fallout" (New York Times Magazine 10/11/87, p. 30). The final para-
graph at the end of 3 columns consisting of dozens of incompleted open
sentences, each one modified by the next, reads as follows: "Since it is
easier to revise and edit with a computer than with a typewriter or pencil,
this amazing machine makes it very hard to stop editing and revising long
enough to write a readable sentence, much less an entire newspaper
column." I am also reminded of the serious concern in Wall Street about
whether the computer has been working so rapidly that the humans scram-
bling in the gamble are unable to keep up with it and direct it reliably. It is
a different kind of entropy—speeding up to an explosion rather than slow-
ing down to a halt.

My colleague, Gunther Geiss, an expert with computers in the human
services, points out that the information explosion is exponential. If information doubles every six years, "in 24 years what you know today will be
less than 10% of what you should know then!" (1987). How can I supply
in this paper, even in small amount, information that social group workers
should know now, based on *presently* available information about "new
populations."

There are two assumptions made, often though not always, by technology experts, that should be considered in our discussion of "information"
in relation to knowledge and knowing for social work practice in general
and group work practice specifically. The first, of course, is that if all the
data can be put in, the machine will be able to do more than what the mind
can do. The second is that it *is* possible for *all* data to be put in, that is data
is finite rather than dynamic and dialectical. Such a stance is deterministic
and linear and does not account for aspects of knowledge generated in our
own minds as we engage with groups or generated collectively as members engage with each other in groups. Getzel states it thus in his paper
presented at the group work symposium VII (1985):

> It is not through a positivist epistemology and rationality that much
> of social work with groups is done. The complexity of individuals,
> their interactions, group-influenced behavior and even our own well
> intended actions preclude a deterministic stance. We group workers
> instantly experience the emergent every time we enter the exhilarat-
> ing chaos of group life. (1985)

The above assumptions in computer technology may account for what
the machine can do with information but they do not take into consideration what knowledge the mind can generate by inferential and creative
powers that the machine cannot. The machine can indeed do things that

the minds of most of us cannot do without intensively developed and highly limiting training and effort, if at all. However, the elaborative and generative skills of thinking about that which transpires in group life represent a different order of the meaning, acquisition, and use of knowledge.

Where then shall we go in our discussion of knowledge for social work practice with groups of "new populations"? Knowledge cannot be accounted for simply as "fact." It is insufficient to define it as "information." How will we look at it in a feasible way that takes into account the infinite aspect of fact and the vastness of information.

KNOWLEDGE AND WORLD VIEW

Let us talk for a moment about a "world view." Imbedded in my comments about "fact" and "information" are notes that are surely representative of a fundamental paradigm, a set of mental comments by which a mind can organize reality and develop ground rules for dealing with life (Babbie, 1986, pg. 32). A world view is a set of beliefs and prioritized notions, conscious or not, extensively developed or not, regarding the nature of reality, the nature of knowledge and essential ethics and values. We are talking here about a world view that influences the creation and use of knowledge in the social and behavioral sciences since the human condition — people engaging in their world — is the domain of our helping efforts.

A WORLD VIEW FOR SOCIAL GROUP WORK

The world view in the context of social work with groups that I am setting forth says as follows:

1. There is a real world that is our domain. It is the world of human interaction taking the form of human groupings. The full range of human problems and strengths, longing and fulfillment, illness and wellness, loneliness and enmeshment is represented and created by members each of whom is struggling with the necessity to adapt in some way to a difficult, all too often, hostile environment. In the real world of the human group the social work interface appears in immediacy.

2. Knowledge in this world has been and continues to be derived by rigorous methods — scientific and empirical — in the study of the group, in the study of human problems and human social experience and in the study of the practice with such groups for social work purposes.

3. The real world, for us the specific group and its members and setting, must be perceived, relevant knowledge sought out, understood and selected for use—all within the unique and individual mental processes of the particular worker. All knowledge that can be available from any source is dialectical as it is filtered through the worker's mind and self, and as it occurs and reoccurs phenomenologically in the particular human interaction in the particular group. All knowledge of the human condition is subject to the mind's knowing, to the cognitive process of each of us, as well as to the quality and authority of the content.

4. Knowledge used in understanding and assessing a human group is lawlike rather than lawful. Sidney Morganbesser, drawing upon the distinction available from the discipline of philosophy, cautioned social workers about this more than 20 years ago. (Murphy, 1964, p. 92-96). "Lawlike" as opposed to "lawful" takes into account the emerging, in vivo, aspect of the human condition.

5. There are other ways of *knowing*, of *developing knowledge* in addition to scientific or empirical means. The extensive literature on social science research often refers to the empirical methods as deductive, since the hypothesis to be proven or disproven dominates the study and as many elements or variables as possible that confound it must be eliminated. On the other hand are the inductive or qualitative methods which seek knowledge by *observation* of the real world, gathering and organizing that which is observable and conceptualing and theorizing from these observations (Glaser and Strauss, 1967).

6. A still further way of knowing is by human intuition by the creative and integrative processes in the mind that one can call wisdom, or insight. These are the non-linear processes that put different elements together in new ways, that utilize the responsiveness of human interaction in such a way that the newness of going into the future is unleashed, valued, in fact delighted in. All human life is new; each moment has never been known before. The past is useful for explanation, the present is real and the future is uncertain and a creative moment. Gale Goldberg and Ruth Middleman have written often, together and separately, about stretching perceptions of the world of the group. (1975, 1985) We have become very cautious and reluctant in recent accountability years about using the concept of "practice wisdom." At one time social workers respected the concept deeply, not only because it accounted for gaps in knowledge which were not available empirically but also because there existed in the profession respect for "other ways" of knowing.

7. In such a "world view" the values and ethics are grounded in love of

the human conditions, individual, group and community, and flow from such a stance. "No man is an island. . . ." "I am my brother's (and sister's) keeper. . . ." and in Hillel's words, "If I am not for myself, who will be for me? And if I am only for myself, what am I? And if not now, when?" I am reminded of a Chinese woman whom I met on the plane from Shanghai. She was wearing a pin with Chinese characters which she translated as "Every human being needs love and assistance."

These world-view ideas, in some instances acknowledged as phenomenological in nature, are inherent in our group work tradition, and re-expressed in our group work literature. Alex Gitterman, at the group work Symposium VIII (1986) wrote about the importance for the group worker to relinquish the need for certainty in order to move empathically into the world of the group. Ruth Middleman and Gale Goldberg (1985), as I have noted earlier, address creativity in the mind of the worker. Getzel (1985) writes about the reflective process of the worker. Howard Goldstein, in an invitational paper that has been published in a special 10th anniversary issue of *Social Work with Groups* (Spring 1988), presents his cognitive-humanistic approach to social work helping (1981) in relation to work with groups. My own work on *Styles of Learning for Direct Social Work Practice* (1978), had as its basic premise that thinking, feeling and doing for the student can be viewed as processes originating in the mind in some kind of balance which creates an individualized approach to learning for practice. Now some years later in a very generalized way, I conceptualize *thinking* and *feeling* as left and right hemisphere functioning, and *doing* as an integrative move of the organism into action.* Harold Lewis discusses the thinking processes of the worker as "tools for thought in a helping profession" (1982). My former Dean, Joseph Vigilante, has been writing and teaching about a phenomenological approach to knowledge building *for social work* for several years (1983). A practice doctoral dissertation by Jerome Sachs (1987) was built upon these notions using a compatible research methodology.

I would like to add that you will find some of these ideas intimated in the editorials that my colleague, Beulah Rothman, and I produce for the

---

*Ruth Middleman has reminded me that the more recent studies of the brain are particularly interested in the viability of various sectors to expand their functions. I am using the hemisphere model here, less technically and more as metaphor, to describe the integrative relationship of thinking-feeling-doing in the human organism.

journal *Social Work With Groups* and in our thoughts on "Issues in Group Work Education" (1986).*

It is important to note examples of work from outside of our profession, though related to it. Notable are the recent papers in *Family Process* by Edgar Auerswald on "Thinking About Thinking in Family Therapy" (1985) and "Epistemological Confusion in Family Therapy and Research" (1987). The recently published works of David Schon of Massachusetts Institute of Technology on the reflective practitioner (1983) and educating the reflective practitioner (1987) are interesting explorations into the way professionals think in action with many insights that social work has been aware of for decades.

In the social sciences the myth of objectivity in empirical studies is widely acknowledged in current and classical writings. Babbie's recent essay on *Observing Ourselves* (1986) is a delightful example.

I would like to comment on the new *Dictionary of Social Work* (1987). My copy arrived as I was writing this paper and I was excited by my anticipation of how helpful it might be. I kept looking for words that represent the contribution of group work methodology to the language of the profession.

There was no listing of "phases of group development," e.g., "preaffiliation phase" or "approach-avoidance." But there was a listing for "phallic phase," "phobia" and many of the DSM III categories. There was a listing for "social control," "social cost," "social causation theory," "social gerontology," "social history," "social inequality," but not "social goals model." There was half a column on "group therapy" and only a few lines on "social group work." There were all the techniques of family therapy but none of the skills of group work. I submit that social work is set back by the new Dictionary and we must find ways to protest and insist on revision. If the Dictionary is based in knowledge the understanding of knowledge by our profession is inadequate.

It is being said then that human knowledge is *content* about the real world developed empirically or by observation or by *process* in the mind of the knower, always anchored in a "world view." Bertrand Russell closed his treatise on *Human Knowledge: Its Scope and Limits* stating that

---

*As an aside I would like to comment that, since this is *my* paper and not *ours*, my colleague has an enviable position. She does not have to agree with what I say today. I, on the other hand, can use what I have gained from my association with her. So perhaps it is I who am the fortunate one this time around.

". . . all human knowledge is *un*certain, *in*exact, and partial. To this doctrine we have not found any limitation whatsoever" (1948, p. 507).

KNOWLEDGE AND ESSENCE

Phenomenologists deal with the uncertainty, inexactness and partialness by struggling with the way in which the content of the knowledge, its physical configuration — either written or oral — is not only influenced by the knowing process but is actually constructed by it. The phenomenologists' concept of "essence" may help us with understanding that aspect of knowledge which is dependent on the mind of the knower, in this instance the social group worker. Essence is that which communicates meaning beyond the constraints of the actual content. It is where the mind of the knower goes in searching out the substance of the knowledge that is presented. The term essence in a phenomenologist's words indicates that which, "in the intimate self-being of an individual *thing* or *entity*, tells us what it really is" (Kockelmans, 1966, p. 80).

Essence in Knowledge for Work with New Cultures

Let us go to the new populations, to see if we can find some aspects of needed knowledge that seem to have a quality that might be called "essence." First let us look at groups where culture and ethnicity are issues.

The classic conception by Kluckholm and Murray (1949) is one example:

> In some ways all humans are like *all* other humans; In some ways all humans are like *some* other humans; and in some ways all humans are like *no* other human. (Degendered by the writer)

This is a remarkably clarifying statement. In working with cultural differences the group worker's mind is continually sorting out basic humanness, cultural prescriptions for behavior, and individuality in each group member. With Kluckholm's conception the worker's assessment processes can be organized in the continuing effort to understand the group, its experiences and its members. The purpose is not to "pigeon-hole" observations and thoughts and interventions but to illuminate one's own thinking processes as one engages with the group while using one's basic methodological knowledge and skill of group work. This I submit is an essence.

I wish to be certain that I am not being accused of stating that this is *enough* knowledge. Rather I assert that cultural knowledge is so extensive

that in the search one must sort and select — and one must do this in relation to purpose or intentionality in using the knowledge. Using the concept of essence, it can be said the Kluckholm statement starts us on the
selecting process for social group work purposes.

Another concept from anthropology, and it is to anthropology that we
must go for this knowledge, is that there is a cultural prescription for much
social behavior but there are also in every culture *ways by which the prescriptions may be altered and modified* (Uko, 1980). This too has a quality of "essence" since our goals as group workers are adaptive goals for
the group members. We wish for the newcomers to be able to understand
the dominant culture since they must become a part of it, survive in it and
contribute to it. However in the spirit of cultural pluralism or bi-cultural-
ism we also have a goal that the newcomers shall be able to hold on to that
part of themselves that sustains identity with those "some other humans"
whom they are like. This bit of cultural knowledge tells us that we can
help the newcomer work through the changes that are being required without loss of identity and with a sense of roots.

Essence in Knowledge for Work with Child Sexual Abuse

Let us look at another kind of new population, new perhaps because it *is*
more prevalent than in past decades, *or* because professionals are listening
and responding rather than turning away — namely, child sexual abuse. An
essential knowledge is that the necessity for denial is enormous for the
abuser because of taboo violation and societal prosecution. There can follow from this denial an overt implication that the child is imagining or
lying in the accusation. Believing the child takes on vital importance, less
self-doubt, self-blame, loss of trust that the adult world will help, and
socialization to the role of victim are added to the actual trauma. These
experiences are carried into adult life often with chilling consequences.

Secondary problems are generated in the triangulation between daugh-
ter, mother and husband/father (or stepfather) and family as a whole.
These considerations must be taken into account in any practice situation
whether it be a group in which an adolescent has shared her plight with
members, or a women's support group in which a member has trusted her
friends and exposed the memory, or a group established explicitly for
abusing fathers/stepfathers, or a group established for adult survivors of
childhood sexual abuse, or a family group, or . . . We remind ourselves as
group workers that in every group which achieves a level of mutual aid
and sharing with trust an unpredictable range of human problems appear.

The dynamic relationship between child sexual abuse, denial by the
abuser, blaming the victim and rejection of spouse becomes an aspect of

knowledge that might be called an essence, whether the knowledge has been established empirically, by experience, or by intuition.

Essence in Knowledge for Work with Adult Children of Alcoholics

Let us consider one more example of essence in seeking knowledge for work with new population groups—this time adult children of alcoholics (ACOAs). Perhaps some essences of knowledge are more difficult to find. Alcoholism and chemical dependence are incredibly complex subjects consisting of biochemical as well as psychological and sociological matters and the helping takes place at many levels of the illness, and in many differing interactional forms of service. The enormity of the "new" problem of ACOAs is apparent in the earnestness with which people flock to the conferences, workshops, and group programs that are widely set up as the awareness of the impact of alcoholism on family members is brought into consciousness. Understanding "the disease concept" is crucial whenever and however alcoholism appears in the lives of our group members. And appear it does—inevitably, since it is estimated that alcohol abuse and addiction will have touched the lives of one in five drinking persons.

There are two concepts that may represent "essence." The first concept is "progression"—progression from social and legal use of alcohol to abuse and on to addiction, progression in the recovering process from abstinence to sobriety, from being dry to being sober; progression in the impact of the illness on the developmental processes of children growing up in families where alcoholism is present; and progression in the family system both in relation to the illness and recovering processes.

The second concept is the spiritual component in the self-help movement, that which in the recovering program represents the paradoxical relationship between independence and dependence. It is a common stumbling block and misconception to assume that the references to a "higher power" in the twelve steps of AA requires any specific traditional theistic affirmation. The meaning is much more complex and individualizing. What is affirmed is "meaning" greater than the self, whatever form it may take in individual minds. This notion *counters* human omnipotence and grandiosity, rooted in early infancy. It challenges the absolutism of a positivist view of the world and says that human responsibility to others lies in growing into maturity wherein one can yield in relation to the needs of one's fellow humans. Gaining the self by giving to others is familiar to group workers. Indeed it is our concept of mutual aid. For the recovering alcoholic it says "I can find self-hood by surrendering to meaning that is greater than myself in the world; I can find my human strength by acknowledging the limits of my control." It is indeed a deeply human paradox related to the paradox of life and death.

In these two concepts, the reality of progression, process, development and growth over time, and the dialectical psychological significance of spirituality, lie "essences" in knowledge required to engage as group workers with members who have experienced in childhood the alcoholism syndrome in their families, and to foster the interactional life in groups in whatever form chemical dependence appears. These essences are surprisingly congenial to the deepest values of our group work traditions.

CONCLUSION

I have wished to discuss several ways of thinking about knowledge and knowing for group work practice with "new," or not new, populations. I have suggested:

- that knowledge is more than fact and information;
- that knowledge is not absolute and is dialectically influenced by the mind of the knower;
- that the "world view" of the knower is crucial in understanding the creation and use of knowledge;
- that the phenomenological concept of "essence," that which takes the mind of the knower beyond the information itself, is helpful in seeking relevant knowledge for practice;
- that such an approach to knowledge is congruent with social group work practice.

I have suggested that a focus on practice principles that flow from such an approach to knowledge and knowing can be seen as group work's special contribution to the profession of social work. I also do suggest that the profession is not yet setting forth or using our knowledge and skills and our special values as explicitly as is required and as our methodological development demands.

Perhaps reviewing more of what is known about knowing can sustain us as we search for knowledge that is needed for practice in the *unknown* of the life process of our groups and members. Perhaps it can free us in sorting out from what in some instances are massive data banks that which can enhance knowing for use and for purposeful practice. Perhaps, too, it can challenge the avidity with which the empirical and accountability race is on within the social work profession by providing new approaches to knowledge building. Perhaps refreshing our minds about these fascinating issues in the nature of knowing can provide distance and richer vantage point from that race with all its excitement, ligitimacy and urgency. Perhaps it can assist group work to claim its rightful place in a profession, the mission of which is the enhancing of human fulfillment, interaction and interdependence at the interface between self and the societal world. As has often been said — where else but in the human group.

BIBLIOGRAPHY

Auerswald, Edgar H. "Thinking About Thinking in Family Therapy." *Family Process* 24 (1), March 1985.

———. "Epistemological Confusion in Family Therapy and Research." *Family Process*, 26 (3), September 1987.

Babbie, Earl. *Observing Ourselves: Essays in Social Research*. Belmont, CA: Wadsworth, Inc., 1986.

Baker, Robert L. *The Social Work Dictionary*. Silver Springs, Md: National Association of Social Workers, 1987.

Baker, Russell. "Computer Fallout." *New York Times Magazine*, October 11, 1987.

Geiss, Gunther. Notes for Doctoral Colloquium, July 1987.

Getzel, George S. "Teaching Group Work Skill Through Reflection in-Action." Paper presented at VII Annual Symposium on Social Work With Groups, Rutgers University, October 1985.

Gitterman, Alex. "Connecting Theory and Practice." Paper presented at VIII Annual Symposium on Social Work With Groups, University of Southern California, Los Angeles, 1986.

Glasser, Barney G. and Strauss, Anselm L. *The Discovery of Grounded Theory*. Chicago: Aldine Publishing Company, 1967.

Goldberg, Gale and Middleman, Ruth. "Visual Teaching." Paper and workshop *Translating Abstract Concepts into Visual Teaching Models*. Annual Program Meeting, Council on Social Work Education, 1975.

Goldberg, Gale. "Breaking the Thought Barriers: New Frontiers in Social Work With Groups." Invitational paper presented at VII Annual Symposium on Social Work With Groups, Rutgers University, 1985.

Goldstein, Howard. *Social Learning and Change: A Cognitive Approach to Human Services*. Columbia, SC: University of South Carolina Press, 1981.

———. "A Cognitive-Humanistic/Social Learning Perspective on Social Group Work Practice." *Social Work With Groups*, 11(2), Spring 1988.

Kluckholm, Clyde and Murray, Henry A. "Personality Formation: The Determinants." *Personality in Nature, Society and Culture*. New York: Knopf, 1949.

Kockelmans, Joseph J., Ed. *The Philosophy of Edmund Husserl and Its Interpretation*. Garden City, NY: Anchor Books, Doubleday Company, Inc., 1967.

Lauer, Quentin. *Phenomenology: Its Genesis and Prospect*. New York: Harper and Row Publishers, Inc., 1965.

Lewis, Harold. *The Intellectual Base of Social Work Practice: Tools for Thought in the Helping Profession.* New York: The Haworth Press, Inc. and the Lois and Samuel Silberman Fund, Inc., 1982.

Middleman, Ruth and Goldberg, Gale. "Maybe It's a Priest or a Lady With A Hat with A Tree On It, Or Is It a Bumble Bee? Teaching Group Workers to See." *Social Work With Groups*, 8(1), Spring 1985.

Murphy, Marjorie, Ed. "Report of the Conference" in *Building Social Work Knowledge.* New York: National Association of Social Workers, 1964. The comments of Dr. Sidney Morgenbesser of Columbia University's Philosophy Department are reported in this monograph, in section subtitled "Law, Lawlike and Lawful Statement."

Papell, Catherine P. "A Study of Styles of Learning for Direct Social Work Practice." DSW Dissertation, Wurzweiler School of Social Work, Yeshiva University, June 1978.

Papell, Catherine P. and Rothman, Beulah. "Issues in Group Work Education," 1986. Invitational paper presented at VII Annual Symposium on Social Work with Groups, University of Southern California, Los Angeles, 1986. To be published in *Proceedings*.

Russell, Bertrand. *Human Knowledge: Its Scope and Limits.* New York: Simon and Schuster, 1948.

Sachs, Jerome. "A Social Phenomenological Investigation of the Practice of Social Work." DSW Dissertation, Adelphi University School of Social Work, May 1987.

Schon, David. *Educating The Reflective Practitioner: How Professionals Think in Action.* New York: Basic Books, 1983.

Vigilante, Joseph L. et al. "Generating Theory for the Human Service Professions: Stage III, A Nucleus." Invitational paper presented at Annual Program Meeting of the Council on Social Work Education, March 1983.

Life with the H-Team:
From Narcissism to Team Spirit:
Social Group Treatment
for the Dually Diagnosed
in Group Homes

Sheldon Blitstein

ICF/MR/DD = Intermediate Care Facility for Mentally Retarded and Developmentally Disabled adults or a community living arrangement that requires intensive staffing because of the severity and complexity of the problems facing these persons.

Westchester Jewish Community Services (WJCS) established its Community Programs division in 1979 to administer the ICF's care facilities. W.J.C.S. is a family mental health and social service, non-profit, non-sectarian voluntary agency providing services to a wealthy suburban New York county with a population of 800,000 people.

Community Programs now operates five intermediate care facilities and offers respite care as well as outpatient treatment for mentally retarded/ developmentally disabled (MR/DD) persons living independently in the community.

Hull House, one of the ICFs, was opened for dually diagnosed young

Sheldon Blitstein, MSW, ACSW, CSW, is Assistant Executive Director, Westchester Jewish Community Services, 141 North Central Avenue, Hartsdale, NY 10530.

adults in 1981. It was specifically designed to deal with young men and women who were mildly to moderately retarded and who also had emotional disabilities. Only one of the ten people admitted was considered to be deinstitutionalized. The other nine came from their homes, although some had spent time in institutions.

Hull House evolved a paradigm of treatment for the dually diagnosed. It's seven-year history is full of trials and tribulations, regressions and progressions, bureaucratic pitfalls and individual successes. It serves as a model for understanding what a group home is and can become. The model is based on other models of residential treatment, milieu therapy, therapeutic community, and token economy.[1] Like any other deinstitutionalized setting, it set out to be a family-style, home-like environment; but how did it "normalize" its residents who were being institutionalized because they were coming from home?

In the beginning, the house was not a home. Ten strangers came to inhabit it. Twenty new staff came to manage it. It was "an aggregate," a collection of people in one place with no history of interrelationships or interactions, with no common bond, without any organization. The development from aggregate through collectivity to group took time.[2] This collection of people began to interact. The interrelationships evolved a degree of social structure and social organization. They were capable of becoming "a group" with a common identity, a sense of unity, and a definitive social structure. This process was stalled. The expectation that this group would become like a family presented certain problems.

CONCEPTUAL FRAMEWORK

What kind of group living is a group home? Garvin[3] explored the differences and similarities between families and groups. The social group of the group home would seem to be a synthesis of both or a "formed natural group." It has the characteristics of a small social unit which functions and develops in a life-space ecology system. As the formed group passes through phases of development, it will take on some family dimensions. The client's need to belong, to be intimate and to be taken care of, will force a response from the caretakers. In this social group, the caretakers will need to take responsibility for the members, like parents for children. This requires highly structured role differentiation and the development of a culture — a tradition of who does what for whom and a set of norms and beliefs about how who does what for whom — the rules of the game. Families have problems with relationships between their members and their members interactions with society change over time. Their functioning depends on the stage of development of the system and the difficulties the members have within the particular stage. The formed natural group interacts and is interdependent with the larger society, from families of origin, to other families, the neighbors, the local community, other agencies who help the clients, the agency which provides the home and governmental regulatory and financial agencies. It must establish boundaries for membership and internal generational boundaries for who's in charge. While normalization took into account the need for a family-style, home-like environment, it did not reckon with the dynamic problems that this formed natural group would engender.

What kind of group was it? It was neither an outpatient group nor an inpatient group. Yalom[4] describes a group as a social microcosm in which its participant members display their maladaptive interpersonal behavior and social patterns.

The group home is the social sphere. The clients live together, but they are not inpatients. They are not likely to be discharged. If left unstructured, their disabilities are likely to recreate a chaotic, distorted, maladaptive and un-normal social microcosm. It would be difficult for the MR/DD person to develop insight into the differences between the maladaptive and disinhibited behaviors learned outside of the group home, in family or institution, and those perpetuated inside the group home. This inpatient is not preparing for life outside of the inpatient setting. This is the life-space for the client.

It is generally accepted that MR/DD people are unable to function as independent members of society; they are considered socially disabled. Rutter's survey of cognitive and behavior symptomatology of brain injury in children concluded that there was an association between brain damage and "social disinhibition."[5] Rutter described children who were socially disinhibited as showing:

> . . . a general lack of regard for social convention. Frequently they made very personal remarks or asked embarrassing questions, and sometimes they undressed in social situations in which this would ordinarily be regarded as unacceptable behavior. Some of these disinhibited patterns also included forgetfulness, overtalkativeness, carelessness in personal hygiene and dress, and impulsiveness.[6]

Normalization requires the development of social inhibition. What is normal then is the development of a superego or conscience — the acquisition and internalization of the rules of social conduct.

The analogy between brain damaged children and MR/DD adults can be made through the use of the concept of mental age. Mental age is a measure of a MR/DD person's cognitive abilities to adapt to the social environment. It should be used as a metaphor. Although the MR/DD person is an adult, she/he functions *as if* she/he were a child mentally, cognitively, and socially. This is not meant pejoratively, as in the view of mentally retarded persons as eternal children. It is a useful way of imagining how a mentally retarded person's mind functions.

If social disinhibition is the diagnosis, then the structure of the ecosystem should be designed to develop social competence. Any competence model is concerned with the effectiveness of an individual's interactions and transactions with the environment.[7] White's model has two components: mastery and efficacy.[8] Mastery involves the intrapsychic and intrapersonal cognitive abilities to develop effective ways to cope with the environment. Effectance, or the feeling of efficacy, involves the abilities to have impact on other people, and that impact, that social intercourse, is satisfying to the person and other others. Normalization[9] is based on the competency model. It is in stark contrast to the defect model of mental retardation. Social competence and normalization are optimistic views that the mentally retarded are human beings capable of changing, learning and developing into effective and skillful persons. However, there are still the cognitive defects inherent in mental retardation. This demands a highly structured ecosystem that instructs, develops and maintains social competency.

Menolascino rated the number-one at-risk factor for producing mental illness in the retarded as the "relative inability to understand the demands of their culture secondary to the presence of intellectual and social-adaptive limitations."[10] Menolascino added the concept of "developmental contingencies"[11] as a concept in assessing mental illness in mentally retarded persons. The relative complexity of evaluating the impact of differential developmental contingencies of physical and personality development in any individual is compounded by the cultural demands of society on the group home environment. While we can ponder the bio-psycho-social, personal and clinical histories of the individuals placed in the group homes, we cannot forget the social-ecological system that impacts, reshapes and influences the developmental contingencies of the life-space situations.

If we use mental and social age as a metaphor, then we have a chance at gaining insight into cognitive development. Piaget[12] examined how children think about moral issues at different ages. Moral issues are social rules and cultural expectations about family and group obligations and responsibilities. Piaget tried to understand where children think rules come from, what they know about the rules and how they decide about fairness and justice. He argued that younger children see rules as emanat-

ing from authority figures who demand compliance and punish wrongdoing; while older children act as members of a social group who cooperate
to maintain the social order. Kohlberg[13] elaborated on Piaget's concept of
levels of moral reasoning and described six stages of moral development.

While our approach was to establish law and order through the establishment of "house rules," we expected that eventually the clients would
enter into a social contract and acknowledge the legitimacy of social rules
for the social welfare. We recognized that each client would respond in a
more primitive, rudimentary and idiosyncratic way about moral standards
and obedience versus punishment. We expected to deal with the responses
through social group treatment.

How do we establish social norms? How do we facilitate the development of social roles within a social context for dually diagnosed people?

Vinter describes group work as social treatment.

> Social treatment through group work practice focuses on ameliorat-
> ing or preventing the adverse conditions of individuals whose behav-
> ior is disapproved or who have been disadvantaged by society. It
> emphasizes manifest, personal and social problems and the rehabili-
> tative potentials of guided group processes to alleviate or avert these
> problems.[14]

This approach recognizes that the group home can be conceived of as a
small social system where potent social forces are at play. While Vinter
entitles his practice social treatment, it could well be called *Social Group
Treatment* to fully encompass all its aspects. *Social* defines the context;
group defines the system and level of intimacy and attachment; *social
group* defines the environmental context of people living together; and,
treatment defines the means by which the social group will be enabled to
become competent.

Vinter's concerns extend to the social contexts that generate and define
the problem behaviors as well as the attributes and capabilities of individual clients. All behavior can, therefore, be changed and/or relearned because it is amenable to the interaction between the individual and the
social environment. Behavior is socially induced and acquired through
learning and training. "Behavior, moreover, is judged, encouraged, or
sanctioned by others within the person's immediate social situations."[15]
Social group treatment clients harnessed the social and personal forces to
train for social inhibition, social competence, and social order in the Hull
House group home.

THE TOKEN ECONOMY AND THE SOCIAL SYSTEM

Hull House had been running for three years. The clients had adjusted to the system in that time, but they were not normalized. They remained socially disinhibited. Their adjustments and maladjustments were idiosyncratic. They had remained a collective. The social group had not developed a sense of identity. The social system was unorganized. Treatment was individually-oriented.

It is not within the purview of this paper to examine each individual client's development through the total treatment environment. Some clients will be used as examples to illustrate the process, but I will attempt to give a flavor of the group as it developed, how the culture was established and maintained, and how the group home, treatment facility and social microcosm can be a model for the social and psychological development of its residents.

The Hull House social system had developed to a rudimentary stage. They had developed a set of rules of conduct, but no one lived by them. They had begun a community meeting which met weekly—all clients and staff attended. It was led by the social worker. Clients could discuss their grievances and negotiate changes. Some clients, when anxious or agitated, were not able to sit through a meeting. Sometimes they were unable to attend. The team would valiantly but ineffectively try to establish the social order by convincing and cajoling the residents to live by house rules. The infractions were multifarious, ingenious, disinhibited and dangerous. There were no consequences.

Everyone was referred to by his/her first name. How did anyone know who was in charge? If no one is, or acts the part, disorganization and chaos will ensue. In this family-style environment, the concept of normalizing was enacted by treating the clients as equals. To normalize meant the abdication of authority and the abstention from parental controls, constraints, discipline, inhibitions, and guidance.[16] Normalization was a euphemism for permissiveness and indulgence.

The development of social inhibition, conscience, and morality were also thwarted by "the kids." Hull House exemplified the "decline of the superego"[17] in this cultural milieu. The superego is built through the social interaction between the ego or self and the environment; initially constructed between parental demands for socially acceptable behavior and the child's demands to be indulged, it continues to develop through interaction with the larger environment and social institutions. Hull House, by labeling its residents "kids," failed to establish socially appropriate norms and roles for its adult clients.

Not only was the superego in decline, not only wasn't it developing into a functional piece of mental apparatus, it was developing holes. Johnson[18] wrote that parental permissiveness and/or inconsistency toward the child produce weaknesses or lacunae in the superego. The ineffectiveness of the staff in establishing social controls gave permission to clients to misbehave.

After this initial assessment, I took a series of steps to establish law and order.

First, I insisted on being called, "Mr. Blitstein." No one was allowed to call me by my first name. As the director, I was the ultimate authority. Everyone, staff and clients, were accountable to me. I took great pains continually and constantly to correct anyone who mistakenly called me "Shelley." I would be no one's friend.

Second, the term "kids," which had been used affectionately, became a diagnostic tool. "Kids" was to mean how we understand the mental age of each client as influencing their functional behavior and how we then treat the social disinhibitions of that developmental age. The center of the interdisciplinary team case conference weekly discussions became the kids' mental ages.

Third, I, as the ultimate authority, took the leadership of the weekly community meeting to establish the rules of conduct. I made the demand that everyone attend. No excuses were acceptable, from clients as well as staff. No opportunity to explore challenges to my authority was lost.

The opportunity to set the social system into order was presented by the crucial event two months later. Karl had to be hospitalized. Karl had been hospitalized twice before—each time he had received a sociopathic diagnosis. He had a history of violence toward himself, others and property. He was our primary window breaker with concomitant self-injury and sutures. This time he had sent another client to the hospital after a violent assault.

Karl's hospitalization became a social event. His previous two hospitalizations had been presented as his individual need for psychiatric attention. Other client's hospitalizations had been presented in a similar fashion. This time, I presented it as a tragedy for Hull House. Hull House had not provided Karl with a "good enough" place to live. Hull House was an "unfit" place to live. Others were as guilty as Karl of delinquent behavior. Hull House would be rehabilitated so that Karl could make it when he returned.

If the goal was to establish a normalized environment for dually diagnosed clients living in a community-based group home, certain dynamic processes needed to be set in motion.

1. What is a group home? If it is a microcosm of a normal social system, then social group treatment is the method of normalization. If the expectation is to establish a social order with a culture that develops and maintains rules of conduct, then there must be a system of consequences, reward for good behavior and discipline for bad behavior. If a token economy is to be established, it cannot be individually-oriented. An economy can only operate within a social system.

2. Do dually diagnosed, MR/DD and psychiatrically impaired, people have egos? If they do, then any social system must take into account their differential developmental ages and their capacities and capabilities of adapting to normal expectations of a social system.

The house rules and token economy system took several months to develop. It was arrived at after hours upon hours of discussion and reviews of clients' behaviors.

The new order was presented to the clients. They were aghast. Their child-like appeals to fairness and their child-like attempts at manipulation of authority were heeded on only one account. If they had to live by the rules, then so did the staff. Each client was given a copy of the house rules. I reviewed it with them at the community meeting. Staff were instructed to review it with them at each community meeting. Staff were instructed to review it with them at every opportunity. A copy was posted for all to see. I went to the hospital to review it with Karl so that he was fully aware of the new social order that he would be returning to.

THE GOOD CITIZENS OF HULL HOUSE

Community meetings were redesigned to develop the social group. In order to develop a group conscience and the individual superego, a group cultural morality and internalized social inhibitions, shame was used as a motivating force. The consequences of all behaviors would be announced publicly. The rewards and punishments would be known to all.

Disgrace and the fear of being exposed in front of the intimate participants in the social group are direct ways of enforcing respect for group standards. They do not leave the responsibility exclusively in the hands of individuals who have not internalized superego mechanisms or mastered social competence.

The identity of the individual is inexorably bound with the identity of the group. The behavior of the individual reflects the identity of the group. Each group member is responsible for and to the group as a whole. It is a burden and a strength that cements the character of a group. Misdeeds discredit the individual and dishonor the group. Public humiliation is embarrassing to the individual and an outrage to the survival of the group. It is a public agony and a private guilt. It demands absolution through punishment and alleviation through atonement. It takes the wrongdoing, inadequacy, deficiency and culpability out of the secrecy of private disability and makes it available for remediation and social learning.[19] Shame is not only vital to superego development; it is crucial to the teaching of social competence. The mind of the retarded person is capable of learning, not only through carefully designed behavior programs with task analysis and methodologies, but in social context and social reality through comprehension, creativity, invention, conventional language and communication, and personal epistemology—developing an internalized model of the environmental ecology.

As the new social order was meeting its first resistances, the state survey team arrived for the annual recertification and relicensure process. Its evaluation cited Hull House for having a dirty house. I seized the opportunity to reemphasize the rules. A community meeting was held after the survey team had completed its deficiency report. In dramatic fashion, I reported the results, grabbed the Operating Certificate from the wall and dashed it to the floor, declaring Hull House an unfit place to live. I was outraged by my sense of shame that the deficiencies of Hull House had been exposed to the state agency designated to recertify the "goodness" of Hull House. As prearranged, the staff requested another chance. The clients begged for absolution. I demanded that they show me. The staff worked diligently with the clients to appease this outraged authority figure. The group response, however, was to begin to develop a sense of pride in the accomplishment of cleaning up Hull House and a sense of identification as a member of the social group called Hull House. The survey team's revisit removed the "dirty" citation and I declared Hull House a fit place to live.

Clients became "good citizens." Good citizen meant that the client lived by the rules for one week and, therefore, received the good citizen award.

At first, the system emphasized the negative. It was what the citizen didn't do that won the award. If the citizen misbehaved, the group took notice. "Lines" were given. If the citizen could write, she/he would write the rule that she/he broke 250 times, thereby insuring that the citizen would remember the rule next time. If the citizen could not write, she/he was to recite the line 50 times in front of an interdisciplinary team member. Until lines were completed, the citizen was on restriction and all privileges were withdrawn. Any infraction resulted in the loss of the weekly good citizen award. All lines were to be verified and submitted to me for review. Breaking rule #1 — no hurting others or oneself — was to be taken so seriously as to be referred to me immediately. No one wanted to deal with "mean Mr. Blitstein."

Joan, whose quest for perfection had led to self-injurious behavior, complained that the new system demanded perfect behavior seven of seven days per week. What chance die she have to become a good citizen? She was right. The team met again and changed the requirements to allow for one mistake per week, but physical aggression, breaking rule #1, would immediately disqualify the good citizen.

Qualification for the good citizen award meant the absence of negative consequences. In order to reinforce good behavior, the Hull House store was created. It was stocked with incidental items and clothing that the citizens would want. The stock was brought out before the good citizen community meeting. The names of the winners were announced and only they were allowed to browse through the store to choose their valuable rewards. The winners were applauded. The losers were left to watch. Each award meeting was ended with an announcement that a new week would now begin with a clean slate with each citizen having a new chance to win.

Resistance to the system was swift and far-reaching. Trish, whose history of manipulation had gotten her thrown out of other facilities, complained to everyone that Hull House had become an institution most like a prison. Betty, who was the newest client recently admitted from home, quickly followed suit. They painted a picture of cruel and unusual punishment in a harsh and uncaring environment.

Their parents and all the other families summoned me to their monthly parent group meeting. They had been meeting with the social worker since their children had been accepted into Hull House. While their complaints had centered around how chaotic Hull House had been, they were not upset at the regimentation the new system required. They accepted the new order because it worked. Hull House had become a good place to live. Their children were learning to be good citizens. The parents quipped that a good parent Hull House citizen award should be awarded for conduct supportive of the group home.

The interdisciplinary team created its own problems. The direct care staff welcomed the new tool for discipline, but they abused it. Everybody got lines for every little thing. We changed the procedure: warning must be given first; work with the clients with therapeutic intent to develop social competence. Result: nobody got lines. More staff training produced a balanced approach. Younger staff, who identified with the clients, recoiled from parental authority and balked at imposing the system. They tended to break some of the rules themselves. Since everyone was accountable to me, citizens and employees alike, all soon complied with the ultimate authority.

Three of the male citizens had histories of violence toward themselves and others. Karl, Sam and Ben all had impulse disorders and had been diagnosed as schizophrenic. All had required psychotropic medications. While the social system developed social order, they needed more than the good citizen award. Before they could internalize superego derivatives, they needed external controls. I was available at a moment's notice to meet with them, read them the riot act, demand restitutive behavior, and maintain the social structure. Karl, Sam and Ben began to feel less anxious and less fearful. If they couldn't be in control, someone else would. The structure would hold.

After the first week of the new system, three were awarded the appellation — good citizen. After the store began, six were awarded. In three months, all ten got it, and thereafter, the average per week was eight.

After three months it was time to use tokens in the token economy. We chose to use theater tickets which were numbered and, therefore, could be kept track of. The citizen's name was written on the back. All winning tickets were sealed in an envelope. During the award meeting, I requested the envelope — à la Academy Awards — from the manager. I read the names aloud. Each citizen came forward for the ticket and a handshake. Everyone applauded each winner. The staff gave hearty applause if all ten had won. The losers were ignored. It was now possible for the citizens to accumulate tickets for awards of increasing value and, thereby, sustain their social learning and competence over increasing lengths of time.

Misdeeds were easily discernible and punished with negative consequences, but we were not "catching our kids being good." In order to give positive rewards for daily good behavior, a star system was initiated. When the citizens returned from day program, the manager would review their behavior for the previous 24 hours. Each person was seen individually and given a star for good behavior. The star was entered into a book by date. By the end of the week, we had a record of the good citizen eligibility, 6 out of 7 possible stars rated the good citizen award. A daily community meeting for all involved was instituted after day program to review the day's events and to plan evening activities. Each citizen got a chance to speak, review the day, make suggestions, register complaints and make decisions about future plans. However, concerns of the social group and Hull House were the primary agenda. Individual concerns were to be discussed privately. It became tradition that the citizens would line up for their daily stars outside the manager's office. One by one, they would enter and privately review their eligibility for the star that day. Special reviews and special community meetings could be called on weekends or during crises which jeopardized the welfare and safety of Hull House.

THE H-TEAM

About 6-months later, something began to happen. Social competence was developing. The social system was operating with expected episodes of regression. There had been no more broken windows. There had been no hospitalizations. Laughter had not been banned, but the ambiance had been serious. Slowly it was becoming fun to live at Hull House. The secure base had evolved. Each citizen was internalizing the structure and the role of good citizen. Each had a sense of belonging—a renewable membership in a socially identifiable and identified group. It showed itself in a humorous way.

One day, when I was late for a community meeting, Sam took my regularly designated chair and attempted to lead the group. He made a valiant effort to imitate me. He tried to talk like me, sit like me, and reprimand like me. The others began to laugh, looked on it as a good-natured pretense, and corrected him to provide a better imitation. Instead of interrupting him, I took his regularly designated seat and tried to imitate him. He was not able to sustain the act, but he had started the process. Each of the clients took turns at leading the group as if she/he were me. We tried to get them to show how they understood the rules and how they would play the game. The process of internalization, incorporation and integration of superego mechanisms with improved ego functioning for the individual was enhanced and supported by the social structure. Play had become the medium between the internal process and the environment. Culture was being invented and created, changed and remodeled.

One year later, it was time for me to withdraw from this intricate involvement with Hull House and establish this kind of social system in the other four ICFs. I was planning to bring in another supervisor, but I would maintain my ultimate authority position as the director. Up to this point, the clients had reacted to each and all losses of key staff as great tragedies from which they would never recover.

At the community meeting to introduce the new supervisor, we reviewed what the normal responses to my departure might be. We discussed how far Hull House had come. Ben volunteered that we had become like a team, like the A-Team (a popular TV adventure series about four men who conquer adversities through cooperation). He was right on target. They were a team, the Hull House Team, "The H-Team." They had the spirit. They had the group identity. They could support and sustain each other. They belonged together. They respected each other. They worked together for the good of the team. They would work for the new coach. I could go on to be general manager.

The new supervisor ordered navy blue T-shirts with the H-Team inscribed in white on the back for the good citizens and the staff. Each shirt had the first name in white on the front. The community meetings became team rallies complete with pep talks, game reviews and game plans. It was still a shame for a team member to have played badly, but now the team was to help that individual get back in the game. Issues that had been private agonies were open to group interventions and social support. The team would understand. Illness and death of natural family members, of staff, of staff's families, of clients in the other group homes in the WJCS family, became the team's social concern. As the team's social competence increased, their epistemology broadened to encompass more of the world. At last, the team asked that its members be allowed the power to distribute the good citizen awards.

SUMMARY

This paper has been about the process of the development of a group home as a treatment facility for the dually diagnosed using social group treatment methodology and various theoretical models. The development required strong leadership, dedicated staff and an agency committed to helping its clients. The ten clients continue to live together. The clients have the trained capacity to cope with life and master its trials and tribulations. They also have the social supports and social group structure to survive in a fast-paced, ever-changing society. They will always need a protected environment because that is the nature of their developmental disabilities. The essence of their protection, however, is not the institution called group home but their self-development of social competence.

I have examined the evolution of the microsystem through the development of the group culture. The normative structure, patterns of acceptable behavior or normal social expectations, evolved from authoritatively imposed rules and standards to the group members involvement in the recreation and internalization of social standards. People were not aware of the rules for everyday life-space activities and this had led to confusion and maladjustment. Clarity, certainty and consistency resolved the moral crisis. Structural control provided by authorative power, regulation and discipline evolved into "group cultural control"[20] through the group process and the interpersonal learning of normal social inhibition.

Germain and Gitterman took an ecological perspective in developing their Life Model approach to practice. They recognized the interdependence, interaction and complex reciprocal interrelationships between people and their environments. They described the interpenetrating interplay between the layers of social and physical environment and the texture of time and space. Their model is concerned with the life space of social interaction.

In person-environment transactions, disturbances often occur between individual needs and capacities, and environmental demands and qualities. These transactional disturbances create problems in living generated by stress arising from three areas of the life space: life transitions; environmental pressures; and maladaptive interpersonal processes.[21]

This paper has been concerned about the life space of 10 dually diagnosed individuals living in a group home. It traced the history of the client — group — home development from the transition of placement and the socially disinhibited maladaptation through to the establishment of a social system that enabled successful adaptation and qualitative growth. The demands of group home living are fraught with problems that can either foster un-normalized living or support human relatedness and community integration. This is one possible way to build an ecological system that is enabling.

REFERENCES

1. See: T. Ayllon and N. H. Azrin, *The Token Economy* (New York: Appleton Press, 1968); T. Douglas, *Group Living* (New York: Tavistock, 1986); G. Dybwad, "Roadblocks to Renewal to Residential Care," in F. J. Menolascino, ed., *Psychiatric Approaches to Mental Retardation*, (New York: Basic Books, 1970), pp. 552-574; P. Lambert, *the ABC's of Child Care Work in Residential Care* (New York: Child Welfare League, 1977); G. L. Paul and R. V. Lentz, *Psychosocial Treatment of Chronic Mental Patients*, (Cambridge, Mass: Harvard University Press, 1977); H. W. Polsky, *Cottage Six* (Walabar, Fla.: Krieger, 1977 Reprint); R. Sovner and A. D. Hurley, "Behavior Modification III: The Token Economy," *Psychiatric Aspects of Mental Retardation Reviews*, 4 (January 1985), pp. 1-4; A. E. Trieschman, J. K. Whittaker and L. K. Brendtro, *The Other 23 Hours* (Chicago: Aldine, 1969); J. K. Whittaker and A. E. Trieschman, *Children Away From Home* (Chicago, Aldine, 1972); I. D. Yalom, *Inpatient Group Psychotherapy* (New York: Basic Books, 1983); and I. D. Yalom, *The Theory*

and Practice of Group Psychotherapy, Third Edition (New York: Basic Books, 1985).

2. N. C. Lang, "Social Work Practice in Small Social Forms: Identifying Collectivity," *Social Work With Groups*, 9 (Winter 1986), pp. 7-32.

3. C. Garvin, "Family Therapy and Group Work: 'Kissing Cousins or Distant Relatives' in Social Work Practice," in M. Parnes, ed., *Innovations in Social Group Work: Feedback From Practice to Theory* (New York: The Haworth Press, Inc., 1986), pp. 1-16.

4. I. D. Yalom, *The Theory and Practice of Group Psychotherapy, Third Edition* p. 30.

5. M. Rutter, "Psychological Sequelae of Brain Damage in Children," *American Journal of Psychiatry*, 139 (October 1981), p. 1541.

6. *Idem.*

7. J. D. Wine and M. D. Snye, eds., *Social Competence* (New York: Guilford Press, 1981).

8. R. W. White, "Motivation Reconsidered—The Concept of Competence," *Psychological Review*, 66 (March 1959), pp. 297-333.

9. W. Wolfensberger, *The Principle of Normalization in Human Services* (Toronto: National Institute on Mental Retardation, 1972), p. 78.

10. F. V. Menolascino, "Overview: Bridging the Gap Between Mental Retardation and Mental Illness," in F. V. Menolascino and B. M. McCann, eds., *Mental Health and Mental Retardation: Bridging the Gap* (Baltimore: University Park Press, 1983), p. 18.

11. *Ibid.*, p. 7.

12. J. Piaget, *The Moral Judgment of the Child*, (New York: Free Press, 1965).

13. L. Kohlberg, "Stage and Sequence: The Cognitive—Developmental Approach to Socialization," in D. A. Gosbin, eds., *Handbook of Socialization Theory and Research* (Chicago: Rand McNally, 1969).

14. R. D. Vinter, "An Approach to Group Work Practice," in M. Seindel, P. Glasser, R. Sarri and R. Vinter, eds., *Individual Change Through Small Group, Second Edition* (New York: The Free Press, 1985), p. 6.

15. *Ibid.*, p. 6.

16. C. Lasch, *The Culture of Narcissism*, (New York: Warner Books, 1979), pp. 301-308.

17. *Ibid.*, p. 305.

18. A. M. Johnson, "Sanctions for Superego Lacunae of Adolescents," reprinted in A. H. Esman, ed., *The Psychology of Adolescence* (New York: International Universities Press, 1975), pp. 245-265.

19. W. Gaylin, *Feelings* (New York: Ballantine Books, 1979), p. 54.

20. T. Douglas, *Group Living*, p. 172.

21. C. B. Germain and A. Gitterman, "The Life Model Approach to Social Work Practice Revisited," in F. J. Turner, ed., *Social Work Treatment: Interlocking Theoretical Approaches, Third Edition*, (New York: The Free Press, 1986), p. 628.

Needs Assessment for Group Work with People of Color: A Conceptual Formulation

Kenneth L. Chau

SUMMARY. Cultural sensitivity in needs assessment is a prerequisite for effective group work practice with ethnically diverse populations. A conceptual framework is presented to explain and assess the nature of psychosocial needs borne out of cultural differences or conflicts, using "sociocultural dissonance" as an orienting concept. Implications for group work are discussed.

The interest in developing understanding, methods, and skills for group work practice with ethnically diverse populations is becoming an important priority for social group work practice (Davis, 1984).

Although advances have been made in recent years to offer culturally alternative services, and to adapt group work approaches and technologies to ethnic factors and minority needs (Chau, 1986; Davis, 1985; Garvin, 1985; Ho, 1984), there is as yet no professional consensus or conceptual clarity regarding the appropriate focus for group work practice with people of color. Questions have been raised about whether the decisions on goals and nature of group work intervention are made without adequate consideration of the unique sociocultural reality confronting these individuals (Chau, 1987; Davis, 1985).

This article aims at developing a conceptual formulation of needs relevant to people of color as well as to professionals committed to understanding and helping ethnic individuals and families through the use of group format. The basic premise of this article is the ecological perspec-

Kenneth L. Chau, PhD, is Associate Professor, Department of Social Work, California State University, 1250 Bellflower Blvd., Long Beach, CA 90840-0902.

53

tive which stresses the importance of interaction between characteristics of people and their environment.

THE STRESS AND STRAIN OF CULTURAL DIFFERENCES: FOCUS FOR NEEDS ASSESSMENT

In group practice as in other methods of social work, needs assessment is considered central to the effectiveness of practice. Almost all group practice approaches stress some form of assessment of what constitutes the client's needs as a basis for defining practice goals, and for developing a plan of intervention.

In a comparative analysis of theoretical approaches of social work with groups, however, Northen and Roberts (1976) noted that among the approaches that subscribe to assessment of individuals for intake and planning, there was little consensus about the dimensions on which the individuals should be assessed (pp. 386-7). Instead, a variety of emphases prevail, ranging from ego assessment to the assessment of social and psychological factors, or past and present experiences, and psychiatric diagnoses. The authors further noted the absence in these approaches of a comprehensive account for the etiology and dynamics of persons seen in their total sociocultural context.

The same situation is also reflected in periodical literature that describes group work services or interventions. With few exceptions, needs assessment relegates the "outer" sociocultural reality to a place of secondary concern, compared to the "inner" world of psychological processes (Davis, 1985). The problems faced by people of color are often defined in terms of psychological dysfunction, and the individual is often targeted for change (Frankel & Sundel, 1978; Paquet-Deehy et al., 1985). Since clinical practice is biased toward a mainstream frame of reference, practitioners have a tendency to ignore the fact that many of the supposed symptoms of "dysfunctional" behavior of people of color may be attempts to influence others in their sociocultural environment. It may be attempts to cope with the stress and strain of adaptation, acculturation or just being different. Or, it may simply be an adaptive response to prejudice, discrimination, or other environmental pressures (Hardy-Fanta, 1986; Smith et al., 1978). The ultimate aim of these efforts is to restore or maintain some kind of social or personal equilibrium.

Therefore, in order effectively to help and empower people of color through the group, needs assessment must be based on their unique sociocultural reality of belonging to two cultures — their ethnic culture and the dominant culture.

The concept that best illuminates this unique sociocultural reality is "sociocultural dissonance" (Chau, 1987). Because of variant cultural beliefs, values, worldviews, behavior patterns and problem-solving methods, people of color are believed to be vulnerable to sociocultural dissonance; i.e., the stress and strain of incongruence between the demands and expectations of the two cultural environments. Sociocultural dissonance occurs as people of color attempt to retain their own culture or aspects of it under the pressure of conforming to the dominant culture. Our tasks of understanding, explaining, and assessing their social psychological needs must, therefore, be viewed in the context of how they cope with the stress and strain of cultural differences, cultural conflicts, and the dual demands and influences of two cultural environments.

The association of stress with psychosocial needs is well documented in the literature. Because of cultural differences or conflicts, and because of societal prejudice and discriminatory institutional practices, people of color, especially those of immigrant and refugee backgrounds, are vulnerable to greater risk of stress (Brody, 1970; Grinberg & Grinberg, 1984). For these people, the processes of adaptation, accommodation, and integration are especially taxing. These processes challenge the resilience of their long-held values, beliefs, patterns of behavior and problem-solving; and require them to make dynamic and synergistic changes not only on an individual level, but in other social and interpersonal realms as well. These challenges and demands represent immeasurable amounts of sociocultural dissonance of which there are three major categories: life changes, role-status changes, and social-structural adjustment. They give rise to psychosocial needs that are manifested at the individual level, intragroup level, intergroup level, and systems level. In exploring the nature and scope of social psychological needs of ethnic minority clients, it requires the practitioner to understand these needs and differentiate them according to the level at which they occur. This allows the practitioner to determine how much his or her client's psychosocial functioning is affected and at what level. This provides a basis for developing a plan of intervention most appropriate to the client.

DIMENSIONS OF PSYCHOSOCIAL NEEDS

Table 1 summarizes the three major categories of sociocultural dissonance and attendant psychosocial needs manifested at the individual level and intragroup level, as well as intergroup and systems levels.

Initially, the concerns the client brings to the worker are often undifferentiated. It is this presenting concern or request for help that provides a

TABLE 1. Sociocultural Dissonance and Psychosocial Needs

Sources Sociocultural Dissonance	Psychosocial Functioning			
	Individual Level	Intragroup Level	Intergroups Level	Systems Level
Life Change Events	Manage stress, anxiety depression. Socialize into new environment & resources. Orientate to new cultural requirements. Help regain self direction and mastery of new life situations.	Manage feelings of loss of affective ties. Foster mutual help. Promote self-help efforts. Develop new social support networks.	Cope with loneliness, isolation & social alienation. Promote intergroups contacts & interactions. Facilitate collaboration between groups.	Address issues of inequity. Cope with unresponsive institutions & resource systems. Promote understanding of minority needs & rights.
Role-Status Changes	Socialize to new roles. Learn to cope with new cultural requirements. Develop & master new areas of interest. Deal with loss of valued roles, captivity in undesired roles...	Promote mutual appreciation of the changed roles. Develop understanding of new definition of authority and cultural traditions. Facilitate intergenerational harmony, relations, inter-actions, & understanding.	Develop understanding of interpersonal relation & communication between groups. Develop understanding of roles and behaviors between groups.	Learn appropriate responses to environmental pressures & expectations. Develop skills to negotiate institutions and systems. Promote understanding of civil and human rights. Cope with imposed inferiority.
Social-Structural Adjustment	Manage emotional distress, low self-concept. Overcome personal disorganization. Maintain balance between own culture and dominant culture. Develop a sense of feeling attached to the soc order.	Foster ethnic consciousness Develop ethnic community resources. Build ethnic organizations and new power bases. Train & develop leadership. Cope with low group identy & feelings of powerlessness	Cope with intergroups tension, distrust, social distance & over-reaction. Engage in collaborative projects. Promote intergroups harmony, acceptance and integration.	Cope with cultural insensitivity. Promote culturally appropriate services. Fight against prejudice and discrimination.

beginning for the process of assessing client needs (Northen, 1987). The following formulation of what might confront people of color should offer a framework for understanding and explaining their psychosocial needs.

Life Change

This dimension refers to stressful life events unique to people of color (such as refugee experience, camp confinement, displacement, dislocation, emigration, separation of family, etc.) that disrupt an individual's usual activities, lifestyle, and established behavioral patterns or sense of self-efficacy. Research indicates that in response to life changes, the individual activates psychological and other coping efforts (Holmes & Rahe, 1967; Rahe & Arthur, 1978). Psychosocial functioning is at higher risk of impairment through refugee experiences and camp confinement (Roberts, Chau, Nishimoto & Mok, 1984), or when the amount of change required overwhelms adaptive coping resources (Dohrenwend, 1973; Eaton, 1978; Miller, Ingham & Davidson, 1976).

The experiencing of stress of life changes is universal. Its impact, however, is greater and more pervasive for people of color than it is for members of dominant groups; and their perception of the change required by various life events differs significantly (Fairbank & Hough, 1981; Janney et al., 1977). For example, people from materially disadvantaged ethnic groups, compared to affluent persons, perceive life events with economic and bodily necessity as more stressful than those events having to do with personal or interpersonal interaction (Ibid.). Blacks, Mexican-Americans, and Asians in Los Angeles, compared to the Anglo population of Northwestern U.S. studied by Holmes and Rahe (1967), rated events quite differently and viewed events having to do with labor, income, and living conditions as requiring more change (Komaroff et al., 1968).

These factors must be taken into account in assessing the psychosocial needs or problems emerging from stressful life changes. On the individual level, it is important to understand and appraise the notion that anxiety and depression are manifestations of the individual's emotional reaction to the changed life situation, to the unfamiliarity of the new environment, to the challenges it poses to the resilience of established behavior, and to the uncertainty in regaining personal competence and direction.

On the intragroup level, feelings of loss of affective and instrumental supports prevail. Potential problems arise as psychosocial functioning and adjustment to stressful events often take place without full recourse to the psychological and material resources of the family or support network from within one's ethnic group. In a sense, the loss or uprooting of one's support networks and family ties occasioned by life changes is itself a stressor, and it affects the person's ability to cope with the changed life situation.

At the intergroup level, psychosocial functioning of people of color is frequently affected by the nature of relationships they have with members of dominant and other ethnic groups. Faced with persistent social alienation, many people of color respond with self-imposed isolation or withdrawal from the social scene. These are convenient, adaptive responses to social alienation, but they often create for these people feelings of loneliness, isolation, and even fear of strangers.

At institutional or systems levels, problems of inequitable access to needed resources are well documented in the literature. Lack of culturally relevant services, insensitive policies and procedures and unresponsiveness of service systems and bureaucracies are often cited as reasons for non-utilization or inappropriate use of services by people of color.

Role-Status Changes

A second dimension for needs assessment focuses on changes in role-status of an individual, and his/her emotional reaction to such changes. Role-status constitutes a basic unit of social behavior; hence, role-status change necessitates adaptation in cognitive, affective and behavioral domains of psychosocial functioning, and is stress-inducing. For example, change to a position of high role-status, as in job promotion, involves achievement-related stress; and change to a low role-status position, as in underemployment or job demotion, induces a threat to one's sense of efficacy or personal security. The loss of valued roles is said to lead to "a mutilated self" (Rose, 1962), and is linked to manifestation of depression, e.g., as in the case of maternal role loss in women (Bart, 1974). Assessing role-status changes will enable the worker to give attention to the nature of the new or modified role-status and its effects on various levels of the person's psychosocial functioning.

Thus, on the individual level, a redefinition of roles occasioned by cultural incongruence may have negative impact on psychosocial functioning, particularly when the individual's restructured cognitions and expectations of the new role are not consistent with prior role and self-concept. The effects of loss of salient or valued roles, or of being a captive in undesired roles must be assessed for intervention planning, as are the effects of redefined roles on people oblivious to the changed definitions.

On the intragroup level, the effects of role-status redefinition are even more pronounced in relationships and interactions among members of family or related groups. Change in sex role-status, for example, may trigger off feelings of loss of control among males, conflict concerning maternal role among females, or confusion about parental roles between spouses, whose prior socialization was based on clear differentiation of sex-role expectations. Intergenerational disharmony often occurs in families where differences in role socialization between parents and children often lead to conflicts concerning what are "right and proper" role behaviors and lifestyles. In many ethnic minority families, where interpersonal relationship is linear and hierarchical and based on a group orientation, redefinitions of role-status based on an egalitarian ideology often impose changes for which people in traditional authority positions in the family system (e.g., the family elders) are ill-prepared. The cultural orientation of role-status, the erosion of the authority of elders and the group orientations of these families, create problems of relationship and communication requiring culture-sensitive solutions.

Some of these problems in relationship and communication also occur in intergroup situations, where discrepant expectations held by each group regarding role sets and norms of behavior can easily cause embarrassment and misunderstanding and discourage inter-cultural contacts and relations.

At the systems level, problems of psychosocial functioning must be assessed in regard to the effects of role-status change on the individual's response to environmental demands. For example, assessment must take into account cultural response to authority as it is manifested in supervisor-subordinate relationships in the workplace. In many incidents, an unwillingness to express differences, to disagree, or be assertive with people in an authority position could be a result of prior cultural expectation rather than an inability to form independent opinion. Assessment must also explore clients' feelings of being like "second class citizens," how this feeling affects their ability to negotiate resource systems for help or services, and how it affects their ability to stand firm on their rights to fair treatment despite the imposed inferior role-status. Similarly, certain role behavior of ethnic groups (such as those based on the virtue of modesty, harmony, Golden Mean, etc.) are often misconstrued as personal weakness, are exploited, or are considered to be at odds with dominant role behavior in the workplace, where self-promotion is the valued means of survival or job advancement. The stress and strain of role-status redefinition and the resultant threat to one's personal security, demand more than changes of cognitions, emotions and customary coping activities by the individuals. They require also sensitive responses from the worker and the social institutions.

Social-Structural Adjustment

This dimension refers to the tasks of adapting and acculturating to new social environment or structure. It also refers to the emotional reactions to these tasks, and to the sociocultural dissonance occasioned by incongruence of cultural beliefs and norms of behavior between the new and the prior social environment.

On the individual level, adaptation and integration demand not just learning a new language but also the nuances of verbal and written language; not just securing employment and housing but developing relationships and familiarity with the new environment as well; not just acquiring and internalizing new social attitudes, but also accepting and adjusting to a lower self-concept. All of these require balancing between ethnic and dominant cultures; relinquishing culturally different habits, customary activities, long-held beliefs and values that may impede adjustment; and retaining those that facilitate social integration. The process of adjustment to cultural differences in the workplace, at home, or other social situations, evokes emotional distress and difficulties and causes intrapsychic confusion, conflicts, personal disorganization, or even anomia — a lack of feeling attached to the social order.

On the intragroup level, psychosocial functioning reflects the family or ethnic group's sense of group identity or cohesion. Often, a self-perceived low group identity or cohesion has the effect of reinforcing the individual's low self-image, social marginality and sense of powerlessness. This "negative self valuation" (Solomon, 1976) or "internalized oppression," can easily reduce minority individuals' effectiveness and ability to control both the internal and external circumstances of their lives.

Adjustment to relationships and communication outside of one's own group on an intergroup level is subject to the influence of many factors. For people of color, however, their "differentness" invites suspicion, fear, stereotyping, or distrust; and may create inter-ethnic tension and conflict (Masuda, 1984). Quite often, the complaints they present to the worker are described as feelings of isolation, loneliness, or depression. These are in fact reactive emotional distress of transition, adjustment and integration; or are consequences of social alienation or psychological ostracism caused by misinformation, misunderstanding, or inappropriate attitudes and behaviors of the dominant group toward cultural differences and toward ethnic minority groups. It could also be results of over-reaction of minority groups to stereotyping or to the cultural insensitivity which they have experienced.

At the systems level, psychosocial needs of adjustment must be assessed in terms of the effects of institutional inequality, prejudice, and discrimination. Social institutions and services are culturally biased toward the needs and problems of the mainstream of society and, as such, they are not equitable to other groups (Cole & Pilisuk, 1976). Evidence suggests that there is inequity in resource distribution, and special groups are assigned to services not on the basis of their unique conditions but on the basis of color or stereotypes about them held by service providers (Kagle & Cowger, 1984).

APPLICATIONS AND IMPLICATIONS FOR GROUP PRACTICE

The above discussion delineates a paradigm of psychosocial needs as sociocultural dissonance experienced by people of color. The paradigm offers a holistic way to view, explain and assess the client's psychosocial functioning at four levels: (1) the individual level—in terms of how an individual adapts to personal inadequacy created by cultural differences in expectations and norms; (2) the intragroup level—how an individual adjusts to minority status and low ethnic identity, and copes with interpersonal relationship within his/her own family or related group; (3) the intergroup level—in terms of interacting and seeking or resisting alliances with dominant or other minority groups; and (4) the systems level—in negotiating environmental resource systems. Each level of functioning addresses the client's emotional reactions to sociocultural dissonance arising out of the demands of life changes, role-status changes and social-structural adjustments in the course of cross-cultural integration into the mainstream of society.

In assessing the needs for group service, it should not be assumed that sociocultural dissonance always leads an ethnic individual to problems of psychosocial functioning. Because of individual variations in response to stress and adversity of cultural differences, some people succumb to these stressors, whereas others emerge from them enriched and strengthened in their coping capability.

Research has indicated the buffering effects of certain "mediating variables" that may affect an individual's ability successfully to cope with the challenges of sociocultural dissonance. They include: (1) salient characteristics of the individuals such as level of acculturation, gender, socioeconomic background (Dohrenwend & Dohrenwend, 1974, 1976; Dohrenwend, 1976); (2) personality features such as self-efficacy or self-esteem (Garmezy, 1985; Masten & Garmezy, 1985); (3) personal resources in terms of coping styles, knowledge and skills, availability and effective use of natural support networks (e.g., family ties, ethnic cohesion, community attachment); and (4) availability of other formal, culturally appropriate external support systems that encourage and reinforce the individual's coping efforts.

Therefore, in assessing ethnic minority client needs based on their presenting complaints or request, the social worker should also assess which of these mediating variables are and are not an asset to the client and to problem-solving, and which of them are also a part of the problems. This understanding will assist the social worker in determining the nature of the client's needs, the level(s) at which the client's psychosocial functioning is most affected, the client's strength and capacity, and societal resources available. This will enable the worker to decide more accurately on the nature and goal of intervention, and strategies.

This paradigm of needs presents important implications for group work practice with ethnic minority populations. In the first place, the extensive nature of these needs suggests that group practice must be broadly based so that a wide spectrum of clients' concerns rather than a narrowly defined interest of the practitioners will be addressed. This follows that group intervention must target not just on changing the clients and their methods of coping, but also on changing the social structural arrangements impinging upon the clients. A broad range of group formats will be necessary, as will group issues, goals, and interventive strategies that will enhance individual, interpersonal, and social processes.

On the individual level of psychosocial functioning, for example, planned group intervention must be sensitive to the individual's emotional responses to the transcultural nature of needs that were created by the three kinds of change, and to his or her psychosocial resilience. Group intervention must be directed at strengthening or validating their coping abilities and adaptation, with the aim of enhancing personal competence and psychological adaptation to cultural differences. Groups most suitable for this purpose are those designed to provide orientation and socialization to the knowledge, resources, and cultural norms and expectations of dominant society. Others include problem-solving groups focused on difficulties of personal nature, and socialization groups for personal growth and social enrichment.

On the intragroup level, the problems of low ethnic cohesion, loss of family ties and support, and the resultant political and social vulnerability of people of color all call for empowerment strategies. They suggest that group intervention must be directed at raising ethnic consciousness and creating new sources of power and ethnic resource bases. Groups designed to enhance ethnic pride, develop leadership potential and foster self-help and mutual-help are especially helpful for raising intragroup identity and strength. By providing a forum for mutual help and encouraging ethnic individuals and groups to develop or utilize their creative capability, group practice empowers ethnic group members to develop their ability and ethnocultural cohesion to deal with new challenges and to control what happens to them.

Cultural insensitivity and stereotyping in intergroup situations also have programatic implications for group practice. Not only must group intervention adopt a reeducative strategy, providing opportunity, such as through dialogue groups and prejudice reduction groups, for correct information and understanding among groups; it must also encourage intergroup contacts and collaborations as a basis to facilitate mutual acceptance and social integration.

The idea that social institutions are culture-bound has implications for group intervention at the systems level. Here, group intervention must assume an advocacy stance aimed at bringing about equity and cultural sensitivity in services and policies. Groups that fall within this practice focus may focus on, but not be limited to, welfare rights or patient rights, mental patients' ward council, and other formats of self-governing, or self-help within an institutional context. These groups help clients to gain greater control over institutional practices, and to ensure that services are more responsive to their needs, more readily available, and easily accessible.

CONCLUSION

This article contends that effective group work with people of color is predicated on cultural sensitivity in needs assessment. By conceptualizing psychosocial needs as sociocultural dissonance, a cognitive restructuring of the nature and scope of psychosocial needs is presented that accommodates the otherwise unique concerns experienced by people of color caught between their cultural background and the traditional ethos of mainstream society.

The three dimensions of sociocultural dissonance occasioned in the course of cross-cultural adaptation to life changes, role-status changes, and social-structural changes, combine to create a useful matrix for understanding, explaining, or assessing psychosocial needs and their manifestations at four levels of psychosocial functioning. Implications of these psychosocial needs for planned group work intervention are discussed, and linked to various group issues or interventive strategies.

REFERENCES

Bart, P. B. The sociology of depression. In Roman, P. M., & Trice, H. M., eds. *Explorations in Psychiatric Sociology*, Philadelphia: F. A. Davis Co., 1974: 139-157.

Brody, E. Migration and adaptation: The nature of the problem. In Brody, E., ed. *Behavior in New Environments: Adaptation of Migrant Populations*. Beverly Hills, Ca.: Sage, 1970.

Chau, Kenneth L. Parameters of group work: A model of practice with special reference to ethnic minority populations. Paper presented at the 8th Annual Symposium for the Advancement of Social Work with Groups, October, 1986, Los Angeles, Ca.

Chau, Kenneth L. Sociocultural dissonance: Locus of concern for group work practice with ethnic minority populations. Paper presented at the Annual Program Meeting, Council on Social Work Education, March, 1987, St. Louis, Missouri.

Cole, J.; and Pilisuk, M. Differences in the provision of mental health service by race. *American Journal of Orthopsychiatry*, 46 (1976), pp. 510-525.

Davis, Larry E., (Guest Editor), Ethnicity in social group work practice. Special issue of *Social Work With Groups*, 7, (Fall, 1984).

Davis, Larry E. Group work practice with ethnic minorities of color. In Sundel, M., Glasser, P., Sarri, R., and Vinter, R., eds., *Individual Change Through Small Groups*, 2nd edition. New York: The Free Press, 1985, pp. 324-343.

Dohrenwend, B. S. Life events as stressors: A methological inquiry. *Journal of Health and Social Behavior*, 14 (1973): 167-175.

Dohrenwend, B. P. Sociocultural and social-psychological factors in the genesis of mental disorders. *Journal of Health and Social Behavior*, 16 (1975): 365-392.

Dohrenwend, B. P.; and Dohrenwend, B. S. Social and cultural influences on psychopathy. *Annual Review of Psychology*, 25 (1974): 417-452.

Dohrenwend, B. P.; and Dohrenwend, B. S. Sex differences and psychiatric disorders. *American Journal of Sociology*, 81 (1976): 1447-1454.

Eaton, W. Life events, social supports, and psychiatric symptoms: A re-analysis of the New Haven data. *Journal of Health and Social Behavior*, 19 (1978): 230-234.

Fairbank, D.; and Hough, R. Cultural differences in the perception of life events. In Dohrenwend, B. S., and Dohrenwend, B. P., eds., *Stressful Life Events and their Contexts*. New York: PRODIST, Neal Watson Academic Publications, 1981, pp. 63-84.

Frankel, A. J.; and Sundel, M. The grope for group: Initiating individual and community change. *Social Work With Groups*, 1 (Winter, 1978).

Gallegos, Joseph S.; and Harris, Olita D. Toward a model for inclusion of ethnic minority content in doctoral social work education. *Journal of Education for Social Work*, 15 (Winter, 1979), pp. 29-35.

Garmezy, N. Stress resistent children: The search for protective factors. In J. Stevenson, ed. *Recent Research in Developmental Psychopathology*. Oxford: Pergamon Press, 1985.

Garvin, Charles D. Work with disadvantaged and oppressed groups. In Sundel, M. et al., eds. *Individual Change . . .* , op cit.

Grinberg, A.; and Grinberg, R. A psychoanalytic study of migration: Its normal and pathological aspects. *Journal of American Psychoanalytic Association*, 32 (1984): 13-38.

Hardy-Fanta, Carol, Social action in Hispanic groups. *Social Work*, (March-April, 1986), pp. 119-123.

Ho, Man Keung, Social group work with Asian/Pacific-Americans. *Social Work With Groups*, 7(3), 1984, pp. 49-61.

Holmes, T.; and Rahe, R. The social readjustment rating scale. *Journal of Psychosomatic Research*, 11 (1967): 213-218.

Janney, J.; Masuda, M.; and Holmes, T. Impact of a natural catastrophe on life events. *Journal of Human Stress*, 3(1977): 22-34.

Kagle, Jill D.; and Cowger, Charles D. Blaming the clients: Implicit agenda in practice research? *Social Work*, (July-August, 1984), pp. 347-351.

Komaroff, A.; Masuda, M.; and Holmes, T. The social readjustment rating scale: A comparative study of Negro, Mexican American and White Americans. *Journal of Psychosomatic Research*, 12(1968): 121-128.

Masten, A. S. and Garmezy, N. Risk, vulnerability, and protective factors in developmental psychopathology. In B. B. Lahey and A. E. Kazdin, eds. *Advances in Clinical Child Psychology*, Vol. 8. New York: Plenum Press, 1985.

Masuda, Robert. Human differentness: A critical variable for international practicum in social work. In Sanders, Daniel S., and Pedersen, Paul. eds. *Education for International Social Welfare*. Council on Social Work Education and University of Hawaii School of Social Work, 1984, pp. 114-122.

Miller, P.; Ingham, J.; and Davison, S. Life events, symptoms and social support. *Journal of Psychosomatic Research*, 20 (1976): 515-522.

Northen, Helen. Assessment in direct practice. In Minahan, Anne et al., eds. *Encyclopedia of Social Work*, 1987, 18th ed., Vol 1, p. 172.

Northen, Helen; and Roberts, Robert W. The status of theory. In Roberts, Robert W., and Northen, Helen. eds. *Theories of Social Work with Groups*. New York: Columbia University Press, 1976.

Paquet-Deehy, Ann; Hopmeyer, Estelle; Home, Alice; and Kislowicz, Linda. A typology of social work practice with groups. *Social Work With Groups*, 8 (Spring, 1985), pp. 65-78.

Rahe, R.; and Arthur, R. Life change and illness studies. *Journal of Human Stress*, 4 (1978): 3-15.

Roberts, Robert W.; Chau, Kenneth L; Nishimoto, Robert; and Mok, Bongho.

Refugees at-risk: Some covariates of mental health. *The Hong Kong Journal of Social Work*, 1984.

Rose, A. A socio-psychological theory of neurosis. In Rose, A., ed., *Human Behavior and Social Processes*. Boston, Houghton-Mifflin Co., 1962, pp. 537-549.

Smith, W.D.; Burlew, A.; Mosley, M.; and Whitney, W. *Minority Issues in Mental Health*. Reading, Mass.: Addison-Wesley, 1979.

Solomon, Barbara. *Black Empowerment: Social Work in Oppressed Communities*. New York: Columbia University Press, 1976.

A Task Centered Group Approach
to Work
with the Chronically Mentally Ill

Charles Garvin

This paper describes our work to develop task-centered group work for the rehabilitation of the chronically mentally ill and empirically to validate this approach. The group members for whom this type of group work has been devised have been classified as chronically mentally ill on the following basis: first, they have been diagnosed as suffering from a serious mental illness, either schizophrenia, a major affective disorder such as manic-depressive psychosis, or organic brain syndrome; second, their disability is severe and involves significant handicaps in fulfilling the requirements of educational, occupational, and familial roles; and third, their disability has existed over a long period of time. While the intensity of this disability is likely to vary, these members may have had their illness for several years during which they have experienced numerous hospitalizations of short duration or a few hospitalizations for longer periods.

The need for new services for this population is great and has been intensified as a result of the process of deinstitutionalization. Prior to this shift in social policy, these individuals were often long-term residents of psychiatric hospitals. They are more likely now to be living in community facilities, including nursing homes, adult foster care homes, single room occupancy dwellings, or with their own families. Many are among the homeless. A recent report estimates their numbers to be between 1.7 and 2.4 million including 900,000 who are institutionalized.[1]

Charles Garvin, PhD, is Professor of Social Work, The University of Michigan, Ann Arbor, MI 48109.

67

GROUPS FOR THE CHRONICALLY MENTALLY ILL

Groups have been used extensively by members of all mental health professions to help meet the needs of the chronically mentally ill. These groups are conducted in hospitals, community mental health centers, day treatment programs, and other in-patient and out-patient facilities. They follow many different models of practice, including all of the contemporary approaches to social work with groups, as well as traditional group psychotherapy, behavior modification, social skills training, and groups oriented to activities such as arts and crafts, music, current events, photography, and so forth. Comprehensive "club house" type agencies such as Fountain House in New York and Fellowship House in Miami, look programmatically very much like the kinds of settlement houses and community centers that played such an important historical role in the evolution of social group work.

This extensive utilization of groups is based on more than nostalgia and ideology. Many research studies have demonstrated the effectiveness of groups in rehabilitating the chronically mentally ill. These studies typically compare outcomes for individuals who receive group services as well as case management and medication with those who do not receive such services. The sample receiving group services almost always fares better than the one that does not. Group services largely focus on education about mental illness, social skills, and discussions of interpersonal problems. Much of the literature implicitly or explicitly favors avoiding the promotion of insight into unconscious material.[2]

Of particular importance to our work was the recent meta-analytic study by Videka-Sherman.[3] She reviewed every controlled study, twenty-three to be specific, of *social work practice* with the chronically mentally ill. On the basis of this, she concluded that the best outcomes are secured by (1) group approaches that are based on (2) structured interventions and that are (3) time limited in nature. This does not imply that the chronically mentally ill can be "cured" in a short time; on the contrary, they are likely to remain as clients of agencies for a long period. Also, their treatment program may be made up of a variety of components including both short-term and long term groups. Thus some of the members of this population participate in long-term groups intended to provide them with ongoing support. This does not preclude their involvement in short-term groups, such as task-centered ones, that focus on highly specific outcome objectives.

TASK-CENTERED GROUP WORK

Task-centered group work shares many features with other task-centered practice approaches that have been derived from the work originally done by Reid and Epstein.[4] These approaches are short term ones and usually consist of six to twelve sessions with the client. During these sessions, the client selects a problem that will serve as the focus of the work. Goals are then chosen whose attainment will help to alleviate the problem. Up to this point, task-centered practice looks very much like other time limited, goal oriented approaches.

The difference between task-centered and other short-term structured approaches such as social skills training lies in the next steps in the process. After a goal has been chosen, the worker helps the group members to help each other to select and carry out tasks in order to reach the goal. A task is, therefore, a course of action that the client thinks will help attain a goal and, thus, ameliorate the problem. The role of the worker at this point is to help the clients to help each other to define the tasks so that they are realistic, appropriate, and clearly enough specified that they can serve as the bases for action. The worker provides help so the group members can help each other in carrying out tasks such as assisting the client to remove barriers to task accomplishment that lie within the client or the environment. The worker may teach the members skills, work with member feelings, and advocate for the members in the environment—all of these interventions are geared to aid the client effectively to carry out tasks.

Many workers, whatever their model, do, in essence, function in this manner. Those who have been most involved in the development of task-centered practice, however, have closely examined the processes of selecting and carrying out tasks with various types of clients so that the techniques that are most facilitative and the clients who are most helped by this approach can be identified. This underscores the idea that task-centered practice is empirically based and its methods and outcomes are subject to scientific measurement.

Several features of the model enhance its attractiveness to many social workers. In addition to its short term nature which coincides with many of the realities of agency services and client wishes, it places a strong emphasis on self-determination in that the client is asked to play an active role in selecting problems, goals, and tasks. In addition, it recognizes the necessity to ground practice in a careful examination of what we as practitioners do as well as in the consequences of our actions.

Early in the development of task-centered practice, this author recognized and wrote about how its ideas could be used, and even enhanced, by social workers working with groups.[5] The dimension that social group work could add to task-centered practice is the way that group members could *help one another* to clarify their problems, select goals, and choose and carry out tasks. Because members share many of life's experiences, they are likely to have ideas regarding appropriate goals and tasks for each other, empathy for the difficulties each may face in carrying out tasks, and ideas about barriers that may be encountered and how these may be overcome.

A number of the features of task-centered group work led to our conviction that it would be a useful component of programs that serve the chronically mentally ill. We shall now examine these.

USE WITH THE CHRONICALLY MENTALLY ILL

As we indicated above, group work has been a useful service with the chronically mentally ill, especially when conducted in a structured and short-term manner. Groups are beneficial because many of the people who suffer from mental illness have severe social deficits. Some may not have had the kinds of socialization experiences that teach one how to interact in a satisfactory manner with others in school, on the job, or during leisure time activities. Others have lost these skills through periods when they were behaving in a psychotic manner and, consequently, were removed from normal social interactions while they lived in institutions. In social work groups, these members have an opportunity to improve their skills in social interaction because these groups provide a safe and accepting setting to acquire and practice social behaviors.

Along with the benefits that all social work groups may offer these members, task-centered groups have additional advantages. One of the concerns frequently voiced by staff members of programs serving the chronically mentally ill is that many clients are poorly motivated to improve their level of functioning and/or they may have difficulty in taking action that will lead to such functioning. The task-centered group provides a structure and a good deal of reinforcement for taking action to attain one's goals. The most important objective of our approach, therefore, is *to enhance the motivation and the skills these members possess to improve their circumstances*.

We do not presume that a short-term group will "cure" mental illness nor remove the need for other services. Rather, we will be satisfied if group members, after the task-centered group experience, are more likely to set goals and engage in activities to attain their goals than they were before. These improvements in their functioning will be evident in the ways they make use of their case managers, other groups, and other therapeutic, educational, recreational, and occupational activities in which they may be engaged.

CARRYING OUT THE PILOT PROJECT

We began the process of what has been called "developmental research"[6] with a pilot project. The purpose of the project was to test the feasibility of task-centered group work with the chronically mentally ill as we initially conceived of it, develop changes in our procedures as they are needed, and create and test ways of measuring both our processes and our outcomes. We successfully secure the cooperation of a county community mental health center in order to accomplish these purposes.

The project was conducted by a team composed of staff members of the community mental health center, field work students, other faculty members of the University of Michigan, and a doctoral student as a research intern. The early stages of the project involved training the team in task-centered methods and consulting with the team regarding adaptation of task-centered group work to this population. The team decided upon a co-worker model and since five staff members and three students were available for direct service, this meant that four groups could be created.

The team agreed that each group should be homogeneous regarding the focal problem as this would enable members to choose to join a group because they wished to work on a specific problem. The members could then quickly move to determining goals, thus making it more likely they would accomplish their work within the time limits that were set.[7] The team, therefore, engaged in a needs assessment in which the types of problems in social functioning of center clients were listed and prioritized. On the basis of this, we created the following groups:

1. A group composed of clients who are among the agency's lowest functioning yet who are capable of agreeing to attend a group and for whom there is a reasonable likelihood of attendance with encouragement and reinforcement. These clients, however, have difficulty acting appropriately in social situations and have minimal social skills. This was viewed as a "pre-task-centered group" as the purposes for the group included helping the members understand such concepts as "goals." It was

also planned that the members tasks would be carried out during the group's meeting times.

2. A group composed primarily of clients diagnosed as schizophrenic who are unemployed and who spend most of their time alone, usually at their residence. These hours are often spent watching television or sleeping. Some of these clients may also be enrolled in a sheltered workshop program but the rest of their time is likely to be spent in solitary, undemanding pursuits. The purpose of the group is to improve their use of leisure time so that they engage in activities that are more social, that represent new interests, that enhance their self-esteem, or that contributes to vocational planning.

3. A group composed of clients who are similar to those described in number 2 above but who also have chemical dependency problems — the so-called dual diagnosed.

4. A group composed of women who, in addition to the social limitations described for the second group, are "trapped" in highly stressful family situations from which they see no escape.

Members were recruited for the groups by presenting the idea of the pilot project and the types of groups to be conducted to the agency's case managers. The managers only had to complete a form with the client's name, address, case number, and phone and to which group the client was referred to effect a referral. These referrals were followed up, however, by a telephone interview with each case manager in which further demographic and clinical data were secured. These data were consequently used for the process of group composition.

The lowest functioning group was allocated six members and the others eight although two more members were assigned to each group to allow for attrition. A balance of men and women (except in the all-women's group) and of Blacks and whites was sought. The group composition procedure described by Garvin was employed.[8] This involved charting salient member characteristics to avoid any one member being extremely different from all other members on too many attributes.

Once members were selected for the groups from the pool created by the referrals from the case managers, the clients were interviewed by their intended group workers to find out whether they were willing to join the group. If so, the ideas behind a task-centered approach were explained to them as well as the specific purposes of their intended group, the time and place of meetings, and the length and number of meetings. They were also helped to think about goals. All of the clients we interviewed agreed at this point to participate.

The team decided that the "low functioning" group would meet twice a week for six weeks as it was hypothesized that the members would need to meet this frequently in order to remember goals and tasks from one session to the next. This turned out to be less of an issue than we had predicted and the team recommended at the end of the project that this type of group should also meet weekly. Groups (2) and (3) met weekly for twelve weeks and group (4) for eight weeks.

The team planned the first two sessions in advance (although it was recognized that even this amount of planning might have to be modified as the members responded to the proposed structure). The program structure of subsequent meetings was determined on a weekly basis based on how rapidly the groups progressed in the task-centered sequence and the suggestions that were proposed by the members during group sessions. Overall, however, the structure the workers sought to implement was as follows:

Meeting 1	Get Acquainted Activities
	Orientation to task-centered work
	Clarification of group purpose
Meetings 2-3	Determining member goals
	Discussion of the idea of tasks
Meetings 4-5	Selection of member tasks
Next 2-5 meetings	Working on tasks
	Learning to overcome barriers to accomplishing tasks
Last meeting	Termination and Evaluation

The groups did proceed in ways that were compatible with the overall program structure outlined above. This presents, however, an oversimplified image of what actually went on inasmuch as the workers employed a variety of program tools to help the members to maintain their interest in the groups and their motivation to participate. Some of these programs were immediately connected to the specific aims of task-centered work and others were more related to group maintenance needs.

An example of programs closely related to the task-centered work was a series of board games devised by the staff. Each board game taught members how to fulfill some aspect of the process such as formulating goals or tasks. In a goal game, for example, members moved their "pieces" around a board and "landed" upon a problem area for which they had to formulate a goal. In a "barrier" game, members also moved pieces around a board through which they encountered "road blocks." They had to devise strategies to move around these blocks which were graphically illustrated as large rock piles. The members enjoyed these games very much and asked to play them again even when the group appeared ready to move to another phase of the process.

Programs that were related to maintenance needs included a variety of trips and parties that were introduced as ways of helping to reward members, and of helping them to reward themselves, as various aspects of the work were accomplished. The workers were convinced that the process of accomplishing tasks had to, at least in part, be fun. In this spirit, every meeting included some refreshments. In addition, within the so-called lower functioning group, many of the individual tasks involved food preparation activities.

An important aspect of working within an empirical model is to be able to document what the intervention was that attained the outcomes that were achieved. Inasmuch as we were working with limited resources and the group workers had many other responsibilities as well, we devised a simple means of accomplishing this. Since we were utilizing a structured approach to work with groups, workers were able to indicate the agenda they planned for the session in some detail. They were asked to number the segments of the agenda and to indicate whether the segment was utilized as planned, modified, or aborted and whether it accomplished its purposes. They were also asked to do selected critical incident recording to elaborate on group processes that they regarded as important.

An example of the type of an agenda was the one devised for the second meeting of group two:

1. Development of individual goals. The idea of the "time line" that was presented at the previous meeting will be reviewed. Each member presents his or her previous day and, with the help of other members, creates a time line on a sheet of paper. Members are asked whether that day was a typical one. If not, a more typical day may be substituted. The member is then asked what might be one way in which his or her use of leisure time on that day might have been enhanced (i.e., what is something he or she would have wished to do that would have been the way he or she wished to spend time). Members give feedback to each other (with help of the workers) in the form of suggestions. Members are asked whether this use of time is the one they wish to make their goal for the group experience. If not, with the help of time lines, other goals are considered. The object, however, is to create the goal in terms of a time line. How the member wishes to spend his or her time may not necessarily be within his or her competency at the time. The purpose is to identify some way that the member will wish to use time at the end of the process. There may be several intermediate steps in the form of tasks; these can be placed on a time line also. It is estimated that the above process may take 10-15 minutes per member so that the group will have to be subdivided into two subgroups of about four members. With this approach, the process will take about an hour. The workers should try to create two subgroups with about equal distribution of members who will approach this process slowly to make it likely that the two groups will finish in about the same time.

2. *"Leisure time experience."* Since members will have been "working," the last 15-30 minutes should be spent in some way that is reinforcing. This should be in the form of refreshments and a game. The game that we recommend is "Leisure Time Trivia." The group is divided into two subgroups. A series of questions have been devised such as the following: name three objects that are necessary for a baseball game; name one movie now playing at a local theater.

3. *Evaluation of session.* The meeting should conclude with some discussion of feelings about the group and how things are going. The plan for the next meeting is described which will include a reaffirmation by the members that they wish to pursue the goals selected at this meeting as well as work on constructing tasks to attain these goals.

OUTCOMES OF THE PILOT PROJECT

In order to use the pilot project to determine the feasibility of task-centered group work with the chronically mentally ill, we utilized several instruments. On one, we recorded the goals established by each member as well as the tasks that were chosen by the member to attain the goals and whether the tasks were carried out. On another we utilized goal attainment scales.[9] Goal attainment scaling involves working with members to identify their goals and then to specify five levels of goal attainment. These levels and the numerical scores we assigned to them are as follows:

- -2 most unfavorable outcome thought likely
- -1 less than expected success
- 0 expected level of success
- $+1$ more than expected success
- $+2$ most favorable outcome thought likely

We also used an inventory completed by members at the beginning and end of the group on which they provided information about their level of social functioning. While the inventories that were completed indicated to us that it is feasible to use this instrument for such research, some workers failed to administer the instrument to all members and we were unable to use it to assess the outcomes attained in this pilot project.[10]

The major findings relevant to outcomes of the pilot project were as follows: a total of 26 clients were served in these groups (Group 1-5; Group 2-9; Group 3-7; Group 4-5). Forty-two percent of the members had a diagnosis of "chronic undifferentiated schizophrenia"; 38 percent, "paranoid schizophrenia"; and 19 percent had other diagnoses.

In three of the groups (excluding the group of members with identified substance abuse problems) 26 goals were selected by the 19 members. For the lower-functioning group, members chose such goals as "start a conversation with another person in the house by the end of the group and "utilize one community resource to spend free time with by the end of the group." The former member chose to carry out such tasks as "say hello to staff member" and the latter such tasks as "investigate one community resource and report about it to the group." As can be seen, despite the assumption made at the beginning by the workers that members of this lower functioning group would only be able to select goals and tasks for behavior within the group, some members did wish to operationalize these outside of the group.

For one of the higher functioning groups, a member chose the goal of "to find a part time job." That member chose a task "to go to S.O.S. (a mental health agency) to look for church work." Another member chose the goal "to become an active player of jazz music." That member chose the task of saving $25.00 a month to buy a trumpet. Another member selected the goal "to work as a volunteer." That member's task was "to ask the adult foster home operator if he could do volunteer work."

The ratings of changes in group member's scores on the goal attainment scale between the beginning and ending of these groups are presented in Table I. This table indicates whether members improved, deteriorated, or sustained their goal attainment scores between the beginning and ending of the group as well as what their final rating was. Nineteen (73 percent) made progress toward attaining their goals. Furthermore, 5 (19 percent) were attained at the "better than expected" level. With all of the limitations on our project in terms of resources, we believe this represents strong support for continuing this program of research into the next stage that we will describe later in this paper.

A less optimistic evaluation must be placed upon our work with the group of members with substance abuse problems. Nine goals were rated and for eight of these no change occurred. For only one was there a

Table I

Change in
Goal Attainment Scores
Between Time-1 and Time-2

	Increase	No Change	Decrease	Total
Final Rating				
-2	—	4	0	4
-1	6	0	1	7
0	8	2	0	10
+1	3	0	0	3
+2	2	0	—	2
Total	19	6	1	26
%	73	23		100

change, this one to the + 1 level. It is possible, of course, that members of this group might have deteriorated without the service but that could not be demonstrated without a control group. We have identified a number of ways that a staff more experienced with the so-called dual diagnosed (mental illness and substance abuse) might have handled group issues differently so as to have achieved better outcomes. In any case, this population is one of the most difficult to serve of all clients with diagnoses of severe mental illness.[11]

PLANS FOR THE EXPERIMENTAL PHASE

In view of the fact that the pilot phase demonstrated the feasibility of task-centered group work with the chronically mentally ill, we have developed a proposal for a major experiment to evaluate the effectiveness of this approach and are seeking funding of this proposal. The following is a brief summary of the major components of the proposal:

Hypotheses

1. Clients who receive task-centered group work at six month follow-up will be more likely than controls to participate in setting specific goals to be achieved through their community mental health center program.
2. Clients who receive task-centered group work at six month follow-up will be more likely than controls to act to attain goals they have contracted with their CMH staff to achieve.
3. Clients who receive task-centered group work at six month follow-up will be functioning at a higher level of self-care and social competence than their controls.
4. Clients who receive task-centered group work will have lower rehospitalization rates and more stable (i.e., fewer changes in) medication histories at six month follow-up than their controls.

Subjects

The subjects will be chosen from among the chronically mentally ill clients at a community mental health center in southeastern Michigan. For a more homogeneous sample we shall only seek referrals of clients whose diagnosis is schizophrenia. In addition all clients in this study will have had at least one hospitalization of six month duration in the last five years or two hospitalizations in the past twelve months.

We shall organize twelve groups and shall recruit eight members for each group. We shall initially seek 160 referrals and shall randomly assign each person to the task-centered group program or a control condition that consists of receiving the typical program of services. We shall need 32 fewer clients than might otherwise be required because that number of control group clients will be promised task-centered group work after a six month waiting period. This is made possible as we will conduct the experiment in three "waves" with only four groups conducted at a time. We can then ascertain by comparing these 32 clients with those not guaranteed task-centered group work whether the presence or absence of such a promise has any impact.

Design

All group work will be conducted by three professionally trained group workers who will be employed by the agency although the agency will be reimbursed through the project budget. Data will be collected from the case managers who refer the members as well as from the members themselves at the time of a pre-group screening interview in order to establish a baseline. Subsequently, data will be secured regarding client goals, goal attainment, tasks, task accomplishment, barriers to task accomplishment, actions to overcome barriers, as well as on a variety of group conditions. Social functioning of clients will also be assessed. The social functioning, investment in goal setting, activities to implement goals, and nature of agency participation will be compared for members of the experimental and control groups during the pre-group interview, at the end of the twelve weeks the group will meet, and at a six month follow-up.

We are particularly interested in finding out whether clients with different attributes, different group workers, and whose groups develop in different ways will have different outcomes. In order to examine this topic, we shall secure data on the demographic characteristics, the history of their mental illness, the therapies they have received, their educational and occupational backgrounds, the nature of their social networks, their living situations, their medication histories, the nature of their psychotic symptoms, and the roles they characteristically assume in groups. We shall also collect data on worker "style." Finally such group conditions as cohesiveness, subgroup patterns, indigenous leadership, and approaches to problem solving will be measured.

CONCLUSION

As the above information should indicate, the process of utilizing research to expand group work knowledge is a difficult yet necessary one with any population and this is certain true of the chronically mentally ill. We strongly believe, nevertheless, that we have reached a stage in our history that this kind of activity is an essential requirement for us in order to play our destined role within social work. We have evolved a powerful way of helping people — one that is based on helping people to help each other. We must use this knowledge and combine it with the powerful tools of scholarship in order to refine, and expand our skills as well as to demonstrate the validity of our convictions about the values of group services.

REFERENCE NOTES

1. Howard H. Goldman, "Epidemiology," in *The Chronic Mental Patient: Five Years Later*, ed. John A. Talbott (Orlando: Grune and Stratton, 1984), p. 22.
2. For a recent summary of this research, see N. Kanas, "Group Therapy with Schizophrenics: A Review of the Controlled Studies," *International Journal of Group Psychotherapy*, July, 1986, pp. 339-352.

3. Lynn Videka-Sherman, "A Meta-Analytic Study of Services to the Chronically Mentally Ill," School of Social Welfare, State University of New York at Albany, 1986.

4. William Reid and Laura Epstein, *Task-centered Casework*, (New York: Columbia University Press, 1972).

5. Charles Garvin, "Task-centered Group Work," *Social Service Review*, 1974, 48, 494-507.

6. For an extended discussion of this way of improving social interventions, see Edwin Thomas, *Designing Interventions for the Helping Professions*, (Beverly Hills: Sage, 1984).

7. As will be explained later, the groups did not all have the same time frame.

8. Charles Garvin, *Contemporary Group Work*, 2nd ed., Englewood Cliffs, N.J.: Prentice-Hall, 1987, pp. 63-72.

9. For details of goal attainment scaling, see T. Kiresuk and G. Garwick, "Basic Goal Attainment Procedures," in B. Compton and G. Galaway, eds, *Social Work Processes, 2nd ed* (Homewood, Ill.: Dorsey Press, 1979.)

10. This inventory was made up of items from two scales: one from L. C. Schneider and E. I. Struening, "SLOF: a Behavioral Rating Scale for Assessing the Mentally Ill," *Social Work Research and Abstracts*, 1983, 19, 9-21; and the other from M. A. Katz and S. B. Lyerly, "Methods for Measuring Adjustment and Social Behavior in the Community: Rationale, Description, Discriminative Validity, and Scale Development," *Psychological Reports*, 1963, 13, 503-535.

11. We are currently at work on a group model for the dually diagnosed that incorporates chemical education and a twelve step model with a skill building group experience.

Group Work with the Bedouin Population of the Negev

Leah Kacen
Jon Anson
Shoshana Nir
No'ah Livneh

SUMMARY. The Bedouin living in the Negev desert, in the south of Israel, are undergoing a rapid and dramatic process of sedenterization. In 1986 a group of social work students surveyed the needs of one of the tribes who were transferred from pastoralism to a new urban settlement when a military airport was built on their old settlement area following the Camp David Peace Treaty. The survey showed a variety of urgent needs, particularly among adolescents about to finish their high school studies. We report here on group interventions with these young men and women, led by Bedouin students, aimed at helping them reach decisions about their future. The groups used the opportunity to discuss and share with others their feelings about marriage, career choice and planning their fu-

---

Leah Kacen has a Masters in Social Work from the Paul Baerwald School of Social Work at the Hebrew University of Jerusalem. In Beer Sheba she teaches group work, and is director of students' field work and the skill development laboratory.

Jon Anson has a Masters in Social Work from the Paul Baerwald School of Social Work at the Hebrew University of Jerusalem and a PhD in Demography from Brown University. At Beer Sheba he teaches ethnic relations and research methodology.

Shoshana Nir has a Masters in Social Work from the Paul Baerwald School of Social Work at the Hebrew University of Jerusalem, and is director of the adult probation service in Beer Sheba. She also teaches Populations at Risk, and coordinates students' projects with special populations.

No'ah Livneh has a Bachelors in Social Work from the University of Haifa. She is a field social worker in the Beer Sheba Municipal Department of Social Services, and lives with a Bedouin tribe. She supervises students' field work, and worked closely with the project described here.

81

ture, though there were clear differences between the dynamics and the content of the male and female groups. We discuss the reasons for these differences, as well as the extent to which the groups were thus able to fulfill the safety valve role of traditional social networks which, because of the turmoil created by the physical and social changes undergone by the community, were unable to fulfill their roles as in the past. We argue that the group formed a stable social resource in a confused environment, characterized by tension between the individual and the society, and an important point of contact on the boundary between the Bedouin and the surrounding society.

How can social work intervene to assist a nomadic population undergoing an accelerated sedenterization process?

The transition from a nomadic to a sedentary form of life involves a total transformation in the mode of existence and in the relations between critical groups in the society. Relations between men and women, between the young and the old and between the group and the broader society around are suddenly transformed; and traditional, accepted patterns of behavior and relationship no longer match the realities of day to day living, and of the control over resources. These dislocations are heavily compounded by changes in mortality, fertility and migration patterns, leading to a rapidly growing population and a changing population structure (Meir, 1986).

We present here a project undertaken by students in their final year in the Spitzer department of Social Work at the Ben Gurion University of the Negev in Beer Sheba, Israel, working with two sets of high school youth in Intiqaal, a newly formed urban Bedouin settlement in the Northern Negev. After describing briefly the changes undergone by the Negev Bedouin in the past half century, we shall consider the special problems faced by the population of Intiqaal, and by the youth in particular, and show how intervention was designed to enable this development of capacities for coping with these exigencies.

THE NEGEV BEDOUIN

In the 1931 Census of Palestine, the Moslem (Bedouin) population living in the Beer Sheba sub district numbered 50,907, of whom nearly 95% were semi-nomadic pastoralists, living from a mixture of extensive agriculture (89%) and goat and sheep herding (11%). Of these, 44% were of pre-pubertal age. If we may judge from the non-nomadic population, about 5% were aged 15-19, and of these 9% of the men and 48% of the women were married (Census 1931). Social organization was in extended, patrilineal families, with the patriarch's power stemming from his control of the family resources and labor power, and the redistribution of land rights and flocks only upon his death (Marx, 1967). After the formation of the State, in 1948, there remained an estimated 13,000 Bedouin in the Israeli Negev. Land rights and nomadic movement were heavily restricted so that, despite the reduction in numbers, a growing proportion of the Bedouin turned to paid employment in the growing Jewish towns and villages. Settlement became more permanent, and two townships were founded during the 1960s and 1970s (Meir, 1984).

As with other populations (Roth, 1985; Meir, 1986) sedenterization led to an increase in fertility, and contact with Israeli social and medical services led to a decrease in mortality. Between 1931 and 1983 total fertility (the number of children the average woman is bearing in her lifetime) rose from seven to eleven, and between 1948 and 1983 the population more than tripled to 44,000, of whom 10% were aged 15-19. Of these youths, fewer than 20% of the women and 5% of the men were married. Of the males aged 15 and over, 57% were in the formal labor force, and of these 35% were in industry and public services (Census, 1961, 1983). We thus see a dramatic transformation of social and population structure, of sources of income and sustenance, and consequently of the relative power of the different age groups, as the population comes to depend less and less on the patriarchal economy, and more and more on earned income brought in from outside (Kressel, 1976).

INTIQAAL (THE RELOCATED)

The Camp David accords of 1979 led to the evacuation by Israel of the Sinai desert, and the relocation of two major airfields into the Israeli Negev. Bedouin who had been living in the area where one of the airfields was to be built were, after lengthy negotiations over compensation, relocated to two new towns which were established in the northern Negev, about 30 miles from Beer Sheba. Housing in these towns was to be built by the Bedouin, using the money received in compensation. However, with no experience of urban living or of building permanent housing, no organized guidance on the best way to use their money, and a galloping inflation, most found their money insufficient to complete building their homes.

In 1984 students from our department interviewed the 61 households comprising one extended family living in one of these towns. Their data give an indication of the changes undergone by this population in the process of relocation, and some of the basic problems they were facing.

a. Population structure. The households comprised 463 individuals, with a median age of 12 years, and an estimated total fertility of 11.5. The population is thus younger, and with an even higher level of fertility, than the population of the Negev Bedouin as a whole.

b. Occupation. Of the 54 male family heads, 12 were over 65, and of the rest only 18 (43%) were employed. Before the relocation they grew crops using traditional extensive methods, and tended goats and sheep. Now they have no skills for urban employment, no land for extensive agriculture, and no water or training for intensive agriculture. Of the 41 youths aged 15-18, 22 were in school, 2 were working, and 17 doing neither.

c. Income. As can be expected from the above figures, only a third of the families are living on earned income. For almost a half, National Insurance Child Allowances were the sole source of income, and over 10% were dependent for support on other family members.

d. Housing. Before relocation a quarter of the households lived in tents, a fifth in corrugated huts, and the rest in wooden shacks. Now 85% live in stone houses, but of these, three quarters are not completed. Forty percent have no running water, 60% have no toilets, and 75% have no electricity. In the whole of Intiqaal there is no central sewage system. It is not surprising, therefore, that a third of the families have a hut by the house which serves as a traditional kitchen, and a further third effectively live in such huts.

e. Satisfaction. Of the 61 families only six had a regular income which they considered adequate and of these six were satisfied with the move to Intiqaal. The rest were not satisfied, and 47 households (77%) considered life to have been better before the relocation.

The survey thus shows that the residents of Intiqaal have problems and needs in just about every sphere of life: basic resources, health, education, inter-generational communication, and inter-familial rivalries and conflicts.

PROBLEMS OF YOUTH

The relocation to Intiqaal destroyed the existing, even if slowly eroding, conditions for a traditional society based on group membership and group survivorship, and forced an immediate coming to terms with life on the periphery of a modern society based on individual achievement. As with all such transitions, a vacuum is created in which traditional norms and modes of behavior break down, and traditional roles lose their meaning, without necessarily being replaced by modern alternatives (Merton, 1971).

Before the relocation, unmarried adolescents were responsible for a variety of tasks in the traditional economy and, because settlement was dispersed, many hours of the day were taken up with the walk to and from school. Since relocation, the school is nearby, and in the absence of agriculture many tasks no longer exist. Before relocation, adolescents were essentially in apprenticeship to their seniors, learning adult roles and behaviors (Tuma, 1955). Since relocation, the whole framework for this apprenticeship has disappeared, and there is no alternative framework for learning these roles and behaviors.

The youth of Intiqaal are thus in a double transition. Not only are they moving from childhood to adulthood, with all that this implies in terms of learning new roles, rights and responsibilities (Ormian, 1975), but they are doing thus under conditions of a very sudden and dramatic social transformation. The traditional roles which they are supposed to take on are no longer meaningful in their new situation, the successful elders of the tribe are no longer meaningful role models, and there is an implicit demand to choose between the values of reference groups in the outside society, and those of the membership group in the tribe.

Under these circumstances, it was felt that high school adolescents would be a suitable, and particularly needy target population for a non-material intervention by social work students (Lippincott, 1978) (though we should mention that the same students were involved in setting up and running a welfare office for the residents of Intiqaal, in order to create a better level of take-up of National Insurance and other benefits). The groups chosen were girls aged 16-17, and boys aged 17-18. These are adolescents in the final years in school, girls tending to leave at the end of compulsory education and boys at the end of high school. A number of them expressed a desire to continue beyond these traditional limits, and it was these adolescents who we felt would be most in conflict between the outside reference and internal membership groups, and who would benefit most from the intervention.

THE MODE OF INTERVENTION

One of the striking features of traditional Bedouin society is that life has traditionally been organized in natural groups. Men and women do not sit together, rather the men of a family would sit in a communal men's tent, and women in the family tents sewing, cooking and looking after the children together. There are few private moments, and life is essentially communal, with the family and the tribe taking precedence over the individual. Poverty, nomadism and constant conflict with other tribes and non-Bedouin led to the individual being defined strictly in terms of his group membership, and to individual self-expression taking place through the fulfillment of roles defined within the group. Within this framework, every individual belongs to a group defined in terms of age and sex, each with its own rights and obligations, and each preparing to move into the succeeding age group. These groups form a natural forum for discussing topics of concern to the group as a whole. In seeking a mode of intervention with Bedouin youth, therefore, it seemed more appropriate to work on a group rather than an individual (case-work) basis (for a discussion of the importance of working within such natural systems, see, e.g., Litwack and Szelenyi, 1965; Taylor and Townsend, 1976). At the same time, it was essential to respect the natural division between male and female groups.

THE INTERVENTION

The intervention was focused on the problem of the identity of Bedouin youth in the Negev, given the conflict discussed above between the internal membership and the external reference groups (Klein, 1972; Runciman, 1966). The aim of the intervention was to strengthen the sense of belonging to the peer membership group while yet increasing their ability to cope with the demands of the external society (Edwards et al., 1978). Decisions taken in a group, we felt, would better enable them to manage living in both worlds simultaneously. When planning the intervention, the following objectives were specified:

a. Acquiring new skills for communicating with parents, in order to reduce inter-generational conflict;
b. Acquiring information about possible alternative life-strategies in the new situation (education, employment, marriage, etc.);
c. Making personal decisions about future plans; and
d. Creating a dialogue with members of the reference group.

Of the 14 young men invited to participate in the group, nine attended regularly. All 21 of the young women invited participated consistently. Each group met eight times for an hour and a half each meeting. The meetings were held in school, at the end of the regular school day. The young men's group was led by a Bedouin student (a man) and a Jewish student (a woman). The young women's group was led by a Bedouin student (a woman), the first Bedouin woman in the Negev to study in the University.

The Male Group

Three major topics were discussed in this group:

a. The transition from the sheltered life of a high school student to making a living in the adult world.
b. Coping with the admissions procedure to post-secondary education.
c. Coping with the exposure to the modern, non-Bedouin society.

Graduation from high school has a number of meanings which were raised in the group. Moving out of Intiqaal, to work or to study, means leaving behind the social security afforded by life in the tribe. This transition is not specific only to Bedouin youth, but it attains particular significance given the overall lack of security of the society as a whole. Group members noted the immediate need to find work, even while they were studying, as their families could not support them, and the group leaders provided information about the opportunities available. During the discussion, one of the members told of friends who had found work with such a good income that they were tempted to work full time rather than study. In this he highlighted the conflict all the group was in, between working now and adding to the meager family budget, and studying for a degree or diploma which would increase the probability of an adequate income in the long run.

Through the group discussions, it became very clear that they had no information concerning the admissions process to higher education. The group leaders provided this information, and discussed the members' ability to meet these requirements. Issues such as: the gap between ambition and ability; the need to make up knowledge before acceptance; the fear of rejection or failure; how their success or failure would be received in the tribe; and what alternatives are available, were discussed. For example, one of the young men wanted to study Law. However, he found he had to make up knowledge in Hebrew and in English before he could even register. The group discussed with him his willingness to make the required effort, and what his alternatives were. Another related that his father expected him to go out to work at once, and finally agreed that his son should study Law or Engineering. After learning in the group of the entrance requirements, it became clear that neither of these was a feasible option, but he did not know how to discuss alternatives with his father. After role playing in the group, he was encouraged to talk it over with his father, who agreed to his studying something else.

A further problem facing these men when they go to study is the loss of the traditional tribal framework, and fitting in to modern urban life. Most of them want to become part of this society, which has served as a reference group until now. But becoming part of urban Israeli society involves moving away from the membership group, and the creation of cultural and educational gaps between them and their erstwhile peers. The group members expressed concern of this process and the decisions they had to take, and together with the leaders they discussed the possibility of living in both worlds, or at least of not severing irreparably their ties with their families. Many examples were given of older brothers and cousins who had studied, and not been able to bridge the gap between the two worlds, some of whom had even emigrated in order to avoid the constant internal conflict.

The Female Group

The young women's group also raised three major topics for discussion, but these were very different from those raised by the men. The major concerns here were:

   a. Father-daughter relations;
   b. Forbidden relationships with young men;
   c. Their future, as set by their parents.

In Bedouin society sons have higher status than daughters. Sons are registered in their fathers' name, whereas daughters are registered in their mothers' name. Fathers, when asked how many children they have, will mention only their sons. Many issues concerning girls' sense of inferiority in their fathers' eyes were discussed. For instance, discussing one's future with one's father is a privilege restricted to sons only, whereas girls have to do as their father decides, without discussion. The discussion was very emotional, with great bitterness concerning this situation. But at the same time they expressed no real desire to change the situation.

Bedouin women enter into marriages which are arranged by the parents, without the partners necessarily being consulted. A young woman caught in illicit meetings with young men is liable to be murdered in order to protect the family's honor. At the same time, exposure to modern Western society and its norms, particularly through television, leads to considerable ambivalence. This topic appeared to be the major preoccupation of young Bedouin women of this age. They wanted to marry a man of their own choosing, not their parents', and they utilized the group framework to discuss (and perhaps seek approval for) the way in which they managed their illicit relationships. The group offered catharsis, but could not offer any practical alternatives to the current situation.

How long a Bedouin woman studies is determined by her father, usually without consulting her. Compulsory education in Israel is up to the end of 10th grade, and after this most young women are required by their families to work in the home, to prepare themselves for marriage, and so on. The growing exposure to Israeli norms has led a growing demand by girls to continue studying, and the group members felt that on this topic they were less helpless than on others. They felt they could discuss the matter with their parents, and even convince them. One of the reasons for this is the change in the major source of income, from crops and herding to wages, with a consequent reduction in the work load in the home, and the gradual introduction of modern home appliances. A further reason is the preference by Bedouin men for a better educated wife, with a consequent increase in the bride-price grooms' families are prepared to pay for a bride who has completed high school. Under these circumstances, whether a girl continues her studies beyond 10th grade or not very much depends on her willingness and ability to demand it of her parents, but the norms of obedience make this very difficult for many of them. One of the major tasks of the group was to encourage and enable those who wished to continue studying to discuss the matter with their parents.

The Group Process

There has been very little professional intervention in Bedouin society, and group work has, to the best of our knowledge, not been tried before. There has been almost no counselling, not even in schools, and it was consequently necessary to spend some time in both groups "learning the rules of the game." One of the major difficulties which the groups had to overcome was in the generation of interaction norms for the group meetings. It was particularly important to differentiate our work from the teacher-led discussion process of the school classroom, and this was particularly problematic as the group meetings were held in school. One sign of the relevance of the intervention was the speed with which these new ground rules were agreed upon (Edwards et al., 1978).

One particular problem which had to be overcome in the men's group was the reflection of inter-family and inter-tribal conflicts in the group discussions and struggles over saliency in, and leadership of, the group. Group members accepted this struggle as a natural extension of daily relationships, and the group leaders decided not to intervene or interfere with this process, in particular as it did not prevent the group from attaining its objectives.

In the women's group, dissociation from school norms was more problematic. The group leader was initially referred to as the teacher, participants raised their hands for permission to talk, and the realization that school rules did not apply led to a degree of anarchy in the group. They spoke all at once, did not pay attention to others, walked around the room, etc. With guidance, the group leader was able to reassert her authority, and to bring out the distinction between having no rules, and having a different set of rules. Only then was the group able to tackle its substantive tasks.

In both groups the leader was a Bedouin who had moved out into higher education, thus offering a natural basis for trust between each group and its respective leader (Schneller, 1984). For the men's group, this presented a positive role-model, and a source of information concerning the member's immediate goals and aspirations. The presence of a Jewish woman as co-leader in the group kept the discussion at a very instrumental level. In the women's group, by contrast, the members saw the (sole) group leader an ally and friendly confessor. The affective direction of the group content threatened, at one point, the authority of the group leader, and part of the reassertion process discussed above involved returning the discussion to the instrumental plane (Davis, 1985).

SUMMARY AND DISCUSSION

The group intervention with young Bedouin men and women took place within the context of the dramatic changes taking place in Israeli Bedouin society, and in Intiqaal in particular. Furthermore, it was focused on late adolescents, people who are in the process of making far reaching decisions concerning their whole life course. Within this double exigency we set seemingly incompatible objectives for the group intervention, namely strengthening the affiliation with the membership group while yet moving closer to the external reference group (Klein, 1972). Our evaluation of the needs of this population brought out the inescapability of this confrontation, and the necessity, for all those who wish to study, of living in both worlds simultaneously. The young people themselves expressed very graphically this sense of being torn between the social-traditional pressures to be Bedouin, and the desire for personal self-fulfillment as an individual in the modern, outside society. Under these circumstances they feel required to choose between belonging and moving out, yet they sense that neither of these is, in itself, an adequate solution. Remaining within the membership group is frustrating, for it involves giving up on the possibility of individual achievement within the already accepted reference group. Moving out, however, is no less frustrating, as the newcomer generally remains an outsider on the fringe of the broader society, without any long lasting, meaningful social networks and relationships (Garvin, 1981). Our aim, therefore, was to suggest a way out of this no-win situation, through helping them find a way to self-realization within the reference group, without cutting the cord which ties them to the membership group, and the source of their own self-identification. At the same time, we felt that a degree of self-awareness was required concerning their own role as agents of change within Bedouin society.

The group process seemed the most appropriate method to attain this goal, under the circumstances. Not only is Bedouin life organized around the group rather than the individual, but also the group acted as a "laboratory" mediating between the two worlds. Furthermore, the peer group is a critical element in adolescent life, which will be a significant resource and source of support during such a multidimensional process of change. Far more than adults, fellow adolescents are facing the same problems and decisions, and can thus offer a far more understanding source of support. At the same time, the differences between the concerns raised by the men and the women brings out how important it was to treat with them in separate groups (Mead, 1950).

The needs of the group members were located at two different levels. On the one hand, there was the need for affiliation, and on the other, for self realization. If we follow Maslow's (1971) scheme, there would appear to be a missing link here, at the level of esteem. This refers to the value of the individual to society, and to the esteem which the society (significant others) accord to the individual's contribution. In this context, the critical questions are: contribution to which society?; and esteem from which society? Unless and until these questions are resolved, self-realization will be impossible. We feel that it is this question of esteem which should be the focus of intervention with adolescent Bedouin groups, and indeed in all groups of this kind intervening in minority populations. By forming a membership group at the boundary between the two societies (of affiliation and reference), the group can act as a laboratory in which they can meet, and where personal encounters with the two can be evaluated.

Males and Females

There were a number of important differences between the two groups with which we worked, beyond the difference in age between them. In part, these relate to the difference in the size of the groups, and in the leadership pattern. In large part, however, they reflect the difference between the roles of men and women in Bedouin society, and to the different meanings and adjustments required in the meeting with the modern, outside world.

Firstly, the anomic interaction which occurred in the women's group, after relaxing the strictness of school discipline, did not occur in the men's group. Bedouin boys live in the shadow of the elder males from a very young age. They hear how matters are discussed, how negotiations are conducted and how decisions are taken. They thus have a considerably greater passive knowledge of how to conduct an instrumental group meeting than do young women, and were able very quickly to settle on a group contract for the running of the group (Tuma, 1955).

Girls, by contrast, have to concentrate on housework and may not, under any circumstances, involve themselves in worldly matters. They do not discuss matters with men, but must submit to their decisions. School reinforces these norms, with most of the teachers being men, and teacher-pupil relations being based on strict authority. The group gave them their first opportunity to discuss matters close to their heart with someone from outside their immediate circle, under conditions of near equality. As soon as they understood this, it was as if a dam had burst, with long pent up emotions and frustrations pouring out, irrespective of whether anyone was listening or not.

A second difference was in the rate of perceptible change in the groups. Among the young women this was particularly slow, largely as a result of the deep rooted patterns of obedience and the sense of helplessness in the face of the father's absolute right of decision concerning their future.

The third and most critical difference between the groups concerns the content of the group discussions. Whereas the men defined their problems in terms of relations with the external reference group, such as moving out of the known framework into the unknown city and acceptance to higher education, the young women defined their problems in terms of dealing with internal relations within the family and the tribe. The women showed a much clearer and unambiguous identification with the traditional membership group, and hence their objectives were focused inward rather than outward, as were the men's objectives.

In general, it would appear the changes undergone by the population of Intiqaal have affected the lives of men and women very differently. For the men the content of the relations with the outside world and the way of earning a living have changed radically, but except for the few who cut themselves off from the tribe and attempt to integrate into the outside society, the form and structure of internal relations has changed very little. The problem of young men is thus to learn how to handle the new circumstances in which the essentially unchanged game may be played. For the women, who previously had no relations with the outside world, and whose roles were defined strictly within the home, a whole new world has opened up. Households and herding tasks have declined, education has opened up a variety of new possibilities outside the home, television has offered the vision of a more egalitarian, "romantic," relationship with men, and the changes in the Bedouin economy have considerably lessened the father's absolute power. These differences in the redefinition of the situation being undergone by Bedouin men and women were very clearly reflected in both the form and content of the two group processes.

CONCLUSION

Bedouin society, a minority within the broader Israeli society, is in the process of transition from a traditional semi-nomadic mode of life to a settled urban mode of living. For some, such as the group we worked with, this process has been suddenly accelerated by an imposed relocation with no opportunity for a gradual adjustment. For Bedouin youth, this social transformation is occurring hand in hand with their personal transition from childhood to adulthood, a transition in which they are expected to determine their personal identity and sense of belonging. However the duality of their being, between a Bedouin membership group in transition which can offer very little guidance to the adolescent, and the urban reference group to which they feel they do not belong, creates considerable conflict and increases the uncertainty of adolescence. In our group intervention, we sought to work with young men and women who, in seeking further education beyond the traditional norm, were signalling their interest in bridging the gap between these two worlds. In the group process we sought to help them reach decisions concerning their relations with both the traditional Bedouin and the modern urban worlds. We trust that in doing so we have helped make the abrupt sedenterization process a little less traumatic, and their self-realization as individuals in the modern urban world a little easier and more feasible.

REFERENCES

Census of Palestine, 1931, Volume II, Part II, *Tables*. Alexandria, 1933.
Census of Population and Housing, 1961, Publication No. 7, *Demographic Characteristics of the Population*, Jerusalem: State of Israel, Central Bureau of Statistics, 1962.
Census of Population and Housing, 1983, Publication No. 3, *Localities, Populations and Households*, Jerusalem: State of Israel, Central Bureau of Statistics, 1984.

Davis, L. E., "Group work practice with ethnic minorities of color," in Sundel, M., Glasser, P., Sarri, R., & Vinter, R. (eds.), *Individual Change through Small Groups*, 2nd edition, New York: Free Press, pp. 324-344. 1985.

Edwards, E., Edwards, M. E., Daines, G. M., & Eddy, F., 1978, "Enhancing self-concept and identification with 'Indianness' of American Indian girls," *Social Work with Groups*, v1:309-318.

Garvin, C. D., 1981, *Contemporary Group Work*. Prentice Hall, pp. 227-239.

Klein, A. F., 1972, *Effective Group Work: An introduction to principle and method*, New York: Association Press, pp. 45-50.

Kressel, G. M., 1976, *Individuality against Tribalism*, Tel Aviv: HaKibbutz Ha-Meuchad (Hebrew).

Lippincott, J. P., 1978, "Reaching the vulnerable people," in N. Brill, *Working with People*, 2nd edition, pp. 178-189.

Litwak, E. & Szelenyi, I., 1965, "Primary group structures and their functions: Kin, neighbors and friends," *American Sociological Review*, v34:465-486.

Marx, E., 1967, *Bedouin of the Negev*, London; Manchester University Press.

Maslow, A., 1971, *The Farther Reaches of Human Nature*, New York: Viking.

Mead, M., 1950, *Sex and Temperament*, New York: Morrow.

Meir, A., 1984, "Demographic transition among the Negev Bedouin in Israel and its planning implications," *Socio-Economic Planning Science*, v18:399-409.

Meir, A., 1986, "Demographic transition theory: A neglected aspect of the nomadism-sedentarism continuum," *Transactions of the Institute of British Geographers*, v11:199-211.

Merton, R. K., 1971, "Social problems and sociological theory," in Merton, R. K. & Nisbet, R. A. (eds.), *Contemporary Social Problems*, New York: Harcourt, Brace & World.

Ormian, H., 1975, *Adolescence*, 3rd edition (Hebrew).

Roth, E. A., 1985, Demographic patterns of sedentary and nomadic Juang of Orissa, *Human Biology*, v57:319-325.

Runciman, W. G., 1966, *Relative Deprivation and Social Justice: A study of attitudes and social inequalities in the 20th century*, London: Routledge.

Schneller, R., 1984, "Empathy and communication in the intercultural encounter," *Society and Welfare*, v5:299-316 (Hebrew).

Taylor, B., & Townsend, R., 1976, "The local 'sense of place' as evidenced in North East England," *Urban Studies*, v13:137-144.

Tuma, E., 1955, "Child rearing in an Arab village," *Megamot*, v6:130-138 (Hebrew).

Social Support Training
for Abusive Mothers

Madeline L. Lovell
Kathy Reid
Cheryl A. Richey

SUMMARY. This paper describes a twelve-week group program designed to help low-income abusive mothers build more effective bases of social support in their daily lives with friends, family and neighbors. The group, conducted at a therapeutic day nursery, was supplemental to ongoing services for maltreated children and their families. The group incorporated training in a range of interpersonal competencies including basic conversational skills, self-protection, and assertion. Sessions were designed around a metaphoric Relationship Roadmap for friendship which visually depicted definitional terms and time frameworks appropriate to various friendship stages. Humor, stress-reduction, and visual aids were components of the teaching process. Individualized goals and skill rehearsal were used to increase relevance and mastery of content. Socialization of mothers to group norms and expectations was enhanced by pregroup induction procedures and by members' previous involvement in an agency-based parenting support group.

Madeline L. Lovell, PhD, is affiliated with the School of Social Work, University of British Columbia, Vancouver, B.C., Canada.

Kathy Reid is affiliated with Behavioral Sciences, Inc., Federal Way, WA.

Cheryl A. Richey is affiliated with the School of Social Work, University of Washington, Seattle, WA.

All correspondence to be addressed to: Dr. Madeline Lovell, School of Social Work, University of British Columbia, 6201 Cecil Green Park Road, Vancouver, B.C., Canada, V6T 1W5.

This research was supported in part by a grant from the University of Washington, School of Social Work, Research Development Fund.

The authors would like to thank Patrick Gogerty and Maggie Edgar of Childhaven, Seattle, WA for their ongoing support and encouragement with this project.

Research in the field of child maltreatment has demonstrated that abusive parents are lonely and isolated in their environment (Garbarino & Gillian, 1980; Polansky et al., 1985). Maltreating parents have been found to have smaller social networks and significantly weaker and less supportive ties with neighbors and friends than would be expected (Salzinger et al., 1985; Gaudin and Pollane, 1983). Furthermore, strong, active social relationships are associated with decreased evidence of destructive behavior in abusive families (Hunter & Kilstrom, 1979) and improved parenting (Wahler, 1980, 1979). The differential stresses and resources among parents at risk for child maltreatment suggest the importance of a range of intervention efforts. For example, Parents Anonymous has been shown to be a singularly effective self-help group for parents able voluntarily to seek assistance (Herbruck, 1980). However, many parents appear to be unmotivated to get help (Smith et al., 1984).

The project reported in this paper was developed in response to prior research evaluating a 6-month parenting and social support group known as the Parent Group designed for mothers whose children were attending a therapeutic day nursery for maltreated preschool children. All Parent Group Members were low-income, involuntary child protective service clients. Weekly group sessions focused on child-rearing and daily living concerns. Agency social work staff expected that participation in this open-ended weekly group would offer mothers the opportunity to develop friendships with other women. However, pre-post evaluation data revealed that the proportion of other group members in mothers' social networks did not increase over time despite a seeming paucity of friends and supportive social contacts (Lovell & Hawkins, in press).

The Parent Group study suggested that mothers' relatively small personal social networks and failure to develop relationships with other group members were related to their relatively low interpersonal skill levels. For example, observational data indicated that it was not uncommon for Parent Group members unwittingly to respond to each other with embarrassing and/or inappropriate comments. They appeared genuinely surprised to learn that their remarks were offensive or hurtful to others. Further, mothers tended to interact with group leaders and not with each other. In general, mothers appeared unable to give and receive social support. Therefore, a 12-week social support training group was offered as a supplemental intervention to mothers currently involved in the comprehensive day nursery program. The group aimed to strengthen prosocial attitudes and skills needed to build more satisfying relationships with friends, neighbors and family.

SELECTION AND INDUCTION OF GROUP MEMBERS

Eight mothers who had attended the Parent Group for a minimum of two months and were identified as needing relationship training were invited by the branch social worker in a personal written invitation to participate in a special social support training project. Prior Parent Group attendance was viewed as important because it socialized mothers to the processes which facilitate group maintenance (Garvin, 1974). For instance, the branch director and social worker encouraged attendance at Parent Group by frequent personal reminders and enquiries. Parents who attended received considerable favorable attention and social support from staff. As a result, mothers developed positive relationships with day nursery staff and became familiar with expectations and norms.

As pointed out by Hartford (1972), a group often develops before the first formal meeting occurs. In this case, important pregroup events included personal written invitations, and individual assessment and goal setting interviews with group leaders. During these initial discussions, leaders emphasized consistently that this "advanced" training group would require considerable commitment and involvement from members, including regular attendance and joining in group activities. Further, participants were compensated $25 to complete all pre-, post- and followup assessments. The mothers recognized that they were being asked to take part in a "bonus" offering at the agency and perceived this involvement as a sign of positive staff regard. Consequently, their motivation to participate was enhanced and all eight agreed to join the group.

The eight mothers had children between infancy and five years of age and had been referred to the day nursery by child welfare officials because they were at high risk for child maltreatment. The women ranged in age from 25 to 42 years with a mean age of 32.5 years. Six were Caucasian, one Asian and one Black. Five of the mothers were living with male partners and three were single parents. Four had histories of mental health problems, notably depression. Four mothers, two of whom were in methadone treatment during this period, had histories of substance abuse. Five reported being victims of physical or sexual abuse in their own childhoods. The black mother missed the first four sessions because of her substance abuse treatment schedule. As bonds between members coalesced rapidly, she was encouraged to remain in Parent Group and consider relationship training again at a future date. Hence, seven mothers participated in social support training.

Both group leaders were Caucasian women, one with a M.S.W. and one with a Ph.D. The group intervention was constructed to reflect the daily living experiences of mothers to minimize any impact of background differences between leaders and members.

COMPONENTS OF THE INTERVENTION MODEL

A fundamental therapeutic task in working with this population of at-risk mothers, who typically appeared unmotivated and resistant to change, was to locate or develop methodologies which could actively engage them in the treatment process. Drawing upon current literature, prior clinical experience, and assessment of individual participants' abilities, learning styles and goals, a 12-week intervention protocol was crafted and refined. In general, these women associated traditional teaching models with embarrassment, criticism and failure. Mothers were extremely hesitant to roleplay difficult situations. Therefore, metaphor, specific stress-reduction procedures, humor, and visual aids formed critical components of the intervention model implemented in this project.

The use of metaphor is particularly beneficial because it is an effective means of establishing rapport, defining the nature of a client's problems in a less intimidating manner than direct communication, and enabling the transfer of learning to new situations (Marlatt & Fromme, 1987; Marlatt & Gordon, 1985; Kopp, 1976). However, metaphor also has been recognized as a powerful means to confront clients' limiting beliefs and rigid perceptions in order to learn radically new concepts (Barker, 1985; Lankton & Lankton, 1983). Abusive parents often have difficulty perceiving the possibility of more social support as, on average, they have poor self-concepts (Anderson & Lauderdale, 1982) and have experienced aversive relationships (Wahler, 1980). Metaphor thus may serve as a means of broadening parents' awareness of their own potential.

An allegorical framework was used to illustratively present important information about forming high quality social relationships. Group sessions were structured around the development and application of a metaphor for friendship, The Relationship Roadmap. The map visually depicted a road connecting five towns. Each town corresponded to a stage in a relationship, e.g., Acquaintanceville, Buddyborough, Friendly City, Personal Friendsville and Partnersburg. Additional time and distance cues conveyed the gradual evolution of intimacy.

Less threatening than direct feedback or confrontation, and less tedious than traditional pedagogical approaches, the use of a visual metaphor with these women greatly accelerated their personal involvement with the material. They quickly began to identify their own patterns and problems in relationships with others. Labeling experiences in roadmap terms such as the "freeway" approach to sexual intimacy allowed difficult experiences to be discussed in an atmosphere of caring. In several respects, the Relationship Roadmap can also be viewed as an "unstructured cognitive game" (Rabin, 1983). This type of game has few, if any, rules; stresses creative expression; and focuses on the attainment of information and insight. Games, like metaphors, can simplify complex phenomena and reduce frustration (Coleman, 1968) and may be particularly useful with difficult-to-teach individuals (Fantuzzi et al., 1986).

Mothers enthusiastically elaborated the map over time as new topics and issues were introduced. For example, confronted with the problem of how to classify their relationship with counselors and social workers, whom they had previously labeled as "friends," they decided after a spirited discussion that "professional friends" should be relegated to an island on the map with ferries running only from the island as these relationship are not reciprocal. Additional analogies were suggested frequently by group members throughout the course of training. For example, conversational exchanges with others were likened to a tennis match, with each participant having to send volleys over the net and avoid putting up barriers which might deflect the message getting sent.

Throughout training, activities were designed to reduce participant stress. Rather than individual members moving to the front of the group to "perform," they remained in their own chairs during exercises and worked in teams to construct and rehearse appropriate responses to difficult situations. Informal, impromptu coaching by leaders and other group members was encouraged during practice activities. The two leaders consistently modeled risk-taking behavior, such as sharing personal information and trying out new skills, before asking members to follow suit. Every positive aspect of members' performance was consistently praised across sessions. Negative or corrective feedback was introduced at the halfway point, during Session 6. It was offered gently, first to members who appeared more socially competent, then to the less skillful, more vulnerable group members. The goal was to establish norms that sharing both positive feedback and critical feedback among members was helpful and that a safe group environment supported risks and mutual aid (Shulman, 1984).

Like metaphor, humor is a powerful therapeutic device to both engage clients and communicate unique concepts (Fry & Salameh, 1987). The use of humor served several functions within the group. Initially, leaders accepted all forms of joking by members, including sarcasm, as these were perceived as possible coping strategies by some to increase comfort in interpersonally tense situations (Bales, 1958). However, shaping through differential leader attention was employed to encourage more appropriate responses over time. Leaders employed humorous examples to render material more enjoyable and relevant to members' daily lives. Finally, shared laughter increased group cohesion. Caution was taken by leaders to avoid such pitfalls as sarcasm or joking that might be hurtful to individual members or represent leaders' attempts to deal with their own anxieties at the expense of group process (Bloch, 1987; Kubie, 1971).

Finally, visual aids were used whenever possible to engage members' attention and facilitate learning. For example, a large drawing of the Relationship Roadmap was posted during each session for easy reference. An 18-inch thermometer facilitated identification of stress levels and accompanying physical symptoms of anxiety. Charts depicting an array of positive and negative feelings, each accompanied by a facial caricature, were posted to help mothers identify and label common emotions that occur in relationships. Additional posters were spontaneously created over the course of training on such topics as danger signals in relationships and steps in assertive behavior. Since, on the average, these mothers had marginal literacy skills, only a minimum of very simply written handouts were distributed to highlight individual goals. Charts and posters depicted material pictorially whenever possible.

SESSION CONTENT

Session 1

The Relationship Roadmap was created in the first session. Participants examined various types of friendships and any time frameworks of which they were aware for developing intimacy. Close attention terms for friendships enabled leaders to incorporate additional labels other than "friend," for example, "buddy" and "pal." It was learned early in the assessment interviews that the term "friend" carried many negative connotations for these women. They reported being repeatedly hurt and taken advantage of by persons they had considered friends.

Members were also encouraged to identify current features or patterns in their own personal social networks, e.g., many acquaintances, few friends. Each was asked to select a stage of friendship in which she wanted to add a network member and to consider potential candidates. This task was difficult for several members. One woman, whose network was particularly small, stared intently at her paper for several minutes and then concluded that she didn't need to add anyone. When she finally agreed to consider increasing her acquaintances, she had no idea of suitable candidates.

Session 2

The second session concentrated on identifying "danger signs" indicative of future relationship problems. Member-generated examples included drug problems, criticism and lying. This list of some 40 danger signs was further divided into "NO WAY'S"—signals warning you to avoid the relationship entirely. An interesting illustration of participants' ambivalence in relationships was the intrapersonal conflict they revealed when the issue of violence arose. While all participants identified violence as a definite "NO WAY," several stated that they would accept violence from others if they had provoked it themselves. In addition, members discriminated among violent acts. Being "hit once when they deserved it" by their partner might be tolerable whereas being "really beaten" would be unacceptable.

Session 3

In Session 3, participants were asked to personalize the danger signs by developing their own cautionary list and by examining the relationship they had targeted to improve in Session 1's homework for any evidence predictive of future relationship distress. These activities revealed a more realistic appraisal of the women's coping patterns in relationships. Whereas in Week 2, participants were in general agreement on the danger signs, in Week 3 many of the women did not incorporate key items in their own personal lists. When the omissions were questioned, two themes emerged. First, while aware of the hazards, for example, in having friends who were using drugs or who had criminal records, many believed that they had the ability to navigate around any obstacles. Second, the relationship often was viewed as unique. For example, a member might comment, "He steals, but he'd never steal from me." Unfortunately, all too often neither belief was accurate.

Session 4

Since many of these women had expressed much distrust of friends as a result of past abusive experiences, it was judged necessary in this session to help group members feel more able to protect themselves from others before asking them to take risks in building new friendships both in and out of the group. The right to feel safe was emphasized. With the aid of the facial illustration and thermometer charts, participants were helped to identify and label the bodily symptoms and inner-emotional experiences of discomfort and fear that often accompanied reactions to abusive or hurtful behavior from others. Observation revealed that, in general, the repertoire of emotions recognized by group members was restricted to "happy," "sad" and "angry." Participants enjoyed discovering names for a range of emotions. Having multiple and confusing feelings in a given situation was normalized.

Protective techniques, e.g., sharing feelings or leaving a situation, were offered and discussed by leaders and members for such common vexatious events as coping with others' drunken behavior and potential violence. The resourcefulness that members demonstrated in creating possible responses to these situations reflected the diversity of members' life experiences. A lively discussion ensued as participants shared common "war stories" and debated the consequences of alternative responses.

Session 5, 6, and 7

These sessions focused on initiating, maintaining and ending conversations to ensure that participants had opportunities to master and refine basic social skills (Gambrill & Richey, 1988).[1] Some members were reluctant to initiate any conversation. Common deficiencies included the inappropriate disclosure of personal information and a lack of small talk. Information was presented on ways of communicating interest or lack of interest nonverbally, differential use of open and closed questions to elicit responsiveness in others, and ways to handle common conversational mishaps such as interruptions and put-downs. The majority of each session was devoted to skill rehearsal. Listening skills were particularly troublesome for participants. They easily slipped into problem-solving attempts without stopping to identify the other's feelings. Leaders began to routinely identify each time clients slipped into premature problem-solving.

Sessions 8 to 11

Situations calling for assertive behavior were the focus of these four sessions. Positive assertions, including giving and receiving compliments (Furman & Henderson, 1984) were targeted since observation suggested that few positively reinforcing statements were exchanged among group members. In fact, clients were frequently heard to make sarcastic comments to others. When probed, speakers frequently reported that such

---

1. This book may be purchased from Behavioral Options, P.O. Box 8118, Berkeley, CA 94707.

comments were meant to be complimentary. Interventions included assessing inhibiting beliefs and self-talk, and developing more effective ways of offering and accepting positive feedback (cf. Galassi & Galassi, 1977). Cognitions that hinder people from paying compliments were generated by the group. For example, praise is unnecessary if someone is "just doing their job." Modesty and low self-esteem were frequently identified obstacles to receiving compliments.

Handling criticism, expressing disagreement, and sharing negative concerns were topics of considerable import to participants. Following suggestions by Gambrill and Richey (1988), teams practiced and demonstrated to the group assertive, aggressive and passive response options to difficult situations. Whenever possible, exercises focused on difficult situations likely to be encountered by participants in their daily lives. Frequently members would raise problematic situations that they would then roleplay for the group. Group leaders modeled assertive responses while explaining their decision-making process when choosing how to react to complex interpersonal situations.

Participants were encouraged to examine the relative utility of habitual responses to difficult situations and practice new techniques which might hold greater promise for problem resolution. The cognitive framework proposed by assertiveness training was new to members. Initially, many believed that an assertive response to aggressive behavior displayed weakness. Group leaders framed assertive responses repeatedly as appropriate adult behavior. Mothers required much practice to overcome patterns of hostility in response to interruptions and criticism.

Session 12

The group's final activity was a shopping expedition. Members were given vouchers to purchase clothing at a discount outlet. This was followed by a luncheon in an inexpensive restaurant. This adult "field trip" allowed members to practice, away from the agency, the interpersonal skills they had learned in the group. It was hoped that practicing in the "real world," and engaging in member-chosen activities that might in the future be shared with friends, would facilitate generalization of training effects. Overall, the mothers participated actively in the outing. However, at times some women behaved anxiously when faced with activities not practiced in the group such as handling service situations with strangers and presenting themselves in public situations including dressing appropriately. A simpler, more friend-oriented activity such as a potluck would have better served learning goals and facilitated group termination.

EVALUATION

Anonymous feedback on participant satisfaction at posttraining indicated a strong positive response to training. Members individually rated their satisfaction with format, content, leadership, and goal attainment. Satisfaction with leadership received the highest mean score (8.8 on a 10-point scale), followed by group format (8.7), content (8.6), skill rehearsal (8.2) and goal attainment (8.0). When asked to indicate what they liked most about the group, members frequently mentioned content and role-plays. Suggestions for improvement included greater opportunity for skills practice and more sessions.

While the small sample size severely limits the generalizability of findings, nonetheless pre-post results were encouraging. Six mothers completed data collection at pretraining, posttraining and followup two months later. After training, members reported improvement in a number of social support indices (Richey, Lovell & Reid, 1987). Significant increases were noted in total network size from a pretraining mean of 19.67 persons (SD = 7.84) to a posttraining mean of 29.67 persons (SD = 10.21) ($t(5)$ = 4.62, p < .01). Members also were asked to rate the quality of their daily contacts on a five-point scale where 1 was "very good" and 5 was "very bad." The quality of contacts was rated significantly better at posttraining (mean = 2.18) as compared to pretraining (mean = 3.33) ($t(5)$ = 2.54, p < .05). Both network size and quality of contacts remained high at followup. Mothers also reported increases in satisfaction with support from friends, in duration of interactions, and in percentage of daily contacts with friends.

CONCLUSIONS AND RECOMMENDATIONS

Social support training appears to offer a promising treatment alternative to help isolated and at-risk individuals develop and more effectively utilize sources of social support. Informal feedback from group members as well as ratings of participant satisfaction suggest that the group was well received. Attendance remained high and consistent throughout the three-month group. Anecdotal evidence suggests that the deliberate utilization of the "Hawthorne Effect" by "selection" for an "advanced" group enhanced member motivation to attend. Induction into group treatment through previous attendance in a parent discussion group facilitated norms for active participation. Prior relationships with members allowed leaders to introduce constructive criticism into the group process relatively quickly. Individual goal-setting interviews before training, leader modeling of openness and risk-taking, and group humor contributed to group cohesion, and behavior and attitude change. On a cautionary note, however, mastery of concepts was slower than anticipated despite the facilitating effects of the Relationship Roadmap. The presentation of material had to be continually tailored to members' actual levels of emotional, cognitive and behavioral readiness.

Recommendations for improving future training to enhance social support among abusive mothers would include more extensive use of personal goal-setting to maximize the individual application of training materials to each client's skill and comfort levels. Homework assignments leading to greater skill mastery outside the group also would be assigned to individual members on a weekly basis. For example, involvement in clubs or volunteer activities could be a therapeutic goal. In this way, training would more clearly reflect a "remedial model" of group work with an emphasis on individual assessment and treatment planning (Papell & Rothman, 1966). Incorporating positive reinforcement procedures more explicitly into training with low-income clients could also enhance outcomes (Landau & Paulson, 1977). For example, Zander and Kindy (1980) used small monetary payments as rewards to increase treatment compliance. Consideration could be given to compensating members for such activities as attendance and homework completion. By client request, training would be extended to allow more time for rehearsing ways to handle criticism from family and friends, and manipulative or abusive behavior from men with whom they form relationships. Finally, an ongoing member-led support group would be a useful adjunct to training by facilitating followup and maintenance of skills over time.

REFERENCES

Anderson, S. C. & Lauderdale, M. (1982). Characteristics of abusive parents: A look at self-esteem. *Child Abuse and Neglect, 6,* 285-293.

Bales, R. F. (1958). Task roles and social roles in problem solving groups. In E. E. Maccoby, T. M. Newcomb, & E. L. Hartley (Eds.), *Readings in social psychology* (3rd Ed.). New York: Holt, Rinehart & Winston.

Barker, P. (1985). *Using metaphors in psychotherapy.* New York: Brunner/Mazel.

Bloch, S. (1987). Humor in group therapy. In W. F. Fry and W. A. Salameh (Eds.), *Handbook of humor and psychotherapy.* Sarasota: Professional Resource Exchange, Inc.

Coleman, J. (1968). Social processes and social stimulation games. In S. Boocock and E. Schild (Eds.), *Stimulation games in learning.* Beverly Hills, CA: Sage.

Fantuzzi, J. W., Wary, L., Hall, R., Goins, C. & Azur, S. (1986). Parent and social skills training for mentally retarded mothers identified as child maltreaters. *American Journal of Mental deficiency,* 91(2), 135-140.

Fry, W. H. & Salameh, W. R. (1987). *Handbook of humor and psychotherapy, Advances in the clinical use of humor.* Sarasota: Professional Resource Exchange, Inc.

Galassi, M. D. & Galassi, J. P. (1977) *Assert yourself!* New York: Human Sciences Press.

Gambrill, E. D. & Richey, C. A. (1988). *Taking charge of your social life.* Berkeley, CA: Behavioral Options.

Garbarino, J. M. & Gillian, G. (1980). *Understanding abusive families.* Lexington, MA: Lexington Books.

Garvin, C. (1974). Group process: Usage and uses in social work practice. In P. Glasser, R. Sarri, and R. Vinter (Eds.), *Individual change through small groups.* New York: Free Press.

Gaudin, J. M. & Pollane, L. (1983). Social networks, stress and child abuse. *Children and Youth Services Review, 5,* 91-102.

Hartford, M. (1972). *Groups in social work.* New York: Columbia University Press.

Herbruch, C. C. (1979). *Breaking the cycle of child abuse.* Minneapolis: Winter Press.

Hunter, R. S. & Kilstrom, N. (1979). Breaking the cycle in abusive families. *American Journal of Psychiatry, 136,* 1320-1322.

Kopp, S. (1971). *Guru: Metaphors from a psychotherapist.* Palo Alto: Science and Behavior Books.

Kubie, L. S. (1971). The destructive potential of humor in psychotherapy. *American Journal of Psychiatry, 127,* 861-866.

Landau, P. & Paulson, T. (1977). Group assertion training for Spanish-speaking Mexican-American mothers. In R. E. Alberti (Ed.), *Assertiveness: Innovations, applications, issues.* San Luis Obispo, CA: Impact Publishers.

Lankton, S. R. & Lankton, C. H. (1983). *The answer within: A clinical framework of Ericksonian hypnotherapy.* New York: Brunner/Mazel.

Lovell, M. L. & Hawkins, D. H. (in press). An evaluation of a group intervention to increase the personal social networks of abusive parents. *Children and Youth Services Review.*

Marlatt, G. A. & Fromme, K. (1987). Metaphors for addiction. *Journal of Drug Issues, 17,* 9-28.

Marlatt, G. A. & Gordon, J. R. (1985). *Relapse prevention: Maintenance strategies in the treatment of addictive behaviors.* New York: Guilford Press.

Papell, C. D. & Rothman, B. (1966). Social group work models: Possession and heritage. *Journal of Education for Social Work,* 2(2), 66-77.

Polansky, N. A., Ammons, P., & Gaudin, J. (1985). Loneliness and isolation in child neglect. *Social Casework,* January, 338-47.

Rabin, C. (1983). Towards the use and development of games for social work practice. *British Journal of Social Work, 13,* 175-196.

Richey, C. A., Lovell, M. L., & Reid, K. (1987, November). Group interpersonal training to enhance social support among women at risk for child maltreatment. Paper presented at the 21st Annual AABT Convention, Boston, MA.

Salzinger, S., Kaflan, S., & Artemyeff, C. (1983). Mothers' personal social networks and child maltreatment. *Journal of Abnormal Psychology*, *922*(1), 68-76.

Shulman, L. (1984). *The skills of helping: Individuals and groups* (2nd Ed.). Itasca, IL: Peacock Press.

Smith, J. E., Rachman, S. J., & Yule, B. (1984). Non-accidental injury to children. III. Methodological problems of evaluative treatment research. *Behavioural Research and Therapy*, *22*, 367-383.

Wahler, R. G. (1980). The insular mother: Her problems in parent/child treatment. *Journal of Applied Behavior Analysis*, *13*(2), 207-219.

Wahler, R. G., Leske, G., & Rogers, E. (1979). The insular family: A deviance support system for oppositional children. In L. A. Hammerlynch (Ed.), *Behavior systems for the developmentally disabled. I. School and family environments*. New York: Brunner/Mazel.

Zander, T. & Kindy, P. (1980). Behavioural group training for welfare parents. In S. D. Rose (Ed.), *A casebook in group therapy*. Englewood Cliffs, NJ: Prentice-Hall, Inc.

Social Group Work with Elders: Linkages and Intergenerational Relationships

Louis Lowy

INTRODUCTION

A substantial literature on social group work with elders has emerged in the last few years (Hartford, Getzel, Saul, Weisman, Lee, Feil, Burnside, Lang, Lowy and many others). This paper will focus primarily on the question: What can social group work as one method and field of social work contribute to provide linkages to older persons with others of their own generation and facilitate intergenerational relationships?

I would go too far afield here to review the demographic changes and their implication for our society as a whole and for families, individuals, for social policies and social organization and institution. In a recently published paper entitled "The Implications of Demographic Trends as they Affect the Elderly," I have discussed some of these aspects and have pointed out that reaching out to older people is becoming an urgent task to avoid their isolation and segregation and to work to enhance their inclusion and integration. Orr summarizes what many authors in the field of gerontology have stated: ". . . the primary developmental task for all older people is to deal with the preponderance of losses which dramatically impact on their lives" (p. 316). Regardless of other events at this stage in the life cycle, the equilibrium of losses and gains becomes upset in favor of an accumulation of losses with which older persons have to cope.

Stanley Cath refers to this phenomenon as an "omniconvergence of losses," be it loss of income, work role, spouse and/or significant others, meaningful relationships, space, physical functioning, opportunities for self-expression, etc. At the same time people experience gains which oc-

---

Louis Lowy, PhD, Professor Emeritus, Boston University, deceased.

109

cur during this period, such as a continuing capacity for growth and learning, freedom from certain role obligations, a new sense of subjective time, new roles of grandparenthood, an overall awareness of "late freedom," as Rosenmayr phrases it (1983). To be able to come to terms with this unbalanced state is the continuous struggle of older persons. This struggle is idiosyncratic and loaded with many variables, such as age, gender, race, ethnicity, previous life experiences, ego-structure, coping capacity etc. Since human beings are social by nature and in need of others to negotiate life's journey, the shifting equilibrium in the late years requires linkages with others who undergo similar struggles and must deal with similar tasks. Social group work can be useful in stimulating and nurturing such linkages with others and thereby help people in coming to terms with these life tasks.

THE PROCESS OF LINKAGES WITH OTHERS
OF THEIR GENERATION

People in their later years are in interaction with others, despite a general assertion that they are frequently isolated, alone and lonely. To be sure, there are times when people at any age feel lonely; ultimately all of us are alone, as Kierkegaard, Sartre and other existentialists have pointed out. It is also true that the type, form and frequency of interactions change as we pass through life and the before-mentioned struggle poses significant challenges. This is why social groupwork knowledge and skills can be useful in meeting these challenges.

It is well-known that social work's engagement with the aging originated in settings where social groupwork was practiced, such as in settlement houses, Ys, community centers (Lowy, 1985). Many older persons felt a need for contact with others as their social world began to shrink; it did not take long before social group workers recognized that their goals, functions and methods were useful in promoting social relationships among the elderly, since social group work's main focus is on group process, collective support and interaction and individualization as a means of enabling individual people to grow, develop and/or achieve a task. Schwartz (1961), Lang (1981), Shulman (1984) characterize the social work group as a unique social form which operates as a mutual aid system that promotes autonomy and benefits individual members through the effective action of the whole group" (Lang, op. cit.).

The question is *how* the processes of linkages of older persons can be facilitated in order to increase the likelihood that the balance of losses and gains be negotiated as successfully as possible.

BALANCING LOSSES AND GAINS
THROUGH INTERACTION AND RELATIONSHIPS

Whatever the setting or milieu in which an encounter takes place, the key concepts are: interaction and relationship. People are engaged with others in the normal course of daily living as spouse, widows, widowers, peers, colleagues, friends, residents, patients, clients, customers, etc. and their interaction varies according to the degree of intensity of relationships from the impersonal, formal and loose to the personal, informal and intense. Interactions also vary as to purposes of the encounter, as well as chance factors. Do they meet because they happen to come together as patients in a long care facility or because they want to participate in an elder hostel program? Allowing for the many variables alluded to, the use of relationships among the participants and the social group worker is a sine qua non of the armamentarium of the social group work process.

"Tuning in" means to be sensitive to the loss-gain balancing struggle; the worker must be able to listen to the direct and indirect signals of the persons in a group situation. At the same time, the worker must be able to empathize and elucidate what it means to risk building new relationships at this stage in life. That is where and how feelings about the characteristics of one's own aging must be examined. "How will I react when I engage in a relationship that may not last long, that may produce pain of renewed losses by the group member and yet demands input of energy which is of limited supply?" Putting oneself into the position of the older person is tough, because many workers, if not most, have not gone through this phase of life and must anticipate feelings and reactions without benefit of past experience. "Tuning-in" means also to be sensitive to the way in which the person struggles in a group that may come into being, to the provisional, the tentativeness of the interaction for fear of impermanence on the one hand and the desire to establish contact and maintain a relationship on the other. While mutual aid places the other person in the position of aiding this "tuning-in process," the other person may not be able to fulfil the role, as he or she finds it hard to cope with the "imbalance of struggle." Therefore it is the worker who is to bridge, the psychological as well as the physical distance, by reaching out to people sensitively and addressing their coping capacities. That is why the initial phase of the linking process is particularly crucial in working with the elderly. The "contracting" stage may indeed be the longest phase and perhaps the only one to exist for the participants and the worker's use of empathic skills of "reaching for feelings, acknowledging feelings and articulating feelings" are especially vital to satisfy older people's needs for affiliation (Shulman, 1984, p. 24). To be sure there are many elderly who join with others readily, who interact without apparent difficulties, who participate in self-help groups, as well as in formal organizations and formed activities. Whether they eventually reach a stage in their lives when they withdraw, become more isolated as they grow older or become functionally ill requires longitudinal research which has not really been undertaken as yet.

Much has been said and written about "reminiscing" as a major task in the later years (Pincus, 1970; Burnside, 1984). Unquestionably the older people get the more they look back "what has been" and ask overtly or covertly: What have I done with my life? What has it been all about? What legacy will I leave? Why survive? Butler considers leaving a legacy as one of the most important elder functions upon which subsequent generations can draw to continue the course of human events (Butler, 1975). Reminiscing or "life review" may bring up the good and the bad, the triumphs and disasters, the victories and defeats. That is why care must be exercised in guiding the "life review" process to avoid excessive recall of traumatic experiences and thereby undo the balance (Lowy, 1962). People who underwent cataclysmic events (such as Holocaust survivors, e.g.) may not experience the needed reconciliation with the past and acceptance of one's life as it has been and therefore "it is questionable that life review serves a similar function of the aged Holocaust survivor" (Rosenbloom, 1985, p. 190). The same comment can apply to veteran groups or survivors of other extraordinary natural or people-made disasters.

In addition to the questions, "what has happened and what have I done with my life so far," older people progressively will ask: "How much time do I still have left?" And the corollary to this question is: "What use shall I or can I make of this unknown?" The group workers' awareness of these time-perception factors must always be present and guide their interventive stances, e.g., in suggesting activities, topics for discussion, social action moves.

When reaching out to older persons, conditions of safety and trust need to be maintained continuously, but most assuredly must be created right at the beginning phase. One of the tools available for workers is to lay open their own losses and feelings about them, as well as their own successes and how they balanced them with their own losses. Anecdotal references serve well; they encourage the group participants to listen, to join in, to risk themselves and to get engaged.

It can happen that some of them tell a younger worker "You really don't understand what it means to lose a wife (or husband)"; or "How can you know what it means to be constantly in pain and take all kinds of medication four times a day?" To be sure, the younger worker may not really understand or know, but he/she can respond by saying: "Although I don't really understand, I really don't know, I will try as best as I possibly can and will look to you to help me with this; let us learn together!" (Falck, 1984).

The "tuning-in" phase can lead eventually to "contracting"; to resolve to learn together can indeed be the initiation of a contract of mutual give and take, sprinkled with issues of "power and control" that raise their heads quite early in the process.

Encouraging the participants—who are not really a group as yet, but an aggregate of individual older persons—to ventilate is another valuable tool to create conditions of safety and trust. This opens doors to relate with one another (with some more than with others) and to talk about losses as well as gains and to continue to meet, although the risk of further losses is hereby increased and resistances are likely to appear stronger. Outreach demands that the worker accepts such resistances and maintains a patient, giving and caring style in all encounters that is being conveyed through verbal and nonverbal behavior.

"Widow to widow groups," especially for those in the later years, have amply demonstrated the beneficial aspects of mutual aid, frequently without the involvement of a social group worker (Silverman, 1974). "All in-the-same-boat phenomenon," support and demands, sharing data and resources have been significant processes in helping widows and widowers (there are fewer widowers than widows; half of all older women in 1985 were widows—over five times as many widows (8 million) as widowers (1.6 million) to cope with bereavement and grieving and to come to terms with their new status. By the way, widow(er) to widow(er) groups may also be viewed on an intergenerational linkage basis, but I wanted to include them also as an illustration of self-help groups along horizontal generational lines.

THE PROCESS OF INTERGENERATIONAL LINKAGES

According to the Spanish philosopher Ortega y Gasset (1958) the relationship between generations is the single most important and controlling influence on our lives and on social change. The inter-generational nature of human life and the role of the elderly on cultural forms to succeeding generations has been well established in the literature as well as in art (McKee and Heta Kauppinen, 1987). Intergenerational exchange consists of giving and receiving. As consumers and producers of foods and services they contribute an economic resource. In the political arena, many are exercising their political responsibilities as vital and active citizens. In the social sphere they act as providers of services, as professionals, paraprofessionals, and as volunteers in many programs that link the old with the old and the old with the young. In educational programs, "in private and public institutions, older adults as learners and teachers, act as example and communicate their life experience, their wisdom as well as their follies, gained in having lived sixty, seventy or eighty years." (Lowy, 1980, p. 218)

Ours is a unique period in history; an increasing number of 3, indeed 4 generations are alive at the same time. An estimated 1/3 of all persons 65 and over have at least one grandchild and 1/4 of persons in the life-range of 58 to 59 have one or more surviving parents. It is not uncommon that of the over 28 million older Americans in 1985 (over 65) — representing 12% of the population, i.e., every 9th person — quite a few older people outlive their offspring (*State of the Families*, 1985). More and more we have a horizontal and vertical system of intergenerational relationships. There is now a burgeoning literature dealing with this demographic phenomenon and their implications (American Association of Retired Persons; The United States Senate, Special Committee on Aging, 1985; United States Senate, Aging Reports, 1985, 1986; Brody, 1981 and 1985).

It is well established that there is a flow of mutual support between generations through kin, friends, neighbors. Those family members, friends and neighbors are important aids to the elderly as they become less capable of functioning on their own (Getzel, 1985). Blenkner in the sixties pointed out that achieving "filial maturity" is a task concerning the relationship between adult children and their aging parents; it is essentially a middle-age developmental task that results from successful resolution of a filial crisis. This crisis occurs when past relationships with family are no longer appropriate or operable — when aging parents require assistance or support of their adult children and their offspring to be available so that parents (or grandparents) can "depend on them to be dependable" (Lowy, 1977, p. 245). Recent research has devoted considerable attention to demands of caregivers, though it is limited to spouses who care for spouses, adult children who care for their parents or kin (Brody, op. cit. 1981; Shanas, 1979; Miller, 1981, and others). Few studies, however, examine older people, notably parents, as caregivers. Jennings has opened up this subject in the latest issue of *Social Work* and has raised a series of questions that call for research, such as: Who are these families and what stresses do they experience? What services do older caregivers request?

How can informal and formal support systems be integrated to provide mutual aid, and many others?

Mutual Aid Groups and Intergenerational Relationships

Because of demographic changes that will become more widespread in this and other countries in the near future, mutual support groups play an important role in dealing with the issues arising from these horizontal and vertical interpersonal systems.

For purposes of this paper I will confine my discussion to the mutual aid process as outlined by Shulman and Gitterman (1986) as it can well apply to such groups and some of the issues in intergenerational relationships that will have to be addressed.

Composition of Intergenerational Support Groups

There are at least eight basic compositions of support groups that can come into existence: (1) Parents of adult children; (2) Adult children with other adult children; (3) Parents of adult children jointly with their adult children; (4) Older widows and widowers; (5) Older widows (widowers) jointly with older widows (widowers); (6) Grandparents with other grandparents; (7) Grandparents with their grandchildren; and (8) Grandchildren with other grandchildren in their respective roles as grandchildren. While this typology focuses on a single status as a major raison d'être for support-group formation (formally or informally), other statuses are likely to play a significant part in the dynamics of such group processes. For example, parents of adult children may also be grandparents and grandchildren are also children of their parents (biological or adopted). This matrix of support groups is made possible by the increase in life expectancies at this juncture of history.

The overt purposes of these groups vary quite distinctly; some people come together as caregivers, others as service providers; others again as friends of neighbors. Some may want to get together to learn about political, economic or social problems and evolve into social action groups; others may engage in learning new skills or brush up on skills that have become rusty over time. Joint ventures, projects or travel may be the outcome of a group that originally met to deal with problems facing them as caregivers to their aging parents. As Greene cites Cohen, 1983; Hartford and Parsons, 1982, some common themes in groups for caregivers include: (1) relocating as person who becomes too frail or dependent to remain in his/her original residence; (2) engaging other relatives of secondary caregivers; (3) making decisions and taking responsibility when an older relative cannot do so alone; (4) dealing with feelings of impatience, frustration, entrapment and guilt; (5) improving communications; (6) reducing conflict; and (7) understanding the biopsychosocial changes of aging (Greene, 1986).

The Mutual Aid Process

The symbiotic relationship between individual and societal needs is inherent in the mutual support group and finds expression in the nine mutual aid processes as outlined by Shulman and Gitterman (1986): "Sharing data, the dialectical process, entering taboo areas, the 'all in the same boat phenomenon,' mutual support, mutual demand, individual problem-solving, rehearsal and the strengthening-in-numbers phenomenon." (op. cit., p. 9). These processes occur at various times, sometimes more pronounced at one stage of a group's development, sometimes repeatedly at another stage and then re-occur as the group moves along in its life.

Let me put my remarks in the context of the "Development of Boston Group Model" (Garland et al., 1969) which essentially postulates five stages with their dominant dynamic characteristics, frames of references, program suggestions and worker focus. The central theme running through all five stages is that of "closeness." From the very first moment that a number of individuals come together tentatively and move towards becoming an aggregate to the dissolution of their common bond "they must struggle with how near they will come to one another emotionally" (p. 29). In the first "pre-affiliative" stage, "exploration" and "approach-avoidance" movements occur when "tuning-in" is the social worker's first and foremost task and requisite skill. While it is of major importance in the initial stages of group life, it has particular relevance when working with any of the combination of support groups in gerontology mentioned before, as "closeness and distance" is one of the recurring themes of intergenerational relationships, whether the people, singly or in groups engage in interpersonal encounters of longer duration or not. Additional major themes in balancing age-vertical relation-age-vertical relationships that I want to allude to are "submission and dominance" and "openness and privacy."

Closeness and Distance

People in their relationships move towards maintaining a certain degree of distance and embracing a certain degree of closeness. When the degree of distance is wider, people feel more disengaged; when the degree of closeness is narrower, people feel more engaged. It is a kind of minuet, moving a few steps forward and a few steps backwards. Too much closeness can engender conflict; that is why "intimacy by distance" has had such an evocative appeal (Rosenmayr, 1986). Research on family patterns in many countries around the world has documented the existence of mutual aid and service between generations under these conditions (Shanas, 1979; Brody, 1981; Palmore, 1982; Rosenmayr and Kockeis, 1968).

Family support is two directional. Older persons are not only passive recipients in a family network; they also provide financial and other forms of help to younger family members. And therefore, for many families, interdependence between the older and younger generations in an arrangement of mutual benefits, and in some cases, outright economic necessity, exists.

"Sharing data" about common concerns brings many adult children as well as their parents together. In fact it is this part of the mutual aid process which leads frequently to the formation of intergenerational groups. "Data" may be factual (e.g., social security), experiential (my father just celebrated his 75th birthday), emotional (I began to feel good about my father's retirement decision). "Sharing data" offers many openings and re-openings for the participants to get engaged, to learn, to ventilate, to interact and the worker can indeed "tune-in" and start building a relationship with individuals. "Approach-avoidance" can get played out and only a tentative commitment to meet again to be made.

This first stage (in the Boston model) may remain for some intergenerational groups the longest-lasting if not the only stage of development and several of the mutual aid processes may be taken up then.

Research on the developmental stages and their dynamic characteristics in intergenerational support groups is sorely needed. Research on the occurrence of several of the nine mutual aid processes relative to the stages of development of such groups and in relation to dealing with issues of "submission and dominance" as well as "openness and privacy" is equally urgent to advance the state of practice.

The "dialectical process" may be initiated when initial trust has been developed. A person states the thesis: "my father feels useless after he was retired from his company"; this comment is followed by an antithesis presented by another individual (member already?): "This does not have to be so, because my father got involved in several community activities through my efforts." Others in the group debate this "solution"; eventually a synthesis can occur that there are different modes for retired people to cope with retirement. The worker acts as a catalyst by pointing our various conditions and personality factors which allow for different modes of adaptation that lead to a synthesis. She also shares additional data and increases the repertoire of potential resources that can strengthen the feelings of support. Gaining "mutual support" is surely a sine qua non of every mutual aid group, but becomes a central theme when "grandparents band together at times when divorce is threatening family ties. In pursuing their legal rights, they are telling us of the meaningfulness of grandparenthood" (Severino, Tensink, Pender, and Bernstein, 1986).

Adult children jointly with their parents find that they are "all in the same boat" and face similar as well as different issues, but essentially they are not alone in facing problems of different generations that co-exist at the same time; a feeling of trust and safety must be achieved before demands can be made without alienating particular persons.

Dominance and Submission

As mentioned already, issues of "dominance and submission" permeate intergenerational relationships, particularly between parents and their adult children. Many unresolved emotional conflicts of the adult child during periods of adolescence with the now aging parent(s) rear their heads at this time. The worker must be sensitively attuned to this and use his emphatic skill to convey genuine understanding without getting entrapped to "solve this problem" now. At the same time he/she needs to be aware that older people need a sense of mastery even though they may be physically constrained and emotionally depleted. They need a sense that they still have a measure of control over their lives, even if it is minimal. As Jahoda has pointed out already in 1958, criteria of "sound mental health" include positive attitudes towards self, reality perception, a sense of autonomy and environmental mastery. To the extent that autonomy expressed through a sense of mastery is present among members of all generations, the need for continued assertion of one's power is decreased (Bengtson and Treas, 1980; Cath, 1971; Neugarten, 1975; Butler, 1975; Lowy, 1986). Here the "power and control" stage may offer opportunities to make demands on one another with the workers ready to lend their balanced support letting people know that they are here and point out realistic limitations.

A group of adult children and their parents may make "assignments" to their parents to bake a cake for the next get-together. Many parents say that this is an undue burden on them. The worker now tries to reduce the burden by suggesting a "division of labor," a re-distribution of the workload between parents *and* their adult children.

As the aggregate of people eventually becomes a "group" — most pronouncedly in the "intimacy" or "familial" stage — "individual problem-solving" is more likely to take place than heretofore, (although people may attempt to do so when they share data and expect to receive answers to a problem by the worker who at that time may be perceived as an expert in this area). Generally, however, solving of a particular intergenerational problem with and via the group presupposes a mutual feeling of trust in one another. Group norms must be accepted by the members; one of these norms is the expectation of mutual trust and a readiness to take risks in presenting a problem openly, with the expectations that the members and the worker are able to help produce a solution. To illustrate:

In a group of families one of the couples is facing the decision to place their mother in a nursing home. They can no longer take care of her in their own home. It is a difficult choice and they experience many of the feelings associated with such a choice; guilt, denial of the need, discomfort, anticipation of alienation, uncertainty about the quality of the institution, etc. (Motenko in Lowy, 1985). The worker now assumes the role of teacher and enabler. He/she helps the couple outline and dissect the issue, asks members whether any had experienced a similar situation, and if so, how they had dealt with it, moving back and forth between the experience of others and the present problem. The worker and/or the members now propose ways and means of finding a suitable long term care facility, the pro's and con's of institutionalization and the avenues available to cope with feelings of the couples and parent. Enlisting understanding, empathy and support of the whole group is at this point the major task.

Role-playing can be a useful technique in facilitating the search for a suitable facility as well as how to present a solution to the parent of the couple. The worker has to be careful though to set limits in a role-play situation to avoid slipping into a role-therapeutic encounter that she/he might not be able to bring under control. Essentially it is a "rehearsal" that can be repeated with group members who are not directly involved "playing out" the situation which will be discussed by the participants and the worker. Affective issues can be tackled and at another meeting of the group the problem might be on the agenda again. Thus the couple get the reassurance that they are not alone and can repeatedly turn to others for help, suggestions and feedback.

Members with or without the worker — depending on group development and contact, can give each other support in bringing up a taboo-subject such as sexual relationships of older persons with younger persons. A courageous member, as Shulman points out (p. 10), may take the initiative in raising the issue and when he/she supports (discussion of the issue) others may join in and discover "their own courage to participate" (op. cit., p. 11).

Here are a few illustrations of collaborative undertakings between older persons and young people, initiated and sponsored by the "National Public-private Intergenerational Initiative" in Washington, D.C., of which the Elvirita Lewis Foundation is the leader for nine projects, presently occurring in several parts of the country.

School child care. By this summer, La Quinta, California will have an intergenerational child care center located adjacent to an elementary school. The older men and women who staff the center will receive training in early childhood development and be encouraged to rejoin the workforce as child care aides, nannies and governesses.

Rural child care. A Western Carolina University project called "Age-Link" is helping local community organizations in 10 rural counties to develop intergenerational child care programs. To date, five counties have established projects in which elders work with children in before and after-school day care programs, in family day care homes or in telephone reassurance programs.

Openness and Privacy

As people grow older, privacy becomes an increasingly precious commodity. Retirement, widowhood, institutionalization create not only separateness but also intrusions into the private sphere. Each person needs a private preserve where he/she can find psychological shelter. It is part of a person's autonomy.

Different generations must be able to define boundaries of openness and privacy, when to be open with one another and when to maintain privacy, not to be confused with secrecy to avoid communication. Communication involves not only the flow of messages, but also the flow of silences. To find the proper balance of openness and privacy is a key aspect of managing intergenerational relationships.

Social workers in working with mutual aid groups need to be conscious of this delicate balance. It is obviously a major factor in the lives of institutionalized older persons. Children, grandchildren, peers, friends have an opportunity to become engaged in change efforts, in seeking redress of grievances when warranted as well as in facilitating communication between staff and residents of short and long-term care facilities. The fight against "hopelessness and despair" of institutionalized aged is not only a task of the residents or patients, but is a joint enterprise of two or three generations, including, of course, those not in the institution. As Berman-Rossi (1986) illustrates, searching out the common ground, challenging obstacles, sharing data and lending a vision had paid off for the group members in that particular facility. An intergenerational group effort is likely to pay off not only for the residents, but also for non-resident family members and friends in experiencing the ups and downs of relationships, of victory and defeat, of feelings of assertiveness, of sharing and reaping towards, of strengthening their egos, of alleviating guilt and anxiety, as we can surmise in the illustrations cited in this paper.

The roles of the worker as enabler, broker, mediator, teacher, therapist, advocate and consultant are indeed a role-bundle that demands knowledge and skills of keen assessment along the bio-psycho-social axis of individuals and groups in their stages of development. It requires interventive skills based on values of human worth and social justice and knowledge of mutual aid processes: when to hold back, when to let go, when to stay in, when to keep out, but above all, how to be there when needed. Based on scientific principles, there is an artistry of the practitioner's performance which, according to Siporin, "is expressed and actualized, first of all, through a personal style, which has distinctive, individualized cognitive and action patterns that express his or her way of relating to others. When well-developed, style includes a discriminating taste and sensitivity and an apt, yet genuine manner of expression" (Siporin, 1987).

Intergenerational Linkages and Social Policy

People all over the country have taken notice of the demographic revolution. Beginning with the awareness of "the greying of the federal budget" (Hudson, 1978) to the emergence of an article in the *Washington Post* in 1986 "The coming conflicts as we soak the young to enrich the old" (Taylor) and Preston's 1984 statement in the *Scientific American* "children and the elderly in the US" (1984), conflict between the generations has now become an issue of public debate. "Most gerontologists in the U.S. believe that the appearance of intergenerational conflict is a fabrication of the Reagan Administration and their powerful supporters as well as such conservative "think tanks" as the Hoover, Manhattan and Enterprise Institutes and the Heritage Foundation which have framed issues in such a way that attention is focused on choices between generations, when choices are really between rich and poor or between domestic and military spending. This point was made vividly at the XIIIth International Congress of Gerontology, held in New York City in July 1985. Independent presentations by five prominent U.S. gerontologists, Robert Binstock, Marjorie Cantor, Robert Morris, Bernice Neugarten and James Schulz, all arrived at the same conclusion: "Intergenerational conflict is a myth, not a reality . . ." (Lowy and O'Conner, 1986).

". . . The increasing tendency in our society to view older persons as 'burdens' can be related to our heavy emphasis on individualism and the assumption that individuals should strive for independence. At times, we seem to forget the social nature of human existence, Aristotle's dictum of a 'zoon politikon,' that humans need to help and support one another in order to assure their very survival as a species. A more appropriate emphasis is of interdependence, on respecting and valuing the individual contributions of all persons to the human group and to society's needs and imperatives for survival. Such a view of human potential recognizes individual autonomy without assuming that individuals who are dependent in some aspects of their lives are any more burdensome or any less human, than anyone else. In the course of a lifetime, we are all mutually dependent. . . ." (Lowy and O'Connor, 1986).

The appearance of intergenerational conflict has been fueled by attacks on the Social Security program, attacks which have undermined public confidence that the program will serve future as well as present generations of older people. At a time when Presidential rhetoric has expressed concern for only the "truly needy," a narrowly defined group which is not assumed to include all those who eat at soup kitchens, the apparent exemption of older adults from a share of federal spending cuts has doubtless caused some ill-feeling among several segments (not only younger ones) of our population. There has not yet been a major public outcry about age-entitlements, but it would be optimistic to assume that the potential for such confrontations has passed. (Lowy and O'Connor, 1987).

Over a hundred nationwide, state, areawide and local organizations, such as the American Association of Retired Persons (26 million persons), "Old and Young Together," "Center for Understanding Aging," "The Executive Office of Elder Affairs in Massachusetts" and other states and "The Youth 2000 Campaign" exist today which promote and motivate intergenerational interests. Programs such as decent dependable and affordable health care and housing for everyone – young, middle aged or older; decent child welfare and employment programs for all economic classes; improved literacy and attainment; lifestyles free from substance abuse; sound long-term care facilities and outreach services for the elderly; mental health programs for all age groups that are preventively oriented; leisure and recreational services that bring the generations together; improved learning and teaching facilities and curriculum for the young and the old, equally for male and female, black, white and brown, Gentile and Jew, urban and rural can be developed and maintained by changing our policy priorities towards a more equitable distribution of our resources.

Recently a coalition of ninety organizations has been formed under the name *Generations United* representing over 30 million Americans. This is certainly one of the largest coalitions, if not the largest ever formed in the United States for any purpose. This alliance has the goal of collaborating in a national effort to forge ties of interdependence and to resist the pressures toward competition and division between generations. It now becomes possible to present a united front on such issues as the need for access by all Americans to quality health are, reform of the welfare system, child and elder abuse and day care for children and dependent adults. No longer does each age-specific interest group have to fight its battles alone. Four working committees; public policy, program development, building state and local support and public education and awareness and a steering committee led by the Executive directors of the National Council of Aging and the Child Welfare League of America respectively, are engaged in moving the coalition towards achieving health, social and economic goals. The prime force towards creating this coalition was the "Center for Understanding Aging." This center originated as a self-help group of older and younger people to deal with intergenerational issues, using social group work as a method, but realized quickly that many of these issues affect a larger segment of the population; indeed these issues are matters of social policy! Thus, a link between micro and macro arenas was formed, a link that is very much in the tradition of social work, particularly social group work (Pratt, 1987).

CODA

Working with members of several generations demands the application of the values, knowledge and skill of social work but also the ability of practioners to establish linkages on the macro level in order to affect social policy by utilizing the appropriate skills for those tasks. This is indeed a merger of the goal model, the reciprocal model and the developmental model of social groupwork. Social action and advocacy can be brought about by applying mutual-aid processes (with or without a social worker), but always keeping in mind the state of development of the group which engages in social change actions and the dynamic nature of these developmental stages when social changes are sought and that appropriate strategies for achieving them are to be devised. What a challenge for knowledge building and knowledge application!

We have to do a great deal of quantitative as well as qualitative research to learn empirically what kinds of specific knowledge and skills are required to work with intergenerational groups as outlined here and to translate this knowledge into action skills on the micro as well as on the macro levels. Intergenerational work of various types of groups — particularly caregiving — is a spectacular challenge and demands not only commitment and engagement of our profession together with other professions, volunteers, members in the community, patients and residents in institutions, clients in various agencies, officials in the bureaucracy, caretakers, families, peers, neighbors, but also the courage to risk new approaches and subject these to repeated empirical testing. At the same time it calls for vision and affirmation that our past has indeed been prologue. Let us now make the prologue the present and participate in building a more socially just and equitable future for *all* generations, old and young together in a saner and more peaceful world!

I want to close by quoting Emerson, appropriately as this 9th Symposium is held in Boston "by the sea," as he interpreted the later years in his book of poetry, *Terminus*:

> As the bird trims her to the gale,
> I trim myself to the storm of time
> I man the rudder, reef the sail,
> Obey the voice at eve obeyed at prime:
> Lowly faithful banish fear,
> Right onward drive unharmed;
> The port, well worth the cruise, is near,
> And every wave is charmed.

REFERENCES

Aging America: Trends and Projections. American Association of Retired Persons and Senate Special Committee on Aging, Washington, D. C. 1985-86, Edition.

America in Transition: An Aging Society 1984-85 Edition. Special Committee on Aging; United States Senate, Washington, D. C. June 1985, Serial No. 99B.

Bengtson, Vern L. and Judith Treas, (1980) "The Changing Family Context of Mental Health and Aging," in James E. Birren and R. Bruce Sloane (eds.) *Handbook of Mental Health and Aging* (Englewood Cliffs, N.J.: Prentice-Hall, 1980), pp. 400-428.

Berman-Rossi, Toby. (1986) The Fight against Hopelessness and Despair: Institutionalized Aged" in Gitterman and Shulman op. cit. chap. 28, pp. 353-355.

Blenkner, Margaret (1965) "Social Work and Family Relationships in Later Life with Some Thoughts on Filial Maturity" in Ethel Shanas and Gordon F. Streib (eds.) *Social Structure and the Family* (Englewood Cliffs, N.J.: Prentice-Hall, pp. 46-59.

Brody, Elaine (1981) "Women in the Middle and Family Help to Older People." *The Gerontologist*, 21 (5) 471-80.

_____ (1985) "Parent Care as a Normative Family Stress," *The Gerontologist*, 25 (1) 19-29.

Burnside, Irene (1984) *Working with the elderly: group process and technique* (2nd edition). Belmont, Calif: Wadsworth Health Sciences Division.

Butler, Robert (1975) *Why Survive? Being old in America*, (New York: Harper & Row.)

Cath, Stanley (1971) "Some Dynamics of Middle and Later Years" *Crisis Intervention* (ed. H. Parad), New York: Family Service Society.

Cohen, P. M. (1983) "A Group Approach for Working Families of the Elderly" *The Gerontologist* 23 (4) 248-250.

Falck, Hans S. (1984) "The Membership Model of Social Work" *Social Work* 29, (155-160).

Feil, Naomi (1983) "Group Work with Disoriented Nursing Home Residents," *Group Work with the Frail Elderly* in S. Saul (ed) op. cit. 57-66.

Garland, James, R. Kolodny and H. Jones (1969). "A Model in Stages or Development of Social Group Work" in Bernstein S. *Exploration in Group Work*, Boston: Charles River Books, Inc.

Getzel, George (1983). "Group with the Kin and Friends Caring for the Elderly," *Group Work with the Frail Elderly* in S. Saul (ed.) *Social Work With Groups*, 5(2), 91-102. (New York: The Haworth Press, Inc.).

Getzel, George S. (1985) "Critical Themes in Social Work Practice" in *Journal of Gerontological Social Work* 8 (3/4).

Getzel, George S. op. cit. p. 8.

Greene, Roberta R. *Social Work with the Aged and Their Families* (1986), New York: Aline de Gruyter. p. 287.

Hartford, Margaret E. and Parsons, R. (1982a) "Groups with Relatives of Dependent Older Adults, *The Gerontologist* 22 (3) 394-398.

Hartford, Margaret, E. (1980) "The Use of Group Methods for Work with the Aged" in J. E. Birren and R. B. Sloane (eds.) *Handbook of Mental Health and Aging*. Englewood Cliffs, NJ: Prentice Hall.

Hudson, Robert (1978). "The Graying of the Federal Budget and Its Consequences," *The Gerontologist* 28, 428-440.

Jahoda, M. (1958) Current Concepts of *Positive Mental Health*, New York: Basic Books. Also quoted in J. Birren and K. B. Sloane. *Handbook of Mental Health and Aging*. Englewood Cliffs, N.J. Prentice Hall, 1980 by James F. Birren and Jayne Renner "Concepts and Issues of Mental Health and Aging," p. 7.

Jennings, Jeanette (1987) "Elderly Parents as Caregivers for their Adult Dependent Children," *Social Work* 32 (5) 430-433.

Lang, N. 1981, "Some Defining Characteristics of the Social Work Group: Unique Social Form" in S. L. Abels and P. Abels (eds.) *Social Work with Groups* Proceedings of 1979 Symposium, Louisville, Kentucky; Committee for the Advancement of Social Work with Groups, 1979; 18-50.

Lee, Juanita A. (1983) "The Group: A Chance at Human Connection for the Mentally Impaired Person," *Group Work with the Frail Elderly* in S. Saul (ed.) op. cit. 43-56.

Lowy, Louis (1955) *Adult Education and Group Work*, New York: Whiteside and William Morrow.

_____ (1977) "Adult Children and Their Parents Dependency or Dependability" *Long Term Care and Health Services Administration Quarterly*, New York: Panel Publishers.

_____ (1962) "The Group in Social Work with the Aging," *Social Work* 7 (4) 43-50.

_____ (1986) Journal of *Geriatric Psychiatry*, Blau and Kahana, (eds.). Madison, Conn. International Universities Press, 19 (2) 149-174.

_____ (1980) *Social Policies and Programs on Aging*, 6th Printing. Lexington, Mass. D.C. Health & Co.

_____ (1985) "*Social Work with the Aging*" 2nd edition. Chapter 12, "Working with Groups of Older Persons" 278-339; White Plains, N.Y.: Longman, Inc.

_____ (1986) "Implications of Demographic Trends as they Affect the Elderly" *Journal of Geriatric Psychiatry*, (Madison, Conn., Vol XIX, 2: 1986).

_____ "Social Group Work with Vulnerable Older Persons: A Theoretical Perspective," *Group Work with the Frail Elderly* in S. Saul (ed.) *op. cit.* 21-32.

Lowy, Louis and Darlene O'Connor (1986) *Why Education in the Later Years*, Lexington, MA. D.C. Heath & Co., pp. 136-137.

McKee, Patrick and Heta Kauppinen (1987) *The Art of Aging: A Celebration of Old Age in Western Art*. New York, Human Sciences Press.

Miller, Dorothy (1981) "The Sandwich Generation: Adult Children of the Aging," *Social Work* 26, 419-423.

Motenko, Aluma (1985) "Working with Families" in Lowy *Social Work with the Aging*, Chapter 11, pp. 242-277.

Neugarten, B. L. (1975) "The Future and the Young-Old," *The Gerontologist* 25, pp. 4-9.

Orr, Alberta (1986) "Dealing with the Death of a Group Member: Visually Impaired Elderly in the Community" in A. Gitterman and L. Shulman (eds.) *Mutual Aid Groups and the Life Cycle*, Kasea, Ill. F. E. Peacock Publishers, Inc.

Ortega Y Gasset (1958) *Man and Crisis*, New York: Norton Publishers.

Palmore, Erdmon R. (1982) "Attitudes Towards the Aged: What We Know and Need to Know," *Research on Aging* 4 (3) 333-348.

Pincus, Allen (1970) "Reminiscence in Aging and Its Implications for Social Work Practice," *Social Work* 15 (4) 42-51.

Pratt, Fran (Winter 1987) Vol. 2, No. 1; (Framingham, MA) Framingham State College, pp. 1-2.

Preston, Samuel H. (1984) "Children and the Elderly in the U.S.," *Scientific American*, Vol. 251, No. 6., December 1984, 44-49.

Rosenbloom, Maria (1985) "The Holocaust Survivor in Late Life" in *Journal of Gerontological Social Work* 8, (3/4) 181-194.

Rosenmayr Leopold and E. Kocheis (1963) "Propositions for a Sociological Theory of Aging and the Family," *International Social Science Journal* 15, 410-426.

Rosenmayr, Leopold (1983) *Die Spate Freiheit (The Late Freedom)* Berlin, W. Germany Severin and Siedler Verlag.

Saul, Shura (1974) *An Album of People Growing Old*, New York: John Wiley and Sons, Inc.

Schwartz, William (1961) "The Social Worker in the Group" in *New Perspectives and Services to Groups: Theory, Organization and Practice*, New York: National Association of Social Workers, 7-34.

Severino, Sally K., J. Paul Tensink, Vivian B. Pender, Anne E. Bernstein. (1986) "Overview: The Psychology of Parenthood" in *Journal of Geriatric Psychiatry*, Blau, Kahana (eds.) 29 (1) p. 15.

Shanas, Ethel (1979) "The Family as a Social Support System in Old Age," *The Gerontologist* 19, 169-174.

Shulman, Lawrence and A. Gitterman (1986) The Life Model, Mutual Aid and the Mediating Function" in Gitterman and Shulman (eds.) *Mutual Aid Groups and the Life Cycle*, 1986. F.E. Peacock Publishers, Itasca, Illinois.

Shulman, Lawrence (1984) *The Skills of Helping Individual and Groups*. (2nd edition), Itasca, Ill. F. E. Peacock Publishers.

Silverman, Phyllis (1974) *Helping Each Other in Widowhood*, New York: Health Science.

Siporin, Max (1987) "The Art in Social Work Practice" presented at the NASW National Conference, New Orleans, LA. (Unpublished copy, p. 10)

Taylor, Paul (1986) "The Coming Conflict as We Soak the Young to Enrich the Old" *The Washington Post*, January 5, 2986, D1, D4.

The State of the Families Study (1984-85) New York: The Family Service of America, 1985.

Weisman, Alia S. (1974) "Does Old Age Make Sense?" *Journal of Geriatric Psychiatry*, 7 (1) 93.

Reaching Inner-City Children:
A Group Work Program Model
for a Public Middle School

David G. Bilides

One of the obstacles faced by community social service agencies is difficulty in attracting adolescents to the services offered them. Adolescents typically do not walk in or keep appointments at outpatient clinics and can be difficult to engage even for outreach programs. One solution to this dilemma is to go where the children are: the public schools.

One of the biggest problems in the Boston public school system is that many students and their families have pressing social, emotional, and physical needs that are not being met outside the school and that adversely

David G. Bilides, LICSW, was affiliated with the School Consultation and Treatment Program, Children's Services, Massachusetts Mental Health Center, 74 Fenwood Rd., Boston, MA 02115. He is presently at the San Mateo City (CA) Mental Health Service.

The author would like to thank the following people for their support in reading and offering suggestions on earlier versions of this paper: Sophia Bilides, Dina Carbonell, Amarilis Carrasquillo-Melendez, Emily Carrington, Melvin Delgado, Jim Garland, Bob Gass, Dannie Mae James, Sarah Newman, and Ceil Parteleno, with special thanks to: Victoria Alexander, E. Thomas Babbin, Denise M. N. Daniel, and Maggie Goodwin.

129

affect their education. The schools are educational institutions, not human service agencies, and they are ill prepared to deal with many of the problems and needs of their students' lives.

In 1984, an independent board composed of representatives from the Boston Public Schools, state, city, and private social service agencies, parents and students, secured funding and formed the Boston Student Human Services Collaborative. The mission of the Collaborative was to supplement and expand support services to the schools. The hope was that such services would free up both children and teachers to invest in each other, thereby increasing learning.

This paper describes the group work component of a Collaborative program at an inner-city school. After a brief look at the inner-city context, the group work program model is presented as a case study, including specific types of groups that have worked well and details of recruitment, composition, goals, activities, and leadership roles. Following this is a discussion of race, color, and ethnicity, and then a list of guiding principles for working with middle school adolescents in groups.

THE INNER-CITY CONTEXT

When participants at a recent East Coast workshop were asked what came to mind when they heard the words "inner-city kids," they generated the following terms: sophistication (streetwise), drugs, gun-toters, street environment, boom boxes, prostitution, Black males aged 10-21, latch key kids, poverty, violence, single-parent households and welfare.

This list is notable for what it excludes: the strengths, resilience and vitality of children's lives in urban areas; demographic factors and stresses (e.g., large and/or increasing Latino and Asian populations and deteriorating and inadequate public schools and municipal services).

In the Boston public schools the majority of students come from what are commonly called "minority" populations. They face race, color, ethnicity, class, language, gender, and economic oppression daily. Group work services for inner-city school children must be modified to deal with the long- and short-term effects of life within this context. There is little in the literature on this topic (see Brown, 1984; Davis, 1984; Delgado & Humm-Delgado, 1984; Gitterman, 1971; and Markward, 1979).

THE BRACETTI COLLABORATIVE

The Mariana Bracetti Middle School (pseudonym) is located in Boston and serves a population of 700 adolescents in grades six through eight. The students, aged 11 to 16, come from many cultural backgrounds. Fifty-five percent are Latino (predominantly Puerto Rican), forty percent are Black (primarily Afro-American with a sizeable Caribbean minority), and the rest are a mix of mostly White (Irish and Greek) and some Asian. The vast majority of students come from inner-city, low income families.

The Bracetti Human Services Collaborative is staffed by social workers from two agencies within walking distance of the school. The four full-time Black, Latino, and White clinicians have office and counseling space in the school. Additional help is provided by staff from the local mental health center, a Latino social service agency and neighborhood health center, and a nearby university and college.

The primary goal of the Bracetti Collaborative is to address those problems faced by students that arise from a variety of psychosocial causes at the earliest possible point of intervention. The social services offered are thereby preventive in nature. They seek to avert the cycle of low achievement, low skills attainment, and concomitant problems such as early school dropout, poor survival skills, teenage pregnancy, and unemployment.

Individual, family, and group counseling services are provided in the school (or at the agencies after school hours). In addition, the Collaborative offers in-school crisis intervention and consultation for school personnel. The latter is especially important, as the Collaborative's philosophy falls along the interactionist lines of Schwartz (1977) and Vinter and Sarri (1965).

THE BRACETTI COLLABORATIVE GROUP WORK PROGRAM

Goals and Limits

The Collaborative's introductory letter states that the goals of group counseling are to help students develop decision-making skills, combat social isolation, clarify values, and promote constructive group behavior. Given these goals, the question arises as to which students should be referred to and served by a Collaborative group.

This is the issue of boundary setting, which permeates all aspects of any school-based program. The worker in the school is constantly faced with setting limits on how much she or he can do and who can be seen. The dilemma is that for credibility a new program must meet the immediate needs of the school (such as crisis intervention and resolution of behavior problems), otherwise it won't be seen as helpful. Thus, the fine art of when and how to say "No," which is essential in working with adolescents, begins to be cultivated in working with school personnel.

Referrals and Recruitment

Students are referred to the Collaborative in different ways. Presenting problems range from low academic achievement and disruptive behavior to child abuse and suicidality. After receiving a referral, the Collaborative staff decides whether individual counseling, group work, or another form of intervention (e.g., family therapy, advocacy, information and referral to another service) is most appropriate.

Teachers and school staff refer to a large number of students throughout the year. The Collaborative's relationship with teachers is critical to its success. They are an important resource for understanding what's going on with students.

Another source of referrals is parents. A parent referral is frequently received after the parent has been called to school to discuss such problems as poor grades, a special education evaluation, or a disciplinary infraction. At these meetings school staff usually describe the Collaborative services and direct interested parents to the Collaborative offices for an intake.

The most fruitful source of group referrals is the students themselves. In the beginning of the school year the Collaborative staff goes to each homeroom and describes the services the Collaborative offers. It is here that the students often first hear about the Collaborative and its group program. A form is passed out after the presentation, and students can check off services they desire and choose from a list of during- and after-school groups those that they are most interested in attending (see McCullagh, 1982, for a similar system). The list includes: activity groups and discussion groups; groups on "serious" topics and "fun" groups; and boys', girls' and co-ed groups. The variety (described in full below) piques the students' interest and helps debunk the stereotype of counseling and therapy as being only for kids who are crazy or bad. The wide range of groups also answers the frequent teacher objection that outside agencies only serve "the bad kids" and ignore "the good kids." This method of group recruitment is so successful that the Collaborative's problem has been too many, rather than too few candidates.

Composition

Once referrals from the various sources have been collected the Collaborative's group work coordinator faces the lengthy task of cataloguing their choices. Each of the hundreds of students who return forms usually checks off between three and six groups of the fifteen offered. What results is a pool of students — anywhere from 20 to 160 — for each group. The students are identified by grade, age, sex, race, and primary language (Spanish or English).

There are a few criteria by which priorities are established for the subsequent interviewing of students. Students referred by teachers, school staff, or parents are matched with the group pools and flagged if they appear. Students who select only one or two groups are also noted, and students who self-refer for a specific group are prioritized as well.

Screening for group members is done through individual interviews and consultation with referral sources. Students are told that they are being interviewed because they have expressed interest in a particular group. The student remembers filling out the form, and this introduction serves the purpose of relieving any anxiety a student might feel about being removed from class to talk with an adult she or he does not know. A Collaborative staff member describes the group to the student and asks whether she or he is still interested in it. A number of students opt out of the process at this stage, but most choose to continue. Questions to the student cover previous group experience, academic progress and problems, school absenteeism, areas of perceived success and strengths, self-image, in-school and extracurricular social activities and interests, family composition, ethnic and cultural background, and degree of comfort with students from different backgrounds. The student is then given time to ask any questions about the group, the interviewer, or the Collaborative. The interview concludes with the student being told that she or he will be notified within two weeks of acceptance into the group or placement on a waiting list.

Selection of group members is based on historical and clinical information gleaned from the interview and on the list of priorities. The group work coordinator tries to balance membership with regard to race or ethnicity, age, and, for co-ed groups, gender. An assessment is also made of each student's readiness for the group, based on past group experience, family situation, and school adjustment.

Students selected for a group are required to return signed parental permission slips within a week. If the group is held during school time, students also have to return forms signed by their teachers, which allow them to miss class once a week with the stipulation that they make up any work missed. This pre-group contracting prepares the student for the formal contracting that will occur at the beginning of their group.

Confidentiality

Students are assured from the initial interview through the life of their group, that what is told to Collaborative staff stays within the Collaborative. They are also told the exceptions to this rule: statements about hurting oneself or someone else; being hurt by someone else (e.g., abused by a family member); or carrying drugs or weapons. The various reporting mechanisms are then described to the students.

Although students appreciate the confidentiality of the groups, it does create some problems with teachers and parents, who often seek information in the interest of better understanding or helping the students. The staff's job is then to explain the purpose of and need for confidentiality and to suggest other ways of helping the students. Some information, conveyed in a general way, which points to specific problem areas, is usually greatly appreciated by teachers.

Types of Groups

The Collaborative groups fall into four categories: support, theme, education, and responsibility. The common caveat that real life group work seldom is so cut and dried applies here also.

Support

As its name implies, this is "your basic support group." It is described to students as a girls' (or boys') group led by a woman (man) where members can "talk about things girls (boys) want to talk about." Structured activities and specific issues predominate in the early meetings, and the goal throughout is to develop social skills. Although the students have contracted for a process-oriented group, their need for structure, containment, and limit setting requires an initial emphasis on a more didactic approach. As the group creates its own structure and trust builds, members can venture into the process realm with less guidance from the leader. One group, for example, initially used an "Ask Beth" column from a local newspaper to come up with their own answers for other teenagers' problems; in later sessions they were able to talk about their own problems. Another group was given stimulus sentences and stories (e.g., "The best thing about being a boy is . . .") to generate discussions.

The role of the leader in the support group is more active than it would be in a similar group for adults. The leader uses techniques such as restating, giving instructions, refocusing, making parallels, modeling, giving opinions when appropriate, and emphasizing the strengths of the members to help them adapt to the group process. Younger adolescents require structured activities throughout the life of the group, while older adolescents are better able to leave the activities behind as they become used to the process format.

The support group is the closest the Collaborative gets to a therapy group. It is similar to Slavson's (1960) group guidance and Mahler's (1969) group counseling models. The group context (in-school, 42 minute period, limited number of sessions), together with the adolescent's aversion to the "therapy" or "mental health" label, mitigates against anything deeper. Nevertheless, a remarkable amount of sharing occurs in these groups. The shift from general discussion to intense personal sharing and back again is characteristic of these Collaborative groups.

Theme

The Collaborative's theme groups have included dance, karate, acting, newspaper, cosmetology, and arts and crafts groups. They are activity groups with a "hidden" agenda. The students have contracted for a group that is action-oriented, in contrast with the process-oriented support group. The group originates with the Collaborative, however, and not with, say, the art teacher or the physical education instructor. Since the Collaborative has the reputation of being a different kind of place in the school, with adults to whom one can talk about "different kinds of things," the students know that the group for which they are signing up is probably going to involve more than the description they were given. The Collaborative staff knows the students realize this, and the students know that the staff knows. What this all adds up to is that the students acquiesce to a "con job"; there is a tacit agreement that the group will entail more than just dancing or putting together a newspaper.

The reason that this can work is that it is not an "anything goes" atmosphere, but instead a careful balancing act on the part of the group leader to respect the overt contract while allowing the group members to explore process issues. Students are encouraged to share their thoughts about various topics, although they are not urged to talk about personal experiences. The use of the third person or the phrase "some people" is acceptable to them. The students enjoy the opportunity to become involved in a process-oriented discussion, but they depend on the clinical judgment of the leader in setting limits on how far that discussion will go.

Seven boys had contracted to publish a newspaper and had chosen the stories to be written. One boy wanted to write an article on "why parents beat up on each other." From this and other references, the boy made it clear to the group leader that his own parents were having physical fights. Over several weeks the worker involved the entire group in helping each member with the articles that she or he had chosen to write. When it was this boy's turn, the group spent the session discussing domestic violence, its causes, effects, prevalence, possible solutions, and so forth. The member in question participated and took notes for his article. The leader kept the discussion general, but accepted examples the boys offered, which were always in the third person.

It would not have been appropriate for the leader to press the group members on revealing their own experiences with domestic violence, nor even to approach the boy individually; none of the members had contracted for that. Yet it was clear from the discussion that the boy experienced some relief talking about the topic, and it is possible that he will grow to trust the leader enough to approach him on his own for help.

The theme group is a safe way for students to try out "talking about things" without having to join a group focused on talking. For instance, group members can tell curious outsiders that they belong to a cosmetology group in which they discuss "fashion." In the group sessions, discussion about fashion may include members' feelings about differences in skin color and its relationship to their perceptions of physical beauty and their own self-esteem. A manicure project can pair members who otherwise might not talk to each other (e.g., Black and Latino girls). Experience becomes the teacher, with the members listening to each other's thoughts and realizing the commonalities in their lives. Students who participate in a theme group one year are good candidates for a support group the next.

Education

Education groups are distinguished from the other Collaborative groups by a format that includes the use of a curriculum. Groups in this category have included career exploration, drug education, prevention of violence, and "Changing Bodies, Changing Selves." The students who join these groups are contracting for a group in which information will be conveyed. The curricula, however, give the members many opportunities to draw from their own experiences. Since the topics discussed are often powerful ones in the members' lives, exercises are used that give the members avenues for discussion in the second person. This can be done with the use of "true stories," an anonymous question box, or other methods.

The group leader's role for these groups is more didactic than in any of the other Collaborative groups. The leader presents a great deal of information and answers most questions directly. She or he may ask the whole group what it thinks about something or take a poll on an issue. Although sensitive to group dynamics and encouraging a healthy group process, the leader does less of a balancing act than in the theme groups and often has to set clear limits on the group's tendencies to overwhelm itself with personal sharing in the emotional areas covered.

> In one violence prevention group, the male and female co-leaders were halfway through a unit on child sexual abuse when one sixth-grade girl began to tell about an incident that happened to her when she was three, involving a man who exposed himself to her. The group members were silent after her story. The leaders handled the situation by calling the incident an example of one type of sexual abuse, generalizing the situation, thanking the girl for her contribution, and moving ahead with the lesson. The group responded well to this intervention but the leaders did not consider the incident closed. After the group meeting, they talked with the girl and offered her an opportunity to discuss her experience in individual counseling.

The foregoing example demonstrates the need for containment, safety, clear guidelines, and structure in the educational groups. The clinician must not succumb to the temptation to "get into it" with the members; they have not contracted for that. They have agreed, however, to discuss difficult issues. The leader can help them do this by creating a safe atmosphere and by helping them over the emotional hurdles (often expressed behaviorally) that crop up. Sensitivity to individual members who demonstrate needs the group cannot meet can result in private conversations and referral for counseling.

Responsibility

The Collaborative's responsibility groups are centered on fulfillment of a behavioral contract. For example, the Boston school system has a program in which students who are two or more years below the appropriate grade level for their age can move up a grade level halfway through the school year and then again at the end of the year, if they meet contract terms. These terms involve behavior, attendance, grades and volunteer work or participation in tutoring. The Collaborative works with students in the program by having them join same-sex and -grade groups. All members know why they are in the group, and they all have the same goal of fulfilling the contract and moving up to the next grade. (See Mintzies (1981) for a similar program.)

The leader's role in these groups is to help each member keep her or his part of the contract and to involve the group members in supporting each other to meet that common goal. Problem solving is frequently done at the first-person level. Members are called on to deal with one aspect of their lives — their schooling — in a very personal way. As a result, responsibility group members often reveal themselves and take risks to a greater extent than members in some of the other Collaborative groups. The task that each member shares with the others, and the group leader's drawing of parallels between them, creates a group atmosphere that allows and encourages members to draw on their own experiences in finding solutions to the problems of individual members. For example, members often have the same teacher for a subject. If a student is having particular difficulty with that teacher, the leader may call on the other members as resources through role play, brainstorming, supportive confrontation, and other techniques to aid the member in need. The creation of this mutual help network in the group raises the self-esteem of the members and builds group cohesion.

The leader also uses the group as a laboratory in which the members can exhibit and change the behavior that has been getting them into trouble in the school. Disruptive behavior is labeled as the kind of action that is keeping members from moving on in school; in other words, the ultimate responsibility for fulfilling the terms of the contract rests solely with the students.

> In one group, as the time limit for the contract was approaching, the leader asked the seven eighth-grade boys who were trying to get into high school how they were going to sabotage the good job that they had been doing. Each member quickly came up with behaviors ("swear at a teacher," "lose my temper and throw a chair," "not show up for school," etc.) that, if carried out, would keep them in eighth grade. The rest of the session was spent figuring out ways to prevent those behaviors.

For those students who do fulfill the first part of the contract and move up a grade halfway through the year, the responsibility group continues in an altered form. Although the main focus is still on completing the terms for the rest of the year, the nature, if not the content, of the group approaches that of support group. Members are told that they can talk about whatever topic they wish, as long as it is related to the primary goal of the group: finishing the contract successfully.

The responsibility group has had a significant impact on the Collaborative program in two ways. First, its creation has destigmatized the program and its staff. Students have seen their friends pull themselves together and graduate earlier than would have been possible without the program. The concrete, positive nature of the service has forced a reevaluation of counseling in the students' minds. No longer is it just a place to go for students who are crazy; it is something worth looking into. Many different mental health services have thereby been made more palatable by their inclusion in a context of groups that have met specific student needs.

Second, the responsibility group has led to the institution of an after-school drop-in center for students. Currently, the center is open only to members of the responsibility groups, who use it to continue their work on developing social skills and practicing the kinds of behavior that will keep them out of trouble in school. The Collaborative staff, however, is also using the center as a pilot program, with the goal of opening it up to all interested students. Most students at the school have no place to socialize after school except the street; the drop-in center is a positive alternative.

RACE, COLOR, AND ETHNICITY CONSIDERATIONS

A complete discussion of race, color, and ethnicity factors in Collaborative groups is beyond the scope of this paper. However, not to spend some time on these issues in a paper dealing with inner-city children would be a glaring omission. What follows is drawn from Collaborative workers' experiences. (A more extensive discussion of this topic, including class issues, can be found in Bilides, 1988.) Also relevant and helpful are Brown (1984), Davis (1984), Delgado and Humm-Delgado (1984), Delgado and Siff (1980), Hardy-Fanta (1982, 1986), and Markward (1979).

Race is always an issue in Collaborative groups. Sometimes it is overt and easy to spot, and sometimes it is submerged, requiring an alert and sensitive group leader to perceive its influence.

In general, differences in adolescent groups engender a struggle for commonality. In racially mixed groups, this struggle is more uncomfortable, and the tendency to form subgroups seems to increase remarkably.

Race is the primary determinant of roles taken by subgroups. These subgroup roles reflect sociocultural patterns and the power structure of the school. For example, in early Collaborative girls' groups, the Latina girls would disappear, figuratively or literally, and the groups would be controlled by the Afro-American girls. Over the next three years the school population changed so that the Latino children became the majority. When the Black children lost control of the school and the Latino students felt more empowered, tensions in all the Collaborative groups increased. White children have no power in the school and don't usually show up for groups unless they have a built-in support system; for example, an alliance with another White subgroup or with a White group leader.

Many groups become microcosms of larger social struggles and prejudices. Black children, resenting the erosion of their power in the school, often have a, "Move over, I haven't got mine yet," reaction to Latino children. Group power struggles become overlaid with race issues: "You Black bear"; "You stupid Puerto Rican girl"; "White people smell like fish." Skin color can enter in on a light-to-dark hierarchy: "Just 'cause you're light, you think you're so good." Ethnic groups acquire negative labels: Dominicans are "criminals," Colombians are "druggies," Cubans are "crazy," and any Black from the West Indian Islands is pejoratively labeled "Jamaican."

For Latino children, language is an important co-factor and its use is emotionally laden. Speaking Spanish often is not simply an avenue of communication. In English monolingual groups it can be a means of forming alliances with some members, excluding others, or protecting oneself. In an analogous way, speaking English can serve a special purpose. A Latino child who is culturally forbidden to be disrespectful or swear in Spanish may choose to do so in English only. On the other hand, a Spanish-speaking child may be uncharacteristically quiet in an English monolingual group because of a self-perceived or real inability to express her/himself in that language.

Group leaders have a difficult task when it comes to race, color, and ethnicity. First and foremost, they must have an awareness not just of racism and cultural issues in general but of how they themselves have been affected by those issues. This self-awareness is of primary importance in any intervention involving these factors. It also helps group leaders deal with both intra-member dynamics and member-leader interactions related to race, color, or ethnicity.

Sensitive and aware group leaders can be sounding posts for group members. The kids can bounce stereotypes and attitudes off leaders different from themselves. For their part, the leaders can share information and help members learn positive ways to deal with the outside world. At the same time, leaders need to prevent or interrupt and encourage exploration of group dynamics that duplicate the day-to-day oppression experienced by the children. The group then becomes a safe place where members can develop new ways of interacting and learning.

The Collaborative has run several groups with co-leaders of different races, color, or ethnicity, providing a good model of cooperation. Of course, if this approach is to be successful, the co-leaders must come to terms with their own differences and stereotypes, as well as the group members' identification of and reactions to those characteristics (see, e.g., Hardy-Fanta [1986]).

GUIDING PRINCIPLES

The experience gleaned by the Collaborative staff from the group work program has generated a list of guiding principles for its work with groups of adolescents in the middle schools. (For other guidelines see Brown, 1984; Davis, 1984; Delgado and Humm-Delgado, 1984; Delgado and Siff, 1980; Levine, 1978; and Ohlsen, 1971.) For the purposes of this paper it can be summarized as follows:

1. Adolescent groups should have a well-defined structure with clear limits. Adolescents in a group need room to bounce around (both behaviorally and verbally), but they also want to make sure that there are established boundaries; otherwise, the risk-taking is too scary;

2. Group leaders must acknowledge and use their power, not only as leaders but as adults. Adolescents want to know what other people think is right and wrong, acceptable and unacceptable. The group leader may be the only adult in the adolescents' lives who can supportively guide them through this maze, who can say "Yes," or "No," in a way they can hear;

3. An emphasis on normalcy is important for adolescent group work. Adolescents desperately want to be normal. They begin with the belief that the Collaborative (or clinic or mental health center) is for abnormal ("crazy," "mental") children. Therefore a group work program has to offer them concrete benefits. Children will buy into almost any kind of group if they think they are going to get something out of it and they can explain it to their peers; the trick is having a wide enough variety. The more a program can sponsor activities that are "normal," the better accepted it will be. Ultimately, the burden of proof is on the program, not the students;

4. The use of the third person and generalizing are important techniques for directing group discussions. In most cases, the leader should avoid zeroing in on what an individual is feeling and instead generalize: "Many people feel . . . ," "Lots of teenage boys . . . ," etc. The Collaborative

staff has found that most adolescents in groups prefer "I think" to "I feel." For adult groups this would be labeled "intellectualizing," but for many of the students in these groups it is the way they express their feelings. The leader needs to recognize that this is a step toward them owning their feelings, and it is important not to dismiss or rush this process. Children who acquire group experience are more likely to be able to tolerate directed discussion about emotions;

5. Group leaders should feel comfortable using themselves and their feelings and opinions in the group process. The leader is a model, simply by virtue of having survived adolescence. Leaders of adolescent groups are often called on to act in ways that run contrary to their training. A leader who is able, when appropriate, to enter a group discussion without joining the group on the students' level is valuable both to the individual members and the group as a whole;

6. Long-term groups (over 15 sessions) seem more useful than short-term groups (8 to 10 sessions). The Collaborative has gradually been extending the life span of its groups. The adolescents' suspicions about the group context, the amount of time they require to settle in and school-life interruptions, have made longer groups necessary. This means that fewer students are served in groups, but they get more out of them.

7. As long as behavior falls within the group's limits, it is important to respect it. It can be used as valuable information about the group's process. For example, there is probably a reason why a student chooses to sit underneath the table during an activity;

8. The use of food in adolescent groups is extremely powerful. The Collaborative uses food at some point in most of its groups, but the timing, frequency, and purpose of its inclusion is well thought out beforehand;

9. To survive these groups, adult leaders must have a clear sense of their own identity, support from their colleagues and their agencies, sufficient emergency backup, good supervision and a sense of humor.

CLOSING REMARKS

Although one frequently hears or reads that "group work is the modality of choice for adolescents," in practice few programs offer comprehensive group work services to teenagers. It is hard even to attract clinicians, let alone children to group programs. Working with adolescents calls for unconventional as well as conventional approaches, and many workers are uncomfortable with groups of teenagers. These problems are compounded when the work is to be done in the inner city. To be sure, adolescents are not the easiest population to work with. Few of them come up to you and say, "Thanks, that was a really great group, I got a lot out of it." One learns to receive nourishment from many small, often non-verbal rewards.

However, the Bracetti Collaborative's group work program demonstrates that one does not have to be a saint to do positive work with adolescents. By enlisting the support of the public school system, educating group leaders about racial, ethnic, and cultural issues, soliciting teenagers' input about what is important to them and providing them with a wide range of concrete and interesting groups, adolescents will come knocking at your door.

REFERENCES

Bilides, D., "Race, color, ethnicity, and class issues in school-based adolescent counseling groups." Unpublished manuscript, 1988.

Brown, J., "Group work with low-income Black youth," *Social Work with Groups*, Vol. 7, No. 3 (1984), pp. 111-124.

Davis, L., "Essential components of group work with Black Americans," *Social Work with Groups*, Vol. 7, No. 3 (Fall 1984), pp. 97-109.

Delgado, M., and Humm-Delgado, D., "Hispanics and group work: a review of the literature," *Social Work with Groups*, Vol. 7, No. 3 (1984), pp. 85-96.

Delgado, M., and Siff, S., "A Hispanic adolescent group in a public school setting: an interagency approach," *Social Work with Groups*, Vol. 3, No. 3 (1980), pp. 73-85.

Gitterman, A., "Group work in the public schools," in Schwartz, W., and Serapio, Z., eds. *The Practice of Group Work*, NY: Columbia University Press, 1971, pp. 45-72.

Hardy-Fanta, C., "Social action in Hispanic groups," *Social Work*, Vol. 31, No. 2 (March-April 1986), pp. 116-123.

Hardy-Fanta, C., and Montana, P., "The Hispanic female adolescent: a group therapy model," *International Journal of Group Psychotherapy*, Vol. 32, No. 3 (July 1982), pp. 351-366.

Levine, B., "Reflections of group psychotherapy with adolescents," *Social Work with Groups*, Vol. 1, No. 2 (1978), pp. 179-194.

Mahler, C., "A framework for group counseling," in Gazda, G., ed., *Theories and Methods of Group Counseling in the Schools*, Springfield, IL: Thomas, 1969, pp. 86-118.

Markward, M., "Group process and Black adolescent identity crisis," *School Social Work Journal*, Vol. 3, No. 2 (1979), pp. 78-84.

McCullagh, J., "Making social work an integral part of the school," *Practice Digest*, Vol. 5, No. 1 (1982), pp. 24-27.

Mintzies, P., "Agency works in schools with problem students," *Practice Digest*, Vol. 4, No. 2 (September 1981), pp. 18-21.

Ohlsen, M., "Counseling children in groups," in Hansen, J., comp., *Group*

Guidance and Counseling in the Schools, NY: Appleton, Century, Crofts, 1971, pp. 297-304.

Schwartz, W., "Social group work: the interactionist approach," in Turner, J., ed., *Encyclopedia of Social Work*, NY: National Association of Social Workers, 1977, pp. 1328-1338.

Slavson, S., "When is a "therapy group" not a therapy group?" *International Journal of Group Psychotherapy*, Vol. 10, No. 1 (January 1960), pp. 3-21.

Vinter, R. and Sarri, R., "Malperformance in the public schools: a group work approach," *Social Work*, Vol. 10, No. 1 (January 1965), pp. 3-13.

The Impact of a Generic Curriculum on the Practice of Graduates: Does Group Work Persist?

Ted Goldberg
Alice E. Lamont

This paper reports on the final phase of a four-year study of curriculum change. In this segment, we sought answers to the question: What happens to the graduate's interest and skill in group work when she/he has experienced an integrated M.S.W. curriculum? Are the outcomes different from those of earlier graduates who specialized in the methods curricula including group work? The decision to seek an answer to this question grew out of discussions of findings of earlier phases of this study presented at previous Symposia on Social Work with Groups, which indicated that having a group work sequence made a difference (Goldberg and Lamont, 1986). The crucial question, some argued was: What do they do after they graduate? We decided to attempt to answer that question, at least for one school and its graduates. In this paper, we summarize findings from the first three phases, discuss the manner in which the fourth phase study was conducted, present findings bearing on the research question and conclude with a discussion of the implications of these findings for educators and practitioners interested in social work with groups.

BACKGROUND

When the faculty of our School agreed to modify the curriculum to feature a generic first year and second year methods tracks in micro or macro practice, the authors decided to monitor the consequences of the change. A five-page, self-administered questionnaire was developed to gather demographic data and information about pre-school and school ex-

Ted Goldberg, EdD, and Alice E. Lamont, PhD, are affiliated with Wayne State University, School of Social Work, Detroit, MI 48202.

periences, perceived skill levels and practice interests. Measures of familiarity with the practice literature were also developed and administered in the classroom courses. The basic data were gathered in each of three phases and participation rates were excellent (over 75%). Respondents were statistically equivalent to the populations studied.

In phase one (1982-83), baseline data were gathered. Students enrolled in the "old"[1] sequence curricula provided data. Essential findings were that group work standards were in place (Goldberg and Lamont, 1986). Group work students were found to be more interested in that modality, were more likely to be practicing it in field work courses, perceived their skill levels as greater and were much more familiar with the group work practice literature than were students specializing in other methods. To be noted is the fact that in this and subsequent phases there was no indication that demographic or other pre-school variables accounted for these differences.

Phases two and three (1983-85) were designed to discover what happened with the introduction of the new curriculum. Findings in these phases reflected a mixture of stability and change. The proportion of students interested in group work did not shift. Nor was there evidence that the amount of practice with groups in the field was significantly different from the baseline year. There was less familiarity with the practice literature in group work ($X^2 = 15.82$, 2 df, $p < .001$), a clear outgrowth of the revised practice courses. There were also trends for the new students to perceive their skill in practice with treatment group as less than that of the old students ($X^2 = 5.7$, 2 df, $p < .10$). Perhaps the major finding was the absence of, or limited amount of change.[2] With respect to the consistency in student interests the authors concluded that a combination of successive years of students who came to this school with comparable career goals and who were taught by class and field faculty who remained relatively constant, appeared to be sufficient to result in practice interests which were the same for new and old students.

METHODOLOGY

The final phase of our study (1985-86), a follow-up of graduates of the new curriculum, began with a review of research reports of follow-up surveys of M.S.W. graduates of this School in earlier years (Auch et al., 1982; Bamberger et al., 1981; Butler et al., 1983; and Johns et al., 1978). The intent was to use these studies to compare the graduates of the integrated curriculum with those from former years. There were some variables reported in each of the prior studies bearing on the focus of this research and they were used for comparison.

A questionnaire was developed for graduates of the new curriculum. It sought information about employment, the nature of their current practice tasks, the kinds of work they most preferred to do, perceptions of their skill levels, and the adequacy of their preparation as well as demographic variables, pre-school and school experiences. We also asked respondents if they would provide the name of a supervisor who knew their work and could be asked to respond to a questionnaire about the new curriculum. The questionnaire was sent to all of the graduates of the new curriculum (May, 1985) and response rates were again quite good — 106 of 147 graduates (73%) returned questionnaires as did 57 of the 75 supervisors (76%) who were identified. Data were analyzed by contrasting the class of 1985 with earlier groups of graduates.

The data from the earlier studies had been collected over a period of ten years from three samples using different instruments. The wording of the questionnaires for some items was very similar to the 1985 instrument. Others varied and in those instances, the wording utilized is given for each sample year so that the reader may compare them. Whenever one of the four studies of the sequence graduates is not referred to when contrasting old and new students, the reader can assume that data were not available from that study concerning a particular variable.

FINDINGS

In this section we present major findings bearing on the research question: Does group work persist? We begin by contrasting the sample group, followed by data on school experiences and post-graduate experiences. The paper concludes with a discussion of the implications of these findings.

Sample Characteristics

Demographically, we found the several samples to be equivalent in most respects: male-female ratios, racial distributions and prior work experience levels. New students were somewhat older, a mean age of 37 in 1985 as opposed to 33 in the earlier studies. The fact that the recent graduates were somewhat older did not lead to a difference in prior work experience levels.

School Experiences

A major question in the implementation of any new curriculum is how it alters the learning experiences of students exposed to it. We knew from our three-year study of students in the old sequence curriculum (82' to '84) and those in the new integrated curriculum ('83 to 85) that classroom content had been altered significantly, leading to a drop in familiarity with group work literature. We also learned in the earlier phases that quantitative levels of experience with groups in the practicum had remained about the same. Now, as we compared the graduates of the integrated program, the class of '85 with the graduates of six to ten years earlier, we were interested in a further test of whether the practicum content had been altered.

Did graduates of the new curriculum have the same opportunities to practice with groups in their field work courses as earlier graduates of the sequence curricula? Table 1 presents findings bearing on this question and other outcomes of this research. It is widely believed that skill and interest in a modality are highly influenced by the availability of "hands on" experiences. Comparative data were available on the field experiences of 1975-76 (Johns et al., 1978) and 1978-79 (Bamberger et al., 1981) sequence graduates. When a comparison was made in the amount of field experience practicing with groups reported by graduates of the old sequence programs and graduates of the new integrated program, a difference emerged between old and new students. As Table 1 illustrates *graduates of earlier years were more likely to say they practiced with groups in*

TABLE 1

IMPACT OF "OLD" AND "NEW" CURRICULA ON GROUP WORK
AS REPORTED BY GRADUATES

Variables	Old	Graduates New
In-school experiences with groups.	More[a]	Less
Work with groups on first jobs.	More[b]	Less
Interest in practice with groups.	Same	Same
Perception of skill/preparation for work with groups compared to classmates.	Same	Same

[a] $p < .02$

[b] $p < .10$

field work "Very Often" (44% vs. 27%) and less likely to say that they had little to no experience with this modality (31% vs. 47%). The differences are statistically significant ($X^2 = 10.46$, 2 df, $p < .02$). We cannot be certain that this "drop" represents a reliable indicator of change in exposure to group work in field courses because of differences in the way the question was asked.[3] It is very likely that at least some of the difference in exposure to groups was an artifact of the way the questions were worded. However, our conclusion is that there was a drop in exposure to practice with groups in the field with the introduction of the new curriculum.

Interests

From the outset of this research, the authors sought to identify respondent interests as an important outcome of any curriculum. Which tasks were they interested in performing/seeking to do in their jobs? We believed that this dimension could be an indicator of the consequences of curriculum change. Data were available on 1982 graduates (Butler et al., 1983) who were compared with graduates of the new curriculum.[4] As Table 1 indicates *no differences in interest in practicing with groups were found between the two samples*. Twenty-four percent of the old graduates listed group work as a task they sought to perform and 21% of the new graduates listed group work as most interesting. This replicates previous findings regarding student interests (Goldberg and Lamont, 1985) that the shift to an integrated practice curriculum does not necessarily lead to a loss of interest in group work.

Perceived Skill Levels

A second variable thought to be susceptible to a longitudinal effect was the perceived skill levels of graduates. How skilled did they think they were in performing the several social work tasks? Would there be differences in outcomes between graduates exposed to differing curricula? In this case, comparative data were found in Johns et al. (1978) for 1975-76 graduates.[5] *There were no significant differences in the responses of the two groups in appraising their skill with groups.* To be noted in connection with these judgments is the fact that respondents were comparing themselves with different student populations, i.e., '75 with '75 graduates and '85 with '85 graduates and it is not known whether these self-ratings reflect similar levels of actual skill. We will discuss this issue in the concluding section of the paper.

Initial Work Assignments

Comparative data were available from the prior research on the initial work tasks assigned to graduates in 1982 (Butler et al., 1983) and in 1978 and 1979 (Bamberger et al., 1981).[6] As Table 1 shows a *trend towards a statistically significant difference was identified in comparing their work with groups*. The new graduates were more likely to report "Hardly at all/None" (42% vs. 31%) and old graduates were more likely to report "More" (69% vs. 58%) initial assignments in practice with groups ($X^2 = 3.20$, 1 df, $p < .10$)

The findings reported in Table 1 suggest that group work does indeed persist in the *interests* of students/graduates and in their *perceptions of skill* with the method in spite of changes in curriculum. It declines in the amount of experience in the field while in school and in the amount of practice with groups upon graduation. The next section summarizes findings for the entire longitudinal study and discusses implications for the future.

SUMMARY

This study was an effort to measure empirically what happens to group work when it is no longer taught in specialized method sequences so typical a few years ago. The authors have been collecting data on student responses to the curricula before and during the modifications and then followed the first group of graduates in their initial job experiences. These respondents to the new curriculum were contrasted with students from earlier years who had specialized in method sequence curricula. As noted, the follow-up studies of earlier graduates were not originally designed for such a comparison. Items were selected which seemed reasonably comparable and relevant to the question guiding this research: Would group work persist? This made for variation in the number of old graduates who could be compared with the new. For some items, all four samples of graduates of the old curricula could be used, for others only one. Even with the limitations posed by this variation and the differences in wording of some of the questions reported above, the comparison seems useful. There is so little evidence of empirical monitoring of curricular effects (Goldberg and Lamont, 1984) a comparison, even with the limitations described here, adds to our knowledge.

Analysis of these data leaves two clear impressions. First, there were differences in their school experiences (See Table 1). Graduates of specialized sequence curricula report more exposure to groups in field work courses than graduates of the new, integrated curriculum.[7] The second indication of program effect is that graduates of the old, specialized programs were more likely to work with groups in their first jobs than were graduates of the new, integrated program. As Table 1 shows, the evidence in this case ($p < .10$) represents a trend towards statistical significance.

In the somewhat more subjective categories, interest in work with groups and perceived levels of skill with that modality, the responses of graduates of the two programs were very similar. With respect to perceptions of skill, it is useful to point out that respondents were asked to compare themselves with *their* classmates. The proportions who saw themselves as more/less skilled were similar. Yet the evidence suggests that the class of '85 may be less skilled. One might expect old graduates who had more experience with groups in school and on their jobs to possess more actual skill. However, the respondents had no way of comparing themselves with other classes. The authors can compare the self-perceptions of skill level in the samples, but cannot make a direct comparison of their actual competence in work with groups. Data from the supervisors of new graduates support comparability in this area. Eighty-seven percent of the supervisors ($N = 47$) rated the preparation of these new graduates for group work practice as at least equal to the preparation of those who had been educated in the earlier sequence programs. Unfortunately, there are no comparable findings from supervisors of graduates of these earlier years.

The cumulative findings of this research project can be summarized in the following statements:

1. Graduates of the old sequence programs report more experience with groups in field work courses.
2. Graduates of the old sequence curricula are more familiar with group work practice literature.
3. Graduates of the old sequence curricula are more likely to be practicing with groups in their first jobs.
4. Altering school programs does not seem to change what graduates *want* to do (their interests) or perceptions of their skill levels (how well they think they perform the tasks in relation to other recent graduates).

We turn next to a discussion of the implications of these findings. What is called for from practitioners and educators knowledgeable about and interested in social work with groups?

IMPLICATIONS

Evidence from our study indicates that even though interest in group work remains constant, we are educating social workers who know less about group work literature, have less experience with groups in school and are less likely to use this modality in practice. And, as Middleman and Goldberg (1987) noted, this was in a school with a long and rich tradition of group work. Tropp (1978) described similar national trends in his article in the first issue of Social Work with Groups. More recently, Lewis (1985) found the scarcity of group work in both B.S.W. and M.S.W. curricula to be widespread. She concluded that ". . . many, if not most, students may graduate without any experience in group leadership, or with very minimal contact with groups" (p. 11). From such evidence our presumption is that the consequences of curriculum change identified in this research are not unlike those in other regions of the country. In the sequence structured programs, we educated *some* social workers who were prepared to practice with groups and who could eventually serve as teachers for other practitioners. Although fewer social workers are being educated to practice with groups now, the current literature identifies many needs for social workers skilled in intervention with both therapeutic and task groups (Jones, 1985; Lewis, 1985; Papell, 1982). A recent survey of field instructors at Boston University indicated that nearly all had practiced with groups since graduation, but only small proportions had formal educational preparation for their practice (Jones, 1985, p. 1). The gap between educational preparation for practice with groups and the need for competence in that area has been identified and seems likely to grow.

Given the decline in educational content about groups in both class and field, and the likely consequences for graduates, what actions should be considered? Proposals in Symposium papers in the last few years cover a broad range: redefining the M.S.W. curriculum to specify practice with non-related groups as one of five basic curricular areas (Glasser, 1985); requiring an introductory course in group work of all students and at least one field experience with a group and educating field instructors in group work (Jones, 1985); reemphasizing the importance of community social work and using the teaching of group work as a means of integrating the professions' individual and social purposes (Lewis, 1985) and offering a specialization in group work together with concentrations in fields of practice (Kurland and Salmon, 1986).

The authors believe that the shift to generalist curricula has made a contribution to social work education.[8] What follows represents a proposal for strengthening the teaching of group work within that framework. Based on our findings and impressions of the feasibility of curriculum reform we see two productive alternatives. The first addresses the generalist framework now in place. It is the hypothesis of the authors that knowledge and skill in social group work can be increased in a generic curriculum by: (1) strengthening basic content on group work in the foundation year; (2) requiring a field experience in group work in at least one year of the practicum, (in programs where such a goal is unreachable, the use of laboratory experiences represents a less desirable alternative); (3) offering elective courses in social group work in the advanced year; and (4) offering additional field and/or laboratory experiences in the advanced year which support the development of competence in group work practice. In addition to the above recommendations, we believe that the planning processes in a generic program can be modified to enhance the fit between student interest in preparing for group work practice and program opportunities which make that possible. Illustratively, field placement planning can attempt to assure that students with interest in group work are placed in settings which provide both opportunities to practice and competent field instruction. That has not always been true since the introduction of the new curriculum. This is but one illustration of how a school can strive to teach group work more effectively as a part of a generalist curriculum.

The challenge to ourselves and our colleagues is to test this hypothesis about teaching group work content in a generalist frame and to report the outcomes. We are currently in the process of attempting to use these findings to support our school's ongoing efforts to improve the effectiveness of the revised curriculum.

A second direction involves considering comprehensive alternatives to the generic curricula in place in most schools of social work. Kurland and Salmon (1986) describe a curriculum in which method sequences are retained and integrated with specializations. Glasser (1985) has proposed that the curriculum include ". . . five basic methods: (1) work with individuals; (2) work with non-related members in groups, including task groups; (3) work with couples and families; (4) community planning; (5) administration." We believe this proposal has merit for strengthening the total curriculum. Both of these options (described in very brief form here) clearly strengthen group work teaching while providing a strong framework for a broad social work education. However, curriculum revision must take into account local circumstances and histories. Not all good ideas are good for all times and places. That is why we have outlined two different approaches both of which we believe offer direction for curriculum improvement in most schools of social work.

All the proposals we have reviewed agree that in the real world of practice, work with groups is expanding. Consequently there is a pressing need to educate students, practitioners and field instructors for practice with groups. As we proceed with this task it is important that we concentrate not on the theme of the loss of group work, but rather on the importance of group work in the education and practice of social workers to better meet client needs.

We close looking forward to reports of revised curricula designed to meet this challenge. We are particularly hopeful that such reports will include empirical data on efforts to evaluate the effectiveness of these programs.

REFERENCE NOTES

1. In this paper "old" refers to students in the old method sequence programs, "new" refers to the students in the integrated practice courses.

2. A fuller discussion of these findings and their implications can be found in Goldberg and Lamont, 1985.

3. The modality was called "direct services in group contexts" in Johns et al., "direct services with groups" in Bamberger et al., and "direct services with groups (clinical)" for the 1985 graduates. In addition, five values were utilized in the most recent survey in contrast with three in two earlier studies. Values were combined in order to make the comparison.

4. Phrasing for 1982 was "Which tasks did you seek to perform on your job?" Graduates of the new curriculum in 1985 were asked: "Which social work tasks do you find most interesting [which may or may not be related to your current assignments]? The phrases describing group work were comparable for the two samples.

5. The '75-'76 graduates were asked: "As you think of your own practice, how would you rate yourself in "direct services in group contexts." Recent graduates were asked: "Comparing yourself with other recent graduates, how well prepared were you to undertake the [following] tasks?" The group modality was listed as "direct services with groups (Clinical)."

6. In 1985, graduates were asked: "To what extent do you perform the following task in your work?" with five response categories listed. "To what extent do you perform the following tasks in your *present* job?" was the question asked in 1982. The question asked of the 1978, 1979 graduates was identical except that "responsibility" replaced "tasks." The latter two studies used three categories and data were combined as described in Note #3.

7. As noted above, data from earlier phases of this research also identified a

significant drop in familiarity with the group work literature. See Goldberg and Lamont, 1986.

8. In the discussion following his paper at the 1979 Symposium, Gitterman (1981) stated his belief that students were being trained to be better *social* workers, although there was clearly a loss in the area of group work. Our experience supports this view.

REFERENCES

Auch, Jean et al. *Further Explorations of the Job Market Experiences of 1978 and 1979 MSW Graduates.* Unpublished Master's Research Report (Detroit, Michigan: Wayne State University), 1982.

Bamberger, Jane et al. *From Graduate School to the Job Market: A Follow-Up Study of 1978 and 1979 MSW Graduates.* Unpublished Master's Research Report (Detroit, Michigan: Wayne State University), 1981.

Butler, Jim et al. *Searching for Jobs: The Experiences of 1982 MSW Graduates.* Unpublished Master's Research Report (Detroit, Michigan: Wayne State University), 1983.

Gitterman, Alex. "Group Work Content in an Integrated Methods Curriculum." In Sonia Leib Abels and Paul Abels (eds.), *Social Work with Groups — Proceedings 1979 Symposium,* 1981, pp. 66-81.

Glasser, Paul H. "The Future of Social Group Work in the Social Work Curriculum." Unpublished paper presented at the Seventh Annual Symposium on Social Work with Groups, New Brunswick, New Jersey, 1985.

Goldberg, Ted and Alice Lamont. "Do Group Work Standards Work? Results from an Empirical Exploration," *Social Work with Groups,* 9(3), 1986, pp. 89-109.

Goldberg, Theodore and Alice Lamont. "Effects of New Integrated Methods Courses on Interest, Knowledge and Skill in Social Group Work: A Three-Year Study." Unpublished paper presented at the Seventh Annual Symposium on Social Work with Groups, New Brunswick, New Jersey, 1985.

Goldberg, Theodore and Alice Lamont. "Searching for Empirical Guidelines for Curriculum Change." Unpublished paper presented at the Annual Program Meeting, Council of Social Work Education, Detroit, Michigan, 1984.

Johns, Carol et al. "Wayne State University Master of Social Work Graduates: Work and Educational Experiences." Unpublished Master's Research Report (Detroit, Michigan: Wayne State University), 1978.

Jones, Hubert. "The Future of Groupwork in the Social Work Curriculum." Unpublished paper presented at the Seventh Annual Symposium on Social Work with Groups, New Brunswick, New Jersey, 1985.

Kurland, Roselle and Robert Salmon. "Concentrations and Methods: Combining Core Content and Specialized Expertise in the Teaching of Group Work."

Unpublished paper presented at the Eighth Annual Symposium on Social Work with Groups. Los Angeles, California, 1986.

Lewis, Elizabeth. "Social Group Work: A Central Component of Social Work Education and Practice." Unpublished paper presented at the Seventh Annual Symposium on Social Work with Groups. New Brunswick, New Jersey, 1985.

Middleman, Ruth R. and Gale Goldberg. "Social Work Practice with Groups." In Anne Minihan (Ed.-in-Chief), *Encyclopedia of Social Work*, 18, Vol. 2. Silver Springs, Maryland: National Association of Social Workers, 1987: 714-729.

Papell, Catherine. "Group Work in the Profession of Social Work: Identity in Context." Unpublished paper presented at the Fourth Annual Symposium on Social Work with Groups. Toronto, Canada, 1982.

Tropp, Emanuel. "Whatever Happened to Group Work?" *Social Work with Groups*, 1978, 1, 85-94.

Retrospective on Reaching Out: Boston's Late Department of Neighborhood Clubs

Ralph Kolodny

The paper which follows disregards an important canon of professional behavior which, for fifty years and more, has dictated that conference speakers avoid sentimentality. Our experiences as social workers are to be shared with colleagues in a crisp, not to say, military manner, that is, they are to be presented as "facts." Whatever their arrangement and usage, when cited, they are to have the ring of medical certainty. And they are never to sound self-serving.

I shall introduce my comments, however, by being unabashedly sentimental, dedicating them to one particular group of worried youngsters whose childhood was too often filled with adult-sized demands. Furthermore, I shall compound that sin by telling a self-serving story of an exchange with one of them, when, at his request, we met for lunch some fifteen years after the group had terminated.

Let me, therefore, begin by remembering now, with affection, Jack, Biff, Ev, Bud, Ducky and Floyd, whose behavior twenty-five years ago I often witnessed with consternation, and whose actual names the professional habits of a lifetime compel me to disguise, even at this distance in time. As a group worker at the Department of Neighborhood Clubs of the Boston Children's Service Association, at the behest of caseworkers in the school system of a nearby industrial town, I worked with this group of emotionally overburdened, and, in large part, economically deprived boys who were failing academically and/or socially in school. Like my colleague, Louise Frey of Boston University, who worked with a similar group of girls from the same system in a parallel effort, I continued with

Ralph Kolodny is Professor Emeritus, Boston University School of Social Work and Consultant, Department of Social Work, Ben Gurion University, Beer Sheva, Israel.

the group for most of three years. Out to the school basement room I came every week with my crafts and my table games and my plans for trips, sustaining a line of "normality' in the midst of nine- and ten- and twelve-year-old lives rent by destructive parental behavior, ranging from the inappropriately infantile to the psychotically punitive and suicidal. I played with group members. I listened to them. I visited their families and their teachers. I became a fixture with them in the bowling alleys and pizza shops of the town. I had little if any ascribed status. I was not a doctor. I went to them where they lived and studied. I said things to them and to their parents and teachers that sometimes sounded downright crazy. Certainly, what I did must have seemed strange. Their lives erupted with violent events, including homosexual rape attempts. I, meanwhile, went about the prosaic task of helping them to invest themselves in becoming a club. I did this in what, undoubtedly, then and today, would seem to some, the vain hope of providing them with a way of assimilating these events without themselves violently or otherwise retreating from life. Then, when I thought I had done all that reasonably could be done, I spent as much time as I could in trying to give them a decent experience in leave-taking and I left.

Fourteen years later, now a teacher of group work, I received a call at my office from Jack. Like all of our former group members, he knew he had access to the staff of my old agency and, through them, to me. He asked if I would come to lunch with him in a nearby town, which I did. Now a devoted, though divorced, father, he had finished the high school technical course with highest honors and had even taken a couple of courses at the local community college. He was considering a job change and wanted to know what I thought. The people at the new job offered many inducements, but Jack did not trust them. I suggested that you could not believe anyone completely. Jack looked up from his dessert and said, simply, "I believe you."

I must say that an experience like this, for me, in and of itself, constitutes sufficient justification for the reach-out approach of the Department of Neighborhood Clubs of Boston's Children's Service Association, which, for thirty-five years, sent its group workers into virtually every neighborhood of Greater Boston in response to the emotional needs of particular neighborhood children. A substantial statistical underpinning may be required by researchers and educators seeking evidence of the efficacy of a particular approach. For the practitioner, immersed in the work itself, however, it is his or her impressions of the potential of the approach, as revealed at moments of its optimum impact on one or more group members, that persuade him or her of its worth. Jack's assertion of trust was one such moment.

The Department of Neighborhood Clubs no longer exists. A casualty of agency administrative changes in the late 1960s, it was seen to be too traditional and "incremental" in its approach by the new administrators. These felt, in line with the spirit of the times, that more sweeping and radical approaches to the problems of troubled youngsters, clinically, as well as in terms of social policy, were demanded. Creative ideas die hard, however, and today, some twenty years later, under enlightened leadership, the Boston Children's Service Association is exploring the possibility of reintroducing social group work along the lines of its venerable Department of Neighborhood Clubs.

What was the Department and what was its approach? The social-psychological target which the Department was designed to attack was social isolation. Its paramount aim was to substantially reduce the social isolation of those emotionally disturbed and severely physically handicapped children who were referred to it for help. It was not clear then, and it is not always clear now, whether, in a particular instance, the social isolation such a child suffers is mainly a result of fearful or hostile avoidance of him by his age peers, or whether it comes about largely because of his own tendency to reject overtures by others toward him. It was clear then, however, and it is clear now that whatever the source of the isolation — rejecting others or being rejected by them — the social isolation of the disturbed or handicapped child, itself, is a psychologically noxious element of profound significance. Rolling it back even if only to reduce the secondary effects of the child's central emotional or medical problem, the social withdrawal and avoidance that accompanies being "sick" in any form, is a task worthy of intense effort. Beyond this, there has always been the hope, viewed by some as a distinct possibility, that once social withdrawal is reversed, important psychological changes will follow. The child may then escape from those circular behavioral patterns in which he is regularly the subject of a self-fulfilling prophecy of social alienation or the object of social attack. The troubled child's escape from what Lawrence Frank, many years ago, called "the hell of alienating people from whom we want acceptance creates the possibility that he will gradually come to behave with less generalized fear and hostility.[1] The more positive experiences in his life following this change in behavior should help him to develop a more rational and balanced appraisal of self and others.

The Department of Neighborhood Clubs sought to achieve this reduction in social isolation by forming social club groups in or close to the neighborhoods of the boys and girls referred to it for group work help. The referred child was to be helped to overcome his inability to become part of the society of those who would otherwise have been his friends and acquaintances, not by being taken out of his neighborhood for treatment with other children in a centralized community mental health or medical facility, but, directly, by having an experience with neighborhood peers, themselves. It was expected that, during the course of this experience, he would engage in all manner of interaction, exhibiting both those of his behaviors that alienated others and whatever social skills he possessed. His clubmates, who would be accessible to him for long periods outside of meetings because of the neighborhood context, would themselves react to his behavior, as well as to each other, with all the warmth and aggression that characterizes childhood interaction. Social learning and emotional growth would take place through emotional testing, the binding and channeling of anxiety, social insight-giving and, above all, through the provision of opportunities for identification with socially positive behavioral models. All of the members would benefit from the interaction. For the isolated child around whom the group was formed, however, its importance could hardly be overstated. For many such isolated children it could represent a last chance, before the turmoil of adolescence intervened, to achieve a degree of emotional stability and capacity for friendship. The Department group worker, by whatever means psychological and sociological understanding, compassion and ingenuity could devise, was to see to it that this chance not be lost.

Two group modes or types were employed by the Department in pursuing its overall goal. One, its more characteristic mode, involved the formation of a small club group whose membership was composed of a socially isolated child referred for group treatment from a particular neighborhood and several other, presumably normal, youngsters from the same neighborhood, whom the Department purposely recruited as members. The other type, called the "all referred" group, was composed entirely of children having relational difficulties. Frequently, all of the members of such an "all referred" group came from the same grade school, where school caseworkers had been treating them, individually. The all-referred type of group represented a departure from the Department's major mode of group formation. Even here, however, an attempt was made to incorporate more positive models for identification among the membership. This was accomplished by including a somewhat less troubled majority of members with a more troubled minority. Also, the neighborhood, its institutions and people, were still used as a major resource in the second type of group.

The practice, which was unique to the Department, that of organizing a group of ordinary neighborhood children around a disturbed child or one with a serious physical problem, must raise a host of questions now, as it did then. In one form or another, most of these questions were addressed in the published writings of Neighborhood Clubs' staff.[2] Several are worth mentioning in the present context: Are the normal children being emotionally exploited for the benefit of the socially isolated child? Must the "referred" child inevitably be regarded as the "preferred" child in the group? Will the difficult behavior of referred children trigger neurotic or anti-social behavior on the part of the other members? Will the behavior of referred children lead them to be permanently scapegoated by others in their groups? How can normal neighborhood children and their parents be persuaded by workers of the value for them of interaction of this sort with a child who is likely to have been a neighborhood outcast? In this connection, what forms of interpretation of service are both honest and useful?

Weeks were spent in building a single group. Initial interpretation to the referred child and his parents of the need for a group and the Department's service was undertaken by the caseworker, psychiatrist, psychologist, physician or educator making the referral for group work. He or she had been briefed by the Department's director as to how he might best describe the service to them at the time that his request for a group for his young client or patient was received. Exploratory and relationship-building interviews with the referred child and his parents in their home followed. Neighborhood acquaintances of the child—he rarely had a friend—were suggested by the parents and/or the child as possible members. Explanatory letters were sent to the parents of suggested members and discussions held with them and their children during home visits. The referred child's social isolation and need for a group was openly discussed at these visits to the homes of potential group members, as had been agreed upon in the interviews with him and with his parents, earlier. What was emphasized, however, was the fact, that once the group began, it was to belong to all of the members, and that the worker, as a social worker, meant to be as responsive as he could to the social and emotional needs of each of them. The process of recruiting members was never an easy one. There may be those who would say that today, in contrast to those "kindlier" times, this approach could not be implemented because of the current climate of suspicion. If so, they should be reminded that the early 1950s, a peak period for the Department in forming new groups, was the era of McCarthyism, when suspicion of anyone from the outside, anyone who was different, ran rampant. What ultimately would convince the parents of non-referred members of the worth of the service was not only their children's reports of group programs, but the group worker's availability to them in the way she or he said he would be in the beginning.[3]

The first group I formed after joining the Department as a worker, for example, was developed around a schizoid nine-year-old boy, with whose parents I was in constant contact. Within weeks after the group began to meet, however, I found myself being asked by another member's mother to help her manage the labyrinth of the administrative system of a local hospital on behalf of a chronically ill family member; helping still another member's parents find clinic resources that might deal with their son's stuttering; and counseling the parents of a third member who were worried that they were devoting too much time to a younger retarded sibling and not enough to him.

Group composition of this type, which brought so-called normal children into such intimate and frequent contact with a different kind of child, one whose negative behavioral reactions were frequently excessive and sometimes bizarre, was challenged, not only by some laymen but sometimes by professional colleagues, as well. Confronted with exaggerated and confusing behavior, "normal" children, they felt, might drive out the referred child, mock his emotional or physical handicap or, alternately, end up imitating his inappropriate behavior. The referred child as scapegoat, on the one hand, or as "trigger" for the acting out of hitherto controlled regressive impulses on the part of the non-referred group members on the other, was an issue which was legitimately raised then and must still be kept in mind.

Marjory Warren, who originated the Department's distinctive approach to group composition in 1936 and who was responsible for the Department's growth to prominence, with twenty-five to thirty groups yearly, during the following twenty-five years, felt that benefits to all outweighed these risks. In the arena of child psychotherapy, Orgel was saying much the same thing in 1941, undergirding his support for the exposure of disturbed and non-disturbed children to each other on a regular basis with theoretical concepts from psychodynamic psychiatry.[4] Ms. Warren's stance came mainly from the experience itself. This experience, on the one hand, suggested that barely restrained, even vicious verbal attacks on a vulnerable referred child and regressive pulls occasioned by his or her behavior had to sometimes be expected. (I still remember being especially taken aback by taunts of "you can't see" hurled at one particularly unpopular blind child by other members.) At the same time, experience taught that, even if the group worker was unable to reduce the tension immediately, or to exploit an incident for purposes of emotional sensitization of the participants, he or she could, by judicious use of programming and verbal intervention over time, prevent unrestrained interpersonal conflict from becoming a way of life in the group.

In every instance Department group workers saw themselves as part of a network of helpers. These included the referring professional, who generally continued individual treatment with the referred child and his family, other professionals in the neighborhood, among whom were those who controlled resources such as buildings in which a group might meet, and school personnel. The network was generally expanded to include still other mental health or recreational workers, as the group worker made himself available to the families of non-referred children in a group. Permission for these contacts was obtained from group members and their families. The Department saw its approach as a form of interagency work, in which the traditional tendency toward possessiveness over cases, which was often characterized social work and mental health agencies, should be consciously confronted and overcome. The Department's group worker was a coordinator of efforts who valued the interdependence of therapeutic personnel over his own independence of action. Intense and time-consuming, the number and nature of these contacts per group dictated that the typical Department worker's group load consist of no more than four clubs.

Interagency contacts sometimes also required immense self-restraint. This became apparent whenever, for example, a collaborating psychologist, who as a doctoral student had led a group for a semester under the famous Dr. X in New York or Detroit, would tell a Department group worker "how to do it better." Perhaps even more disconcerting sometimes was the behavior of collaterals presumably trying to be helpful in more direct fashion. Thus, the director of a branch YMCA in which my group of ten-year olds was meeting rushed into the club room to berate the members for shoving each other in the hallway. "Ralph comes all the way out here from downtown every week just to help you have a good time," he shouted as I tried to slink out of sight, "And this is how you thank him!"

Contacts of this unfortunate sort, however, were more than compensated for by phone calls such as that I received in 1976. The call came from a psychiatrist who, in 1960, as a resident, had referred a young patient for group services. After referral for group, he continued to treat this child, who was in desperate emotional straits, using every means, including hour-long telephone interviews. I, meanwhile, tried to help the youngster maintain some semblance of social relationships in a neighborhood group, in the face of his constant impulse to flee them. I would very soon receive an invitation from Jimmy, now married and a father, to visit him in his new apartment, the collaborating psychiatrist informed me, "I just talked with him," he exulted, "You won't believe what Jimmy's like. Ralph, we saved that kid from psychosis."

Department clubs really did come to belong to the neighborhood and not to the referred child alone. Once a club was formed and began to meet, even if the referred child could not sustain contact, as occasionally happened, and proved unable to remain a member, the group continued to meet, at least until the end of the school year, in order to fulfill the Department's pledge to the other members. Such a group also attended the three week session at the agency's overnight summer camp, available to all Department Clubs.[5] Actually, the Department had every reason to continue many of those groups which had "lost" their original referred member, as problems exhibited by the so-called "normal" members clearly needed to be addressed. (I was amused, whenever I asked a colleague to read an entry in a Department process record, to see how often he was unable to pick out the referred child from among all of those whose behavior was being described.) Non-referred members, naturally, reflected in their outlook and behavior the social characteristics of the referred child's neighborhood. "Normal" is always a relative term. If the neighborhood from which a troubled child was referred for help was characterized by a high rate of delinquency, for example, anti-social acting out was likely to be an acceptable, and on occasion, preferred form of behavior on the part of the normal members of the club formed around him or her. If the club that was drawn about the child came from a neighborhood undergoing racial or ethnic population changes, the normal members would almost inevitably reflect the intensely antagonistic attitudes of their own particular in-group. Aside from this, the problems aroused by the intimacies of interaction among any combination of members often placed a considerable demand on the therapeutic repertoire of the Department group worker, whether or not the referred child was present or continued as a member.

To illustrate: in the early 1960s, I led a group formed around an eleven-year-old boy whose mother was frequently hospitalized because of paranoid delusions and who was regularly savaged by a disciplinarian father. Like the referred child, the club members were white, lower-middle class and working-class. Almost all were Roman Catholic and ethnically Irish. The referred youngster's absences were frequent, but, even without the time spent in efforts to persuade him to come on any given day, I had considerable to do. On one particular afternoon when the referred child was absent the group went to a bowling alley. One of the members, athletic, persistently aggressive and complaining, became upset over his low score. He was beside himself when, in addition to this, he had to watch while I presented a birthday card, signed by the other members, to a member whose birthday it was, this being a regular practice in the group. The recipient, as luck would have it, was next to the lowest man on the totem pole in the group by reason of obesity and the extremely openly protective behavior of his parents toward him. Whenever the designated scapegoat, the referred child, was absent, this youngster could count on being pressed to take his place as the major target of the group's scapegoating activity. The pent-up fury of the most aggressive member, who had failed at bowling, was now directed at him. Epithets and an exchange of blows followed, which I was able to manage by stepping between the combatants. (At age 38 one still has a physical advantage over eleven-year olds!) The group then entered the car to return to the neighborhood.

Driving back, the verbal battle was revived, with all the members now participating. Finally, the supreme insult was hurled at the birthday lad. "Your mother cleans houses for Jew-ladies!" A flurry of invective involving Jews and their obviously unpleasant characteristics followed. After some five minutes of ventilation by the group, I wondered aloud how the Jews happened to get mixed up in their fight? As if suddenly remembering that their group worker who had been with them for two years was a Jew, they shifted their attack to blacks. At one very busy rotary—it was now five o'clock—they rolled down the windows to scream the most obscene racist slogans they could devise at all and sundry whom we passed, black and white alike. I was firm about their rolling the windows up. "You can say anything you want about how you feel when you're inside the clubroom or when the car's closed up, but you've got no right to dump it on anyone outside." The windows went up, but the swearing and expressions of hatred continued, punctuated only by the members' stopping to cross themselves every time we passed a Catholic church. They were at the age when they were receiving instruction prior to being confirmed. (I have never, then or since, quite been able to rid my mind of the image of Nazi soldiers singing Christmas Carols, in thinking about this behavior.)

As the violent group diatribe continued, I kept asking them to lower the screaming and tell me about their contacts with Black people. This had the effect of relaxing the atmosphere slightly as they paused momentarily in order to organize their stories while trying to outdo each other with tales of bad things Blacks had done to them. It goes without saying that the original fight had long been forgotten and that group unity had been purchased in the good old-fashioned way, by focusing on an external enemy. I said that it sounded like they were pretty scared of Black people, and I was sorry about that. As they knew, however, from past conversations with me, I really did not go along with the lousy things they and their buddies usually said about Blacks. By now we were coming to the neighborhood corner where they were to be left off, and, following the practice which they and the members of other club groups often mimicked—one of my groups called it "talking 'mental' like a social worker"—I left them with something to think about. I said I wondered if all this nasty talk about Jews and Blacks wasn't a way of trying to get me angry. Maybe they had wanted me to "blow my stack" about the fight outside the bowling alley and in that way to show them I could control things. I hadn't done so, and I guessed they were worried about this. The members climbed out of the car angrily, without replying, muttering threats of never coming back to this "goddamn club." They did, of course, come back. So, by the way, did the referred child. Clearly, however, it was not only his emotional problems which called for the group worker's attention. Hardly less urgent were those of his fellow club members and the neighborhood culture which had shaped their attitudes.

In this same connection, I am still bemused by the comments made to a colleague by another former referred child regarding my benign influence on the youth culture of his particular neighborhood. Unfortunately, group work was not to have much of an impact on this boy's core psychological problem. Nevertheless, the caseworker he saw some years after the group's termination told me of the lad's admiration, in retrospect, for my group leadership abilities. "Why, after a few months with Ralph the kids even gave up their favorite activity, "fencing stolen tires." I accepted this tribute with becoming modesty, but with considerable bewilderment. Stealing tires and selling them through a friendly receiver of stolen goods had been a custom of the group members of which I had been totally unaware during three gruelling years of work with the group.

The process of interaction in Neighborhood Clubs groups and the outcome of attempts at social integration for which this process was designed have been described over the years in papers published by Department staff members in a variety of professional journals.[6] What was, however, never sufficiently described in these publications is something most group workers who work outside agency walls experience, but few discuss. This was Neighborhood Clubs' workers' constant exposure to embarrassment and loss of face in public. The attempt by these workers to make positive use of this vulnerability whenever possible should be of particular interest to practitioners planning to function extramurally.

Numerous instances could be cited. One which I vividly recollect occurred when I took a group on an outing during our third year together. We had gone to a zoo and wildlife refuge frequented by many children's groups in the area. The three hours we had spent had apparently been enjoyed by all. An unfortunate corollary of the enjoyment was, of course, that nobody wanted to leave. I attempted to cajole the members into the van, as, all about us, cars and buses filled with children and their adult leaders came and went in the parking lot. Next to the lot was a huge field and next to this a number of cages filled with birds and fowl of various types. In the field, drawn up in military formation, stood several troops of nine- and ten-year-old Brownies, who were being addressed by a severe looking young woman from the Audubon Society, whose manner reminded me of nothing so much as my old drill sergeant, with stentorian voice to match. Just as I thought I had all of the youngsters in the van, three of them ran pell-mell for the cages, and, with wild yelps, opened them. Pigeons, pheasants, their exotic cousins and distant relatives flew madly out of the cages and directly at the woman from the Audubon Society who was in the middle of her address to the Brownies. The reactions of all assembled, the girls, their troopleaders, everyone, can be imagined. I stood crestfallen, with upturned palms, while my young charges ran back to the van for protection. After a feeble and futile gesture in the direction of capturing the birds I sneaked back to the van myself and drove off with the group.

After about three minutes of silence, during which I attempted to maintain my composure, the club members began to whisper to each other. "He's mad now," as if I could not hear them. They continued this for some time until one of them, plucking up his courage, asked me directly, "You're mad ain't ya?" "No, I'm not mad," I said, meanwhile seething with rage. "I'm just sorry that you guys spoiled a good time for yourselves." The lie deceived no one. It simply confused the members and left them silent for another few minutes. I finally decided that none of this was helpful, but that perhaps, strangely enough, my obvious dissembling could be made use of, clinically. "What I just said was not true," I said, loudly. "You guys made me feel like an awful damn fool out there and I was mad as hell at you for it, but I did not want to show it." Silence again followed, and shortly afterwards, agitated whispers. A number of these youngsters came from backgrounds in which adults in their lives were constantly angry at each other, separating and sometimes leaving forever.

This suggested to me the tack I should take. I repeated that I had been real mad and still was, but that, at the same time, I was wondering what they thought was going to happen now that I had gotten mad. The answer came back, almost in chorus, "You're gonna stop the club." "You ain't coming back after today." I wondered aloud whether people absolutely had to leave each other whenever they got mad at each other. For the next half hour, and a number of times during subsequent meetings, this was a question we considered together. At one particular meeting, finally, new and old ideas and feelings were put to the test. One member had made an accusation of stealing against another. When this was followed by a hard slap across the face the group split into two warring camps, one staying in the clubroom and the other rushing into the lavatory down the hall. Both sub-groups put on their coats and said they were leaving. "This club sucks and we ain't ever coming back." I shuttled between both groups, recognizing with them the reason for their anger and their right to be angry. The big question right now, however, was not who was right and who was wrong, and how lousy they felt about staying, I said. It was whether, no matter how mad they were, they were strong enough to keep the club together. Still fuming, they stayed.

To return, finally, to the question of outcomes: What did the Department of Neighborhood Clubs actually do for those who were the subject of its ministrations? When I think of a response to this question my thoughts, oddly enough, do not run to before and after studies of attitudes and behavior, experimental and control groups, or even to the modest pre-evaluative studies which we undertook as a Department staff.[7] What comes to my mind is a brief set of events which followed the death of a former Neighborhood Clubs' referred child. When he was nine years old a club had been formed around the youngster after referral by one of the doctors who had been treating him for hemophilia. Group work had terminated when he was twelve. He died from severe hemorrhaging at sixteen.

I had met weekly with the group for three years in the kitchen of this youngster's home, he being completely homebound. I had also devised program activities in which I tried to reconcile the needs of the members, including the referred child, for expressing aggression with the limitations on aggressive behavior dictated by the child's dangerous condition.[8] The club had met under the watchful eye of his mother, who had remained in the living-room during meetings but would customarily come in to serve refreshments and chat with the boys at the meeting's end.

I was called by the family during the youngster's final hospitalization and remained with them until close to the hour of his death. Shortly thereafter I was a bit surprised to have the mother call and ask me if I could possibly get in touch with the five other former group members. She had not seen them in several years, most of them having moved far from the neighborhood. She wanted so much to see them. Through one of the former members who still lived nearby I was able to make contact with the others, now well into their teens, and, a week after the funeral, we met on the corner outside the house. They had not seen me in some four years, and a couple of them, lanky sixteen year olders, laughed and said, "Ralph, you shrank." We went into the house and sat in the kitchen with the mother. Her tears were matched by the warmth of her greeting. Where she found the emotional resources I do not know, but when I left the house she was still sitting with the boys and reminiscing about some of the lively and humorous incidents that had occurred in the group, four years and more before. I really don't have any idea of the outcome measures which one would use in evaluating the meaning of this behavior and the Department's contribution to it. All I know is that thirty-one years later, as I recite these facts, I continue to be deeply moved.

REFERENCE NOTES

1. Lawrence K. Frank, "Change Through Group Experience," *Social Welfare Forum*, 1958. National Conference on Social Welfare and Columbia University Press, New York, p. 261.

2. See, for example, Richard Bond, Virginia Burns, Ralph Kolodny and Marjory Warren, "The Neighborhood Peer Group," *The Group*, Vol. 17, no. 1, October, 1954, pp. 1-8; Ralph Kolodny and Samuel Waldfogel, "Modifying Tensions Between the Handicapped and Their Normal Peers," *Child Welfare*, Vol. 36, No. 1, January, 1967, pp. 30-37; James Garland, Ralph Kolodny and Samuel waldfogel, "The Use of Social Group Work as Adjunctive Treatment for Disturbed Adolescents," *American Journal of Orthopsychiatry*, Vol. 32, No. 4, August, 1962, pp. 691-706.

3. See Ralph Kolodny, *Peer-Oriented Group Work for the Physically Handicapped Child*, Charles River Books, Boston, 1976, pp. 60-69.

4. S. Z. Orgel, "Identification As A Socializing and Therapeutic Force," *American Journal of Orthopsychiatry*, Vol. 11, No. 1, January, 1941, pp. 118-125.

5. See Virginia Burns and Ralph Kolodny, "Group Work with Physically and Emotionally Handicapped Children in a Summer Camp," *Social Work with Groups*, 1958, National Association of Social Workers, New York, 1958.

6. See Bond *et al.*, *op. cit.*, Garland *et al.*, *op. cit.*, James Garland and Ralph Kolodny, "Characteristics and Resolution of Scapegoating," *Social Work Practice*, 1967 Columbia University Press, New York, 1967 and Ralph Kolodny,

"The Impact of Peer Group Activity on the Alienated Child," *Smith College Studies in Social Work*, Vol. 37, No. 1, February, 1967, pp. 30-37.

7. See Ralph Kolodny, "Research Planning and Group Work Practice," *Mental Hygiene*, Vol. 42, No. 1, January, 1958, pp. 121-132.

8. See Kolodny, *Peer Oriented Group Work for the Physically Handicapped Child, op. cit.*, pp. 97-98.

The Group-in-Institution as the Unit of Attention: Recapturing and Refining a Social Work Tradition

Edith E. Moore
Audrey J. Starkes

All social workers in America are keenly aware of the continuing thrust towards de-institutionalization. They are equally familiar with the promotion of the community's responsibility for the so-called deviant populations in our society. Many may not be so aware, however, of a paradoxical trend that is occurring simultaneously. The use made by these populations of a great variety of residential facilities is on the increase. Nevertheless, indications are that these facilities are being used differently to achieve quite different aims now than in the past.

For example, periods of admission to institutions are shorter and more frequent. Temporary admissions for many are often arranged to give some relief to their family members or other caregivers. Further, two different types of institutionalized populations are emerging as: (a) those who become socialized to the institution because of repeated or long-term admissions, and (b) those who become dependent on the institution almost immediately upon their admission to it. Thus, if institutions are to become more than merely custodial services, these trends forecast the need for a more differentiated practice by the social workers who work in them (Anthony & Farkas, 1982; Mercier, 1986; Toews & Barnes, 1986).

Edith Moore, PhD, is Associate Professor, School of Social Work, Carleton University, Colonel By Drive, Ottawa, Canada K1S 5B6. Audrey Starkes, MSW, is with Royal Ottawa Hospital, 1145 Carling Avenue, Ottawa, Canada K1Z 8N3.

This paper asserts that group practice with individuals residing in institutions contributes significantly to the constructive use they make of institutional services. Not only does the group provide a therapeutic milieu to its members for the resolution of psychosocial problems through interactions within the group. The group is also a powerful influence on the institutional environment of the group, as well as on the external community of each of its individual members.

It is further contended that there are special competencies inherent in this kind of practice with groups whose members reside in institutions. Thus the impact of institutional services on members and staff is explored in order to identify the salient practice issues. In the light of these issues the external influence of the group is conceptualized. This conceptualization is then tested against the realities of practice with groups in two contrasting institutional contexts.

THE NATURE OF INSTITUTIONS
AS SERVICE DELIVERY SYSTEMS

An institution is a type of human service organization in which a number of like-situated individuals are removed from their natural life situation and live together in a formally administered round of life. The purpose is generally to socialize or resocialize the population with which it works (Anderson, 1978:73).

There are three types of institutional settings: those which are hospitals or medically oriented; those which are residential/service centres; and those which are custodial/corrective facilities. All provide some mix of custody and treatment and have some key features in common: they are living units in which the inhabitants are totally immersed; in which the boundaries between them and the larger environment are clearly drawn; in which the total milieu is implicated in the service delivery process; and which is formally organized by executive and operational employees.

Historically the institutional structure represented a kind of social engineering which originated in the mid-1800s in Canada with the beginning of industrialization. It sought to provide a corrective milieu of "kindness and firmness" to deal with what was considered to be inadequate family upbringing (Moore, 1980). Rothman's (1971) illumination of the "cult of the asylum" in the United States points out that the institution was also an attempt to compensate for public disorder; was a beginning recognition of the social causes of poverty, crime and insanity; and was seen as a panacea for undifferentiated deviant populations who had to be removed from the chaotic conditions which caused their illness. In essence the original declared intent of institutionalized services was to induce the "inmates" to conform to the discipline and order of the institutional system and hence to an external social order.

An analysis of these beginnings suggests a number of historical themes which continue to resonate in present-day institutional services. There are continuing issues around the concepts of status, philosophy of care, social control, banishment and differentiation of service.

A subsequent pattern was that of the deinstitutionalization of deviant populations—the "paupers," the "insane," the mentally handicapped, the physically disabled, the criminals, the elderly. This pattern represented a trend toward more pluralistic services. As well, it represented a trend toward a community-based service delivery system. A dominant impetus has been the economic consideration based on the fact that institutional care is more costly than that for which the community assumes responsibility. Consequently the institutional milieu was being used more differentially, more specifically and for shorter periods of residence. Correspondingly there also evolved more variation in the structure of institutions.

Currently the issue of locus of care is being replaced by the issue of continuity of care. Rather than choosing between institutional or community-based care, the continuity-of-care perspective views institutionalization as one aspect of treatment, rather than the whole treatment or as something to be shunned (Toews & Barnes, 1986:3). Consequently the emerging patterns of admission tend to be periodic, temporary, frequent, and short-term.

Goffman (1973) in his study of asylums described them as "total institutions" which:

- cut off residents from the greater society,
- formally administer and direct maximal aspects of inhabitants' lives,
- provide a life of sameness for most participants,
- dispense their authority from above through a formal system of rules and regulations.

Later writers, however, specify totality as a relative condition, thus pointing to the variability of institutional forms.

The lower the totalistic features of an institution the more congruence is possible with the needs of an individual resident and the more exchange with the community outside. Size is no longer a differentiating factor in bureaucratic inflexibility (Rai, 1983). But greater technological complexity gives rise to greater specialization and greater delegation of executive power (Street et al., 1974:207). Furthermore there is evidence that specialized institutions are "total" for residents and "minimal" for employees; whereas structurally unspecialized institutions are "minimal" for residents and "total" for employees (Rosengren, 1974:407).

At present therefore there is a range of institutional forms providing a range of differentiated services to a range of target populations. All have some degree of totality. There are clear consequences therefore for all who are resident in institutions.

While institutionalization per se has an impact on all residents, one cannot conclude that the nature of that impact is the same for each. There is evidence to suggest that if the occupants have personality traits that are congruent with environmental demands, they will experience less stress (Berman-Rossi, 1986:337). This is in contrast to the earlier view that institutionalization is solely a function of time spent in institutions.

In fact Toews and Barnes (1986:3) have identified the "new chronic patient" who shows all the characteristics of institutionalization early in the admission to the institution. This patient (smaller in number than the rest of the patient population) will return to institutional life regardless of the adequacy of the milieu and its programs.

Thus the nature of institutional dependency is different for each resident. This more complex view of the effects of institutionalization makes more complex the defining and operationalizing of an optimum milieu for each resident.

Nevertheless there is a basic need of each person to be in charge of one's own life. All institutions by their very nature curtail the satisfaction of this need in all residents, but do so to varying extents. In general residents are overwhelmed by their own vulnerability and relative powerlessness, often ignorant of their rights and lacking skill in negotiation. Frequently they have limited psychological resources, fewer family supports and find themselves in an institutional environment that is not supportive to their needs.

Berman-Rossi (1986:339) likens them to immigrants who are strangers in a strange land. "Entering alone without status and with a predominance of liabilities, new residents find an uncertain future requiring the tasks of establishing friendships, becoming oriented to surroundings, establishing role identities and responding to the unequal balance of power between care-givers and care-receivers."

In essence the plight of residents in institutions is a combination of four sets of interrelated factors:

1. Individual predicaments which predate institutionalization but which are brought into institutional life by the residents. At some level these predicaments are social in nature.
2. The consequences of relocation — predominantly those experiences and feelings related to loss — loss of role, freedom, independence, privacy.
3. Individual responses to the process of socialization to the new role of institution resident.
4. Individual responses to the specifically therapeutic processes within the institution.

Ultimately, since institutions are a group living situation, consisting of a network of groups, the residents find themselves by choice or assignment, in many groups. The social worker in an institution practices in many of these groups.

SOCIAL WORK WITH GROUPS IN INSTITUTIONS

Tom Douglas (1983:203) makes the point that all groups are embedded in larger groups. All members of groups are members of other groups. The influence of the other groups is always present. In his later writing about group living the notion of imbedding is highlighted as a more salient feature of institutional contexts. The constraints that imbedding can create are often not recognized. "Thus consequences arising as a result of external factors are often unfortunately ascribed to influences operating within the group" (Douglas, 1986:158). Embedding only shows up when a group tries to create for itself patterns of behaviour that are manifestly incomparable with the accepted and acceptable behaviour patterns of the larger system.

Yalom (1983:1), writing about group psychotherapy notes that, unlike other groups, groups in institutions are not "free-standing," but always part of a larger therapeutic system. While social work groups have never conceived of themselves as freestanding, it is nevertheless true that social work groups in institutions are more imbedded in their organizational auspices than those in non-institutional human service organizations.

The autonomy of the group, like that of the resident and the worker, is more immediately curtailed by the institution. The institution has long-standing heavily invested and predetermined structures for changing behaviour in a patterned way by arranging and ordering the living unit and its inherent relationships according to a cultural system of values and goals.

This culturally-shaped pattern is reflected in processes which occur in parallel fashion at each interface between systems and subsystems. Each system therefore is constrained towards becoming a microcosm of the larger one.

Logically then the role of the group would be to attain as much autonomy as possible under these contextual circumstances. The residents' over-riding need is to exercise control over their own lives. The commonality of this need is greater by virtue of the fact that they all share the institutional living environment of the group. This common need is more likely to be met by means of the collective action of the group than by actions of individuals.

Logically also, the role of the group vis à vis its institutional context would be to sustain those aspects of institutional life which further the goals of the group in the interests of its members; as well as to act as a countervailing force with respect to those aspects of institutional life which inhibit the realization of these goals.

The institutional response to this external role of the group has often been to institute a type of group, frequently labelled a "milieu group," whose explicit purpose is to deal with external issues. This type of group is in contrast with the treatment group whose purpose is to meet the individual needs of its members. Berman-Rossi (1986:342) aptly describes the two types as resembling town meetings or intimate family gatherings. While this may be an organizationally efficient means of managing problems in the institution, it also formalizes an artificial "split" in the essentially social nature of the helping endeavour. It fails to see the interconnectedness between the residents' situations predating institutionalization, the institutions's contribution to the residents' treatment in the institution, the treatment group's embeddedness in the institution, and the treatment group's role in creating its own environment. By containing each type of group within these organizational structures the residents can more easily be induced to conform to the institution.

Our position is that this organizational dichotomization of groups into those which are externally oriented and those which are internally oriented is unrealistic in practice. Our argument is that all groups have their own particular purposes, and that all of these purposes have both an internal and an external dimension. The individual treatment of residents in groups is imbedded in the lives of those residents outside of the group. Furthermore the common interests of residents, and their shared living arrangements, also predispose groups in institutions to a blurring of boundaries between individual and collective concerns, both of which have an internal and external dimension.

In fact groups for residents in institutions have been rationalized in many ways. Though a claim cannot be made for a systematic study of a representative sample of recent literature, there seems to be sufficient evidence to support some tentative impressions regarding the purposes of social work practice with groups in institutions. When stated purposes of groups for residents were listed and then grouped, the distribution was as follows:

- Purposes which facilitate the operation of the institution: 21 statements.
- Purposes which are in the interests of the residents: 16 statements.
- Purposes which are directed to institutional change: 5 statements.
- Purposes which are directed to both individual and institutional change: 5 statements.
- Purposes which relate to residents' situations outside the institution: 5 statements.
- Purposes which are directed to buffering the impact of the institution on the residents: 2.

From this it appears that group services in institutions are an integrated part of institutional life. They are also most often conceptualized in terms of their contribution to that institutional "world" of the resident. The externality of the group is defined predominantly in terms of the institution, with only minor attention to the world outside the institution, particularly the situations to which the resident will return. The dominant impression conveyed is that the group is in the service of the institution, with only minor recognition of a role for the group in rendering the institution more congruent with resident needs. At best the group is seen as a "buffer" for the anti-therapeutic effects of the institution.

In general then the group is conceptualized as an extension of the espoused treatment objectives of the institution. This is a valid perspective if it can be assumed that the institutional structures and processes adhere to these objectives and are entirely in the interests of all of the residents. However there appears to be no operational attention to the fact that all organizations have a life of their own, that the survival of the organization supersedes all other considerations, and that residents are in a relatively powerless position with very few legitimized rights in a living unit more removed from public scrutiny than other, more structurally open organizations.

There is some focussed attention to pre-discharge or re-entry groups. These appear to be a response to the finding that the gains of institutional treatment are speedily eroded if residents are not helped with the return to their natural living units. In some respects this appears to be another institutional mechanism for dealing with a systemic problem. Re-entry should be an integral concern at entry, and throughout the time in residence, rather than the "tacking on" of a compartmentalized service in the final few weeks of residence. Furthermore, the community and social systems and networks of the residents play a significant part in the creation, sustaining or resolving of the resident's need of institutionalization, and are in need of active involvement from the point of entry, rather than being "handed" the institutionally processed resident at the point of exit. One must acknowledge that institutions do vary with respect to the extent of permeability of their boundaries, but at the same time point out that all institutions by their very nature are more closed than other service organizations.

Given the foregoing analysis of institutions, their impact on the residents, and the place of groups in them, what is the role of the social worker in the group? To begin to answer this question we must first define the role of the social worker in the institution at large.

The complexities and contradictions inherent in institutions along with the differing needs and responses of residents to institutionalization make it difficult for any intervenor to define a service role. Mercier (1986:16) points out the contradiction between improving the quality of life in institutions while at the same time discouraging dependency on the institution. Her survey of staff in a psychiatric hospital concluded that "interveners are squeezed by a model of organization of services which contrasts active treatment rehabilitation with quality of life, whereas the needs of their clientele are manifested simultaneously at both of these levels."

With respect to social work practice there appears to be a shift in the way an institution-based social worker's role is defined. Earlier definitions saw the social worker much more directly engaged in activities outside the institutions in the interests of residents. However as Hasenfeld (1974:311) points out, the worker is not likely to pursue client problems to which the institution does not have the resources to respond.

In effect there is a tendency for the staff also to become institutionalized just as they may become socialized to any organization (Parsons, 1974:89). Institutions being "total" organizations have a stronger hold on their members. Furthermore, being based inside the institution, rather than on the boundary of the institution, is more advantageous from the point of view of turf consciousness and protectionism. In a situation of unequal power and resources, professionals latch on to what is considered high status work and often drop their own unique professional skills.

The current trends in institutional care, however, suggest the need for a return to the earlier role of social workers in institutions. The debate is no longer one of the preferred locus of care (i.e., the community *or* the institution) but rather one of continuity of care. Therefore institutional boundaries must be bridged, with respect to both the service network and the residents life-space of origin.

Parsons (1974:78) emphasizes that institutional services are simultaneously services to the resident and to the social groups of which he is a member, notably his family. This emphasis is in tension with the custodial nature of institutions. Personnel in close operative relations with the daily lives of residents have a strong vested interest in the smooth functioning of the institution, or at least their part of the institution. Residents who are well-socialized to such an institutional community may become too well-adjusted to be brought over a therapeutic hump. In effect both care receivers and caregivers are prone to institutionalization.

In the light of these complexities of institutional life, Yalom's view of inpatient group psychotherapy may be subject to qualification. He avers (1983:162) that the over-riding principle is that the therapist must act in such a way as to facilitate the group's attaining its goals for the members. But he also advocates (p.3) the use of the group to facilitate the functioning of the ward. This dual perspective is based on the dubious assumption that the functioning of the ward is completely congruent with the needs of all residents.

One is reminded of the parent of a child in a residential treatment centre who observed that she "had to become a bit crazy" herself in order to get some attention for her child. The implication was that in order to be "heard" by the institution she had to adopt a role which the institution recognized and to which it could respond. Clearly this institution did not have a community-centered orientation.

The social work literature presents some varying viewpoints as to the role of the social worker in institutions.

Hans Falck (1964) takes the position that effective social functioning of the members inside and eventually outside the group is the goal of social work in general and of the social group work method in particular. "Outside the group" is taken to mean the life-space of the client, not in the institutional milieu, but in the "world" from which the client came and to which s/he will presumably return.

Nevertheless such well-known writers as Shulman, espousing the mediating model state that the professional task is "to find the viable operational connection between the institution's need for a tight ship and the client's need to develop autonomy and to negotiate within and among the various systems (Gitterman & Shulman, 1986:143). The social work function in engaging the system offers assistance to both the institution and the client, siding with neither, focussing on the dialogue and seeking to lessen the distance between the two (p. 355).

The hazards of this mediating approach are particularly salient in institutions where the needs of the institution and the needs of the resident are frequently incompatible, and where power and status differences are firmly entrenched. In these situations, as Douglas points out (1986:176) "mediation tends to reward the more aggressive and intransigent of those involved as the mediators seek concessions from the more amenable of conflictors. Thus the whole purpose of mediation is frustrated as the aggressive party can only gain by continuing to be intransigent."

Given the propensity of all organizations to be a microcosm of the larger society, a neutral, mediating role for the worker is problematical. Nor does such a role seem possible in face of the institutionalizing influences to which staff and residents alike are subjected.

Furthermore workers are less autonomous in their practice in institutions. Institutional factors are accentuated in developing and delivering services. Multiple staff members interact regularly with residents. In most instances also the worker has dual accountability—to the executive and to the operative lines of service delivery, i.e., to the administrative head of the institution and to the professional or service head of the living unit.

While recognizing the constraints and complexities, our bias is that the social worker needs to induce and stimulate changes in the organization before effectively achieving changes in the client. A less comfortable, but perhaps more effective role for the worker might be to assume a more pivotal role on the boundary between the resident and the institution, and between the group and the institution, and between the institution and the environment of the institution. This role always assumes an imperfect environment and is perhaps more difficult and crucial in practice within an institutional context because the system is, by virtue of its structure, more closed than that of other service organizations. The centripetal force of the institution on its members—residents and staff alike—require a continuous countervailing watchfulness on the part of workers who are clear about their role and function, and self-aware with respect to their institution-based practice.

This boundary role is comprised of both direct and indirect service activities. The direct service is that practice which intervenes with the resident as well as with the social situation outside the institution in which the resident's non-institutional life is imbedded. The indirect service is that practice which seeks to influence the institution towards greater congruence with residents' individual and collective needs.

Thus the social worker in the group is also in a difficult but pivotal position if she chooses her rightful place on the boundary as a bridge-builder between group and institution and between resident and institution and community. That boundary position cannot be neutral. Professionally and structurally it requires that resident interests be placed ahead of those of the institution.

In beginning with a conception of the place of the group in the institution the social worker confronts the following questions:

• Is the group an extension of the institution?
• Is the group both integrated with and differentiated from the whole of the institutional service?
• Is it an agent acting for the institution?
• Is it a buffer against the counterproductive aspects of institutional life?
• Is it a countervailing force in active opposition to the counterproductive aspects of institutional life?
• Does it seek to ameliorate institutional conditions as they impact on the service to group members individually?
• Does it have a role in changing institutional conditions as they affect the members individually and the group as a whole?
• Does it have a role in linking with the external life of the institution?
• Does it have a role in linking with the life of the resident-members external to the institution?

The literature pertaining to practice has very little to say about these critical interfaces.

THE EXTERNAL INFLUENCE OF GROUPS IN INSTITUTIONS

We have borrowed the term "environmental competence" to capture the notion of the group's ability to intervene in the situations of the group and its members in the interests of the group and its members (Moore, 1984). In effect we are attempting to operationalize the role of the group with respect to its own externality. The nature of that external environment varies. Therefore the group's competence to deal with it consists of some abilities specific to that particular environment. In this instance we are presenting some practice guidelines which have particular relevance for groups in an institutional environment.

The environmental competence of groups in institutions is directed outward and upward, that is it attempts to bridge with salient situations outside the institution in the interests of its members (outward influence); and it attempts to bridge with the institutional hierarchy in the interests of the groups and its members (upward influence).

It is proposed therefore that external influence is composed of outward influence and upward influence. External influence as we are using it is not the same as the concept of group influence as it appears in the literature pertaining to group theory. Group influence as found in group theory refers to the influence of the group on its members. By external influence we mean the deliberate impact of the group on those situations outside of the group which affect the group and its individual members.

In the literature on group practice there is a continuum of perspectives on externality. The position of this paper is closest to that of Trecker (1972 quoted in Whickham and Cowan 1986:100) who, among other criteria thinks that "good group work results when:

- a group develops not only consciousness of its own self but also wholesome relationships with other groups in the agency and the community;
- a group shows evidence of a developing social consciousness which enables it to take responsibility for leadership in the vital affairs of the community."

This is interpreted to mean that a fully developed group is an environmentally competent group; furthermore, that a less than fully developed group is environmentally competent in less refined and less concerted ways.

This view is juxtaposed by Yalom (1983:178,227-9) who, in writing about inpatient group psychotherapy considers "externalization" to be a form of resistance — a failure to take responsibility for one's role in creating one's own distress. Furthermore he states that "responsibility refers to ownership." Attempts by the group to problem-solve around members' outside problems are "always unsuccessful because the data are presented to the group by a demoralized, biased observer." Despite our respect for the humane contribution of this author to our knowledge of working with people in groups, we cannot but speculate that this view of externalization as a defensive maneuver tends to blame the victim.

Between these two positions there is a third position which appears in some of the social work literature. Systems theory is used to locate the group within a context. A recent text (Wickham & Cowan, 1986:16) referred to this theory but stated that "The question to be addressed is: how does each aspect of the [context] affect the worker and his work with groups?" This text noted the "interdependence" between the group and its context. But when it came to identifying the action at this interface it was all unidirectional. That is, the notion of *exchange* between the group and its situation was not recognized and hence there was no attention to the impact (potential or otherwise) of the group on its context. Thus the operationalization of systems theory is incomplete in much of the practice literature.

Our position is that social work practice with groups encompasses both intervention within the group and intervention outside the group, i.e., that the group is both a context and an instrument of change involving actions by the group and its members inside group meetings as well as actions by the group and its members in situations outside the group.

Externality is being addressed in the recent emphasis on rehabilitation (Anthony & Farkas, 1982; Mercier, 1986; Toews & Barnes, 1986). Strategies and technologies are being formalized and evaluated for the deinstitutionalization of residents. These strategies have been influenced by the earlier models developed for the rehabilitation of the physically disabled. They emphasize the behavior change of residents by means of skill training. The skill training is said to take place in groups.

This recent rehabilitation focus does represent the institution's recognition of the need to encompass the community outside the institution. However its underlying assumptions are not entirely congruent with those of social work with groups.

Anthony and Farkas (1982:14) for instance question the goal of deinstitutionalization as an end in itself, and believe that it is achieved at the expense of other outcomes. They cite research which suggests that residents as a result of a rehabilitation program are discharged with more interpersonal skills, but are also rated as more anxious than those who have not acquired these skills.

In these programs the group is used as a vehicle for training residents individually to be able to cope outside of the institution. This is in contrast to an approach which develops the group competence as a division of labor for the purpose of intervening in the situations of the group and its members. In fact skill training is replacing the earlier emphasis on developing a support system for the resident on discharge. The emphasis on support system was faulted for not increasing the resident's skills. The assumption seems to be that the solution to the problem of re-integrating the resident into the community lies in enhancing the skills of the resident. By contrast, our focus on the environmental competence or external influence of the group is based on the view that resident's problems require more than one locus of intervention.

Furthermore these medically-based rehabilitation programs stress compliance as a major factor in the prevention of re-admission. Compliance was initially restricted to schizophrenic patients and their medication. However the concept is now being generalized to include compliance with a range of social and behavioral "prescriptions" on discharge (Toews & Barnes, 1986:3). The consequence is seen to be a trend toward "institutions without walls—the stigmatization and ghettoization of chronically institutionalized populations."

Our definition of environmental competence, then, extends beyond a narrow focus on individual change to include the empowerment of people individually and collectively to change factors in their situations which impede their self-actualization. Competence must always be conceptualized within an ecological framework.

How then does one begin to operationalize the external influence of the group?

The group of course is well suited to its task. It has more visibility than the individual. It elicits more attention from the institution and the community. It affords some protection to the individual member by representing common concerns and for acting on behalf of a member. It is a vehicle for both developing and deploying the environmental competence of the group and its members.

The over-riding concern of residents in institutions is "the negotiation of one's world." The task of the group therefore is first of all the creation of environments, both inside and outside the institution which allow the influence of residents. Assertion is required for survival. The group can be instrumental in opening up opportunities for the members to satisfy their need to be in charge of their lives.

Secondly, the group's task is to empower its members and the group as a whole to negotiate those worlds inside and outside the institution. In effect the development of environmental competence empowers the group to negotiate these worlds. This competence is exercised in the form of external influence. External influence, as we have said, is comprised of outward influence and upward influence.

The goals of outward influence are to ensure those social arrangements and situational conditions which would permit the group member, on discharge from the institution, to assume his/her rightful place in society.

This activity is frequently compartmentalized organizationally as discharge planning. However if institutional boundaries are permeable and continuous with their community contexts, the exchange between the institution and community should be continuous from the point of entry of the resident. That is, the direct involvement of significant others and the preparation for discharge should begin at the time of the resident's admission to the institution. The group is an effective vehicle for keeping those avenues to the community open by actively assisting its individual members with their life situation of origin.

The goals of upward influence are more complex than those of outward influence. This is in part due to the fact that the institution has to meet two often contradictory resident needs. On the one hand there is a need for a therapeutic milieu which would be conducive to the treatment of the resident — an environment which is individualizing and supportive. On the other hand there is a need for a milieu which enhances the ability of the resident to cope with the less than therapeutic world outside the institution.

Research in the field of education suggests that an optimum learning environment consists of a combination of those conditions which satisfy the learner and those conditions which stimulate the learner. Expectations of the learner should be set at a level within reach, but just beyond where the learner is presently functioning (Hunt, 1971). Ideally the institution would be capable of radiating and modulating those environments which both support and challenge each resident differentially.

The upward influence of the group therefore is directed towards achieving institutional arrangements which protect and nurture its members as well as incite and enable them to come to grips with the less than ideal social realities outside the institution.

In effect the group seeks institutional environments which allow as much as possible the influence of residents as a mitigating force against institutional totality. The upward direction of the influence derives from the fact that there is a concentration of power in the staff of the institution and a consequent loss of decision-making on the part of the residents. As a hierarchically ordered structure, reflecting the larger society, the institution is subject to the abuse of power.

The task then is to articulate the ways by which the group-in-institution can be effective in achieving these goals of outward and upward influence.

Group work is fundamentally based on using real work, reflecting the reality of members' lives, to develop new roles and abilities. In this instance the real work of the group is located in two places: the members real life environment outside the institution, and the institutional environment.

Social work is also fundamentally based in the principle of building on strengths. Members enter the group with some real or potential competencies, which need to be actualized and concerted. Further competence to engage in the real work of environmental intervention is developed by developing members' ability to be assertive; second by doing real work which in the process develops competence; and thirdly by having opportunities to make decisions about their own lives. Thus the environmental competence of the group and its members is acquired by means of an experiential learning process.

The worker listens for the primary concerns of the members with respect to the environment. Since institutions socialize their residents, and tend to reward conformity, these concerns are not always readily apparent. However there are usually some points of resistance which are frequently indicators of the need for environmental intervention. Beginning where the group is, and responding with commitment and self-awareness, the whole spectrum of issues — both private and public — inside and outside the institution, of concern to this particular group will emerge over time.

The worker identifies and clarifies these issues with the group, then presents them as potential items of group business. The shared institutional environment of the group makes some of these issues obvious. The more critical task is that of broadening the horizons of the group to see these issues as the legitimate work of the group. This interpretation is particularly critical if the group was formed initially to meet member objectives inside the group.

Nevertheless the readiness of the group members will be a factor in this movement to action. The practitioner has a responsibility not to impose her agenda on the group. At the same time, however, since she also spends her working life in this institution, she must remain open to "seeing" and considering environmental issues as legitimate areas of social work practice with groups.

The environmental issue or concern is then converted and partialized into tasks. Task group methods can then be applied by the group in order to arrive at strategies for action. Toseland and Rivas (1984) have elucidated the strengths and weaknesses of a range of task group methods such as problem solving, brainstorming, nominal group technique and social judgement analysis.

The environmental competence of the group is a division of labor composed of individual and group competencies. The ability to function in groups is in itself a key component of environmental competence. Other competencies are required on a contingency basis to implement the strategies associated with the tasks. Motamedi (1977) for example has used Trist's classification of environments as contingencies for the selection of actions to be undertaken by social systems. The four environment types are "placid randomized," "placid clustered," "disturbed reactive," and "turbulent field." The actions applied selectively in relation to these environments include "conforming, resisting, opposing, arresting, resolving, stalling."

Those actions associated with outward influence draw heavily on natural helping processes. The group and its members therefore need to recognize the competence they already possess in this area. Swenson's study found that natural helpers were effective in helping with needs ranging from practical matters, to relationships with organizations and with other people, to developmental tasks, to feelings about the self. The skills they used included sustaining emotionally, helping with problem-solving, mediating with organizations and individuals, providing tangible services, sharing material resources.

Some competencies may need to be developed or acquired by the group in order to be able to carry out its environmental intervention. Drawing on andragogical principles, the members are helped to take responsibility for their own learning and, through the skills acquired in doing so, to become lifelong self-directed learners. The members are assisted to name their learning through praxis: action plus reflection (Herman, 1983).

Finally the group members need to be aware of and prepared for the constraints and limitations which will inevitably confront them as they carry out their efforts to intervene in their environment. There are those constraints which inhere in the participatory process of the group; as well as those which are based in the environment they are intent on changing. Realistic expectations and early success ensure sustained effort. Change most often occurs as a result of an accumulation of influences which capitalize on unforeseen opportunities. It seldom proceeds undeterred in linear, step-by-step fashion.

CRITICAL INCIDENTS OF EXTRA-GROUP INTERVENTION

Until now this paper has used a deductive approach to arrive at practice guidelines for dealing with the externality of groups in institutions. We now propose to ground these conceptualizations by examining actual instances in which groups in institutions have been able to exert upward and outward influence.

The following grid is designed to specify those actions outside of group meetings by group members in the interests of group members or other client populations.

EXTRA-GROUP INTERVENTION

			IN THE INTEREST OF:			
	MEMBER	GROUP AS A WHOLE	POPULATION REPRESENTED BY MEMBER	POPULATION REPRESENTED BY WHOLE GROUP	NON-AFFILIATED	
					INDIVIDUAL	POPULATION
WORKER ACTIONS						
MEMBER ACTIONS						
COLLECTIVE ACTIONS						

The associate author, who has been a social worker in groups in two contrasting institutions, identified critical incidents which illustrate each category of the grid. The insights gained as a result of this exercise further elucidate the nature of externality in practice with groups.

CONCLUSION

This exploration of the significance of the institution as a context for practice with groups is the latest in a series of papers which have explored other contexts of practice with groups (Moore, 1978, 1983, 1984, 1985, 1985). In each paper, the concept of group externality has been analyzed with a view to articulating the environmental competence of the group.

This journey of discovery has led to the conclusion that all groups in all contexts must actively intervene outside of themselves in order to achieve their purposes. There is no such entity as a "freestanding" group. However we have also concluded that the issues relating to environmental intervention are more salient for groups in institutions than for groups in any other context we have explored.

The reasons for this are to be found in the service delivery systems, with respect to permeability of boundaries, socialization of residents, status relationships and embeddedness of the group. In fact there is some question as to whether a group can ever function democratically in an institutional milieu. But one fact is certain: the more such a group functions according to egalitarian principles the more it is bound to engage with the external environment of the group as a whole, as well as that of its individual members.

It is urgent therefore that we develop the necessary tools for effectively implementing this social work tradition.

SELECTED REFERENCES

Social Work with Groups

Douglas, Tom, *Group Living: The Application of Group Dynamics in Residential Settings*, New York: Tavistock Publications, 1986.
Douglas, Tom, *Groups: Understanding People Gathered Together*, New York: Tavistock Publications, 1983.
Garvin, Charles, *Contemporary Group Work*. Englewood Cliffs, N.J.: Prentice-Hall Inc., 1981.
Garvin, Charles, "The Changing Contexts of Group Work Practice: Challenge and Opportunity," *Social Work with Groups*, Vol. 7, No. 1, Spring, 1984, pp. 3-19.
Gitterman, Alex and Shulman, Lawrence, eds., *Mutual Aid Groups and the Life Cycle*, Itasca, Ill.: F. E. Peacock, Publications, 1986.
Glasser, P., Sarri, R. and Vinter, R., *Individual Change Through Small Groups*, New York: The Free Press, 1974.
Konopka, Gisela, Book Review of "Therapeutic Communities: Reflections and Progress," Hinshelwood and Nick Manning, eds., London: Routledge and Kegan Paul, 1979; in *Social Work with Groups*, Vol. 6, No. 2, Summer 1983, pp. 95-97.
Konopka, Gisela, "Group Treatment of the Mentally Ill: Education for Life," *Canada's Mental Health Supplement*. January-April 1967.
Wickham, E. and Cowan, B., *Group Treatment: An Integration of Theory and Practice*, Guelph, Ontario: Raithby House, University of Guelph, 1986.
Yalom, Irvin, *Inpatient Group Psycho-Therapy*. New York: Basic Books, 1983.

The Institutional Context

Anderson, R., and Carter, I., *Human Behaviour and the Social Environment: A Social Systems Approach*, Chicago: Aldine Pub. Co., 1978.
Berman-Rossi, T., "The Fight Against Hopelessness and Despair: The Institutionalized Aged," *Mutual Aid Groups and the Life Cycle*, Gitterman A. and Shulman, L., eds., Itasca, Ill.: F. E. Peacock, Publications, 1986, pp. 333-358.
Cumming, John and Cumming, Elaine, *Ego and Milieu: Theory and Practice of Environmental Therapy*, New York: Allerton Press, 1962.
Goffman, Erving, *Asylums: Essays on the Social Situations of Mental Patients and Other Inmates*, New York: Doubleday, 1973.

Gubrium, Jaber, *Living and Dying at Murray Manor*, New York: St. Martin's Press, 1975.

Hasenfeld, Y., and English, R., eds., *Human Service Organizations*, Ann Arbor: University of Michigan Press, 1975.

Hasenfeld, Y., "Organizational Factors in Services to Groups," *Individual Change Through Small Groups*, Glasser, P., Sarri, R., and Vinter, R., eds., New York: The Free Press, 1974, pp. 307-322.

Holland, Thomas and Cook, Martha, "Organizations and Values in Human Services," *Social Service Review*, March 1983, pp. 59-77.

Moore, Edith E., "Mental Health Services in Ontario to 1926: Historical Antecedents of the Community Mental Health Movement," Unpublished paper, 1980.

Parsons, T., "The Mental Hospital as a Type of Organization," *Human Service Organizations*, Hasenfeld, Y. and English, R., eds., Ann Arbor: University of Michigan Press, 1974, pp. 72-97.

Rosengren, W., "Structure, Policy and Style: Strategies of Organizational Control," *Human Service Organizations*, Hasenfeld, Y. and English, R., eds., Ann Arbor: University of Michigan Press, 1974, pp. 391-412.

Rothman, David, *The Discovery of the Asylum*, Boston: Little, Brown and Co., 1971.

Steele, F., *Physical Settings and Organization Development*, Don Mills, Ont.: Addison-Wesley Pub. Co., 1973.

Street, D., Vinter, R., and Perrow, C., "Executiveship in Juvenile Correctional Institutions," *Human Service Organizations*, Hasenfeld, Y. and English, R., eds., Ann Arbor: University of Michigan Press, 1974, pp. 199-209.

Developing Environmental Competence

Baker, Paul, "The Division of Labour: Interdependence, Isolation and Cohesion in Small Groups," *Small Group Behaviour*, Vol. 12, No. 1, February 1981, pp. 93-106.

Bass, Bernard, "Team Productivity and Individual Member Competence," *Small Group Behaviour*, Vol. 11, No. 4, November 1980, pp. 431-504.

Brown, Leonard, "Mutual Help Staff Groups to Manage Work Stress," *Social Work with Groups*, Vol. 7, No. 2, Summer 1984, pp. 55-66.

Evans, N., and Jarvis, P., "Group Cohesion: A Review and Re-evaluation," *Small Group Behaviour*, Vol. 11, No. 4, November 1980, pp. 359-370.

Galinsky, M., and Schopler, J., "Group Goal Formulation in Social Work Practice," *Social Work Practice*, 1971, pp. 24-32.

Gambrill, Eileen, *Casework: A Competency-Based Approach*, Englewood Cliffs, N.J.: Prentice-Hall, Inc., 1983.

Herman, Reg., "Intervening in Groups: A Repertoire and Language of Group Skills for Self-Directed Learning in Decision-Making Groups," *Small Group Behaviour*, Vol. 14, No. 4, November 1983, pp. 445-464.

Hewitt, John P., *Self and Society: A Symbolic-Interactionist Social Psychology*, Boston: Allyn and Bacon, 1976.

Hunt, D., *Matching Models in Education: The Coordinator of Teaching Methods with Student Characteristics*, Toronto: Ontario Institute for Studies in Education, 1971.

Jurma, Wm., "Leadership Structuring Style, Task Ambiguity, and Group Member Satisfaction," *Small Behaviour*, Vol. 9, No. 1, February 1978, pp. 124-134.

Liebowitz, S., and De Meuse, K., "The Application of Team Building," *Human Relations*, Vol. 35, No. 1, 1982, pp. 1-18.

Maluccio, Anthony, ed., *Promoting Competence in Clients: A New/Old Approach to Social Work Practice*, New York: The Free Press, 1961.

Short, Ronald, "Competency Education and Evaluation: Issues and Dilemmas," *Group and Organization Studies*, Vol. 2, No. 1, March 1977, pp. 75-87.

Toseland, Ronald and Rivas, Robert, "Structured Methods for Working with Task Groups," *Administration in Social Work*, Vol. 8, (2), Summer 1984, pp. 49-58.

Upward and Outward Influence

Anthony, Wm., and Farkas, Marianne, "A Client Outcome Planning Model for Assessing Psychiatric Rehabilitation Interventions," *Schizophrenia Bulletin*, Vol. 8, No. 1, 1982, pp. 13-38.

Brass, Daniel, "Being in the Right Place: A Structural Analysis of Individual Influence in An Organization," *Administrative Science Quarterly*, 27, 1982, 304-316.

Cooper, L. and Gustafson, J., "Family-Group Development: Planning in Organizations," *Human Relations*, Vol. 34, No. 8, 1981, pp. 705-730.

Falck, Hans, "Social Group Work and Planned Change," *Social Work Practice*, 1964, pp. 209-220.

Friedlander, F. and Green, P., "Life Styles and Conflict-Coping Structures," *Group and Organization Studies*, Vol. 2, No. 1, March 1977, pp. 101-111.

Likert, R., and Likert, J., "A Method for Coping with Conflict in Problem-Solving Groups," *Group and Organization Studies*, Vol. 3, No. 4, December 1978, pp. 427-434.

Mastenbroek, W., "Negotiating: A Conceptual Model," *Group and Organization Studies*, Vol. 5, No. 3, September 1980, pp. 324, 339.

Mercier, Celine, "Intervention in the Psychiatric Hospital in the Era of De-institutionalization," *Canada's Mental Health*, Vol. 34, No. 3, 1986, pp. 13-17.

Motamedi, K., "Adaptability and Copability: A Study of Social Systems, Their Environment, and Survival," *Group and Organization Studies*, Vol. 2, No. 4, December 1977, pp. 480-490.

Papell, C., and Rothman, B., "Group Work's Contribution to a Common Method," *Social Work Practice*, 1966, pp. 32-43.

Rai, G., "Reducing Bureaucratic Inflexibility," *Social Service Review*, March 1983, pp. 44-57.

Ramsay, Richard, "Influencing Political Systems: A Look at the Hospital Structure," *The Social Worker*, Vol. 50, No. 4, Winter 1982, pp. 157-160.

Schilit, Warren and Locke, Edwin, "A Study of Upward Influence in an Organization," *Administrative Science Quarterly*, 27, 1982, pp. 304-316.
Specht, H. and Vickery, A., eds., *Integrating Social Work Methods*, London: George Allen and Unwin, 1977.
Swenson, Carol, "Natural Helping Processes," Doctoral Dissertation, Columbia University School of Social Work, 1983.
Toews, John and Barnes, Gordon, "The Chronic Mental Patient and Community Psychiatry: A System in Trouble," *Canada's Mental Health*, Vol. 34, No. 2, June 1986, pp. 2-7.
Whittaker, James K., "Family Involvement in Residential Treatment: A Support System for Parents," *Department of Health and Human Services Publication No. 81-30308*, April 1981.

Critical Incident Approach

Cohen, A. and Smith, R., "The Critical Incident in Growth Groups: Theory and Technique," La Jolla, Calif.: University Association Incorporated, 1976, pp. 114-134.
Gooderich, D., and Boomer, D., "Some Concepts about Therapeutic Interventions with Hyperaggressive Children," *Exemplars of Social Research*, Fellin, Tripodi and Meyer, eds., Itasca, Ill.: Peacock Publications, 1969, pp. 285-304.
Lang, N., "A Method of Linking Practice Theory with the Actualities of Group Interaction and Worker Intervention in Social Work with Groups." Paper presented at Group Symposium, November 1980.

Papers in This Series

Moore, Edith E., "The Implications of System Network for Social Work with Groups: Literature and Experience," *Social Work with Groups*, Vol. 1, No. 2, Summer 1978, pp. 133-143.
———, "The Group-in-Situation as the Unit of Attention in Social Work with Groups," *Social Work with Groups*, Vol. 6, No. 2, Summer 1983, pp. 19-31.
———, "The Group-in-Organization as the Unit of Attention in Conceptualizing Social Work with Groups," *1983 Symposium Papers*, University of Michigan, Detroit, 1984.
———, "The Group-in-Community as the Unit of Attention in Conceptualizing Social Work with Groups," *Social Work with Groups Annual, 1984*, New York: The Haworth Press, Inc., 1985.
———, "The Member-in-Situation as the Unit of Attention in Conceptualizing Social Work with Groups." Presented at Symposium on Social Work with Groups, Rutgers University, 1985.

Group Work Practice
in Neighborhood Centers Today

John H. Ramey

INTRODUCTION

Much of group work practice originated in the settlements and neighborhood centers through the first half of the twentieth century. Club work, social action and adult education groups were the core community structures through which the people could get involved, provide leadership for and take control of their mostly immigrant or minority, disadvantaged communities.

Group work, along with social action and adult education, dominated neighborhood centers through the mid-sixties. Then with the development of other action strategies, the loss of separate identity for group work within social work, the emphasis on other, individualistic helping strategies and methods, and many other factors, group work lost its centrality and its visibility in the centers and the larger social welfare service community.

But group work is alive in many neighborhood centers throughout the U.S. It is not always conceived of in terms of social work services, nor is it evenly developed. It is a significant part of what many centers are doing today when many of the action strategies of the sixties and seventies have diminished in popularity. The interest here is in the what, why, where and how of group work in neighborhood centers today.

QUESTIONS BEING INVESTIGATED

This paper will emphasize the group work content of neighborhood centers' programs. It is part of a plan for a larger, ongoing study of the services, structures, and other aspects of centers throughout the U.S. and

---

John H. Ramey, ACSW, LISW, is Associate Professor Emeritus of Social Work, Department of Social Work, The University of Akron, Akron, OH 44325-8001.

Canada. In this paper we will focus on developing the group work themes for the study.

At the most general level, the inquiry was directed toward finding out if group work still exists in centers, and, if so, to what extent, in what forms and whether it is a central or peripheral function of the centers.

The inquiry has sought information more specifically on several subsidiary and supportive areas of concern. First, there was a methodological and content interest in the extent to which the respondents are knowledgeable about group work in other centers in their cities and elsewhere. Second, a line of questioning concerned the populations being served, the settings in which groups are meeting, and the activities (the program content) of the groups. Third, the inquiry focused on the purposes for the centers' work with groups, the models and styles of group work, and the extent to which groups are seen as a means of developing indigenous leadership for social concerns. Fourth, questions were asked about staffing patterns, undergraduate and graduate education for group work in centers, involvement of volunteers in worker roles, involvement of students in training, and the development of in-service and other training workshops. Fifth, information was gathered about funding patterns and other sources of support. Sixth, there is the concern about formal research and evaluation of the effectiveness of group work within centers. Finally, statements were solicited about specific problems encountered and recommendations.

These questions were explored in order that we might assist professionals involved with social work with groups in understanding and contributing once again to neighborhood centers and to having the center movement once again firmly ally itself with social work with groups.

GENERAL BACKGROUND OF THE STUDY

Not since Arthur Hillman's *Neighborhood Centers Today* (1960) has there been a major study of the exact characteristics and dimensions of the neighborhood center movement in North America. St. Clair Drake (1966) explored center work in race relations. Street gang and other aspects of the work were described in national publications. In the intervening years Chambers (1963), Reid (1981), Davis (1967), Hall (1971), Berry (1986), Trolander (1987) and others have all written primarily from a historical perspective.

In her conclusion Trolander (1987) provides a summary of the various influences which in her opinion have changed the "settlements" into "neighborhood centers" and altered their character. She has concluded there is a somewhat distant relationship between the social work profession and settlements and suggests that, as they are early now in their second century, the settlements might well be given recognition and help by the social work profession which they helped create. We hope that this exploratory study will help give some direction to one of the ways in which social work may once again become central to the functioning of neighborhood centers, that is through the further development of group work services with the utilization of social workers with appropriate education and experience in group work.

METHODOLOGY

A complete survey of all centers has not been undertaken for this report. The method of gathering data has been the interview with key informants throughout the country. The writer has used personal contacts and the leads provided by these contacts along with key persons listed in the literature. In some cases the interviews were in person at the centers. In other cases they were telephone interviews. Written materials provided by the centers have also been used. The key themes and general nature of the conclusions were confirmed by the developing similarity of responses as the inquiry progressed. Current published literature and other information resources have been surveyed.

FINDINGS: DESCRIPTIONS OF THE VARIOUS KINDS AND DIMENSIONS OF GROUP WORK FOUND TO DATE IN THE SURVEY

The findings of this survey will be described by quoting, paraphrasing and summarizing the responses which were obtained from interviews in relation to each of the areas of questioning outlined above and by generalizing and drawing conclusions from them.

The most general conclusions need to be stated first. First is that in relation to any of our questions, responses were widely divergent. Second, in spite of much opinion to the contrary, group work is an integral part of the operations of many if not most neighborhood centers today.

Does Group Work Still Exist and, If So, How Much and Where?

When asked "How much group work is taking place in your center," responses ranged from "Don't I wish?" (meaning "nothing,"), and "not much going on as we knew it," through "it very much depends on the programs," to "still very much involved with groups, absolutely not dead." One executive said "As close to real group work as one can come, we're doing it." Another said "Very much (group work is going on.) Group work is absolutely vital if one is prepared to deal with the consequences of people and groups working out their own destinies. If not, leave it alone. The profound consequences must be dealt with."

Regarding the concern about the extent to which the respondents would be knowledgeable about group work in other centers in their cities and elsewhere, there was a wide range of responses. As one would expect, most were reasonably familiar with other centers in their cities but less familiar with the nature of group work in centers elsewhere. Several, however, could really only speak about their own centers. This appears to be related to the extent to which the highly decentralized and independent, often isolated centers no longer come together regularly through their federations in contrast to other more centralized systems such as the mental health centers. This really is the genesis of our concern about the extent of sharing of knowledge, and will be a theme to be discussed later.

Information shared by the majority about what was happening elsewhere included the idea that group work practice was "spotty," or that "there are still groups, but very few trained people working with them." Another executive (same large midwestern city) said that many agencies were still involved, that some were specialized, but that there was much ferment in neighborhood centers to develop new ways of working with their communities. One worker was providing consultation for the development of a center in another city and including group work as a central focus. One worker stated what it appears most would agree on, that "Informal group-work-as-recreation is very much diminished in emphasis."

Populations Being Served, Settings, and Activities

As one might expect there was a wide range of populations being served, settings in which groups were meeting, and activities as the program content of the groups. There were groups of all ages. Most were specialized. Teen drop-in centers, which might look traditional and generalized, were focused on helping teens with their transitions, the "passages," or their specific problems. Children's groups were no longer after school in one center, but held in the school for those children who were referred by the school or other agencies. Substance abuse groups for teens were common, in one case supported by contract with the court. For young parents there were groups serving educational and mutual support needs. Children's day care has been paralleled by adult day care in recent years. There are groups for helping children do their homework. One center says that while "there are no gangs in the area," they "work with groups in difficulty." The center is "noted for it." There are many activity, support and educational groups for the elderly.

Among the innovations and adaptations to the times, one center had developed an AIDS support group, another had groups for those with dual diagnosis of mental illness and mental retardation, and another a support group for handicapped residents of a housing project.

Most of the groups met in agency facilities, but others met in school during class time, in churches, or other community facilities. Several centers still operated resident or day camps.

Purposes, Models, Leadership Development

There were some very interesting and informative responses when the inquiry focused on the purposes for the centers' work with groups, the models and styles of group work, and the extent to which groups were seen as a means of developing indigenous leadership for social concerns.

On one level centers were responding to the United Way service profiles as a means of securing funding. Groups were viewed as personal services and defined as "group social development" which had a low priority rating, or "group social adjustment" which had a high priority rating. The impact of these service profiles is to focus the work of centers toward impacting, changing individuals within a group context while ignoring the importance of the group as a unit of society and its functions in relation to empowerment and social change. This has profound implications in relation to the central purposes of neighborhood centers and will be discussed below.

Another center was very clear that group work was vital and central. The groups were organized around problems confronted in various life stages, the challenges of transitions for pre-school children, for teens and for young adults. These were termed "transaction groups." This appeared to be a highly coherent approach and program.

In another center it was stated that there was no consensus within the staff on any particular model. "Practice varies with who does it." But groups were still seen as the central theme of the center's program orientation.

A similar response from another center indicated that groups were mostly developmental, but some were therapeutic. There is a psychologist on this center's staff. Thus there were many referrals to the center whose participants included neglected children and youth. Still it was suggested that the inquiry about a model of group practice be directed to the program director and in a general summation it was expressed that the model used by a particular worker depends on worker training and experience.

One center director stated that money was coming through mental health channels to provide prevention services. The model therefore was mental health prevention even though group workers knew what that was and were doing it long ago before the term was invented.

It was clear to most that the traditional service of informal group work as recreation is considerably diminished in emphasis. One director spoke of problem-oriented groups combined with individual counseling. There is no loner any "club" program. The one or two afternoon or evening drop-in programs were carefully staffed with MSW group workers and oriented toward children and teens with known problems.

One center was actively concerned about finding and developing new models of community practice. The assessment by this director was that "we are dealing with a new reality in the waning years of this century and the old ways just don't really help any longer."

Groups in relation to community organization efforts were mentioned. One center spoke of neighborhood groups with community organization workers. Another stated that community organization was on the decline. Yet another stated that there was some serious political action group activity.

In relation to the related issue of development of community leadership for social issues, there was a wide range of orientations. One center emphasized community leadership training with a focus on youth. Another said there was no work on leadership development although some adult groups were organized around a self-help model. One center's workshop trainer had on the same day of our inquiry been trying to help staff understand the need for and the benefits of leadership development among teens. In another center however the generalization was made that "really the professionals provide the leadership; there is no real client participation." The only leadership development was a senior citizens' executive committee.

What is obvious here is that while there are groups in centers, there is no coherent model, theme or direction among centers, or often even within individual centers. Thirty of more years ago, while there were differences among group workers in centers, at least there was an attempt to develop, apply and test various theoretical perspectives and models, and to share such information and skills.

Staffing Patterns, Education, Training, Students, and Volunteers

Staffing patterns showed a similar wide range of responses. As reported above, one center employed only staff with MSWs or Masters in Special Education. In other centers a more usual response was that MSWs are the executives or, at best, head up program units. There were several center camps with MSW's as director. One executive was looking for a program director but had little hope that anyone with an MSW would be found. The day of our inquiry one large urban center had a new program director who had a Bachelor of Education degree. All staff under that person's supervision were described as paraprofessionals, though one person had a BSW.

In one large program there were only three full-time group workers. The rest of the staff were students from two nearby theological seminaries. Another had ten full-time group work staff, all licensed by the state and with BSWs from a large, local, combined BSW-MSW-PhD granting School of Social Work, even though there was no specific group work education there. The center took it upon itself to provide the necessary additional training. The center executive and the program director had MSW degrees. There was one student in field placement. The director stated that "we don't hire MSW's; the salaries are not all that great. They don't want to work until 9:30 every evening, and they resign too soon."

One executive stated that while there are still groups, there are few trained people and few of the trainers are even trained. Another stated plaintively "There are jobs. Why doesn't the School of Social Work prepare people for them?"

In general the prospect of professional education for group work in centers was the least encouraging facet of this inquiry. Typically, the response was that the school is clinically oriented, that group work faculty are retiring and not being replaced, that where there are group work faculty they are not teaching group work, that there is no group work sequence, and that there are no students in field placements. One executive talked with the dean of the school of which the person was an alumnus about the state of group work education and was simply asked to write a letter. The dean wasn't really interested. In one school it was stated that the only experienced group work instructor is "off the wall, abstract and clinical!" Fortunately at the other end of the spectrum, there were some areas in which there were still students graduating with specific preparation for group work in centers.

As reported above, students in centers were often not social work, let alone group work oriented. One center had many seminary students. Another had a group work student from Germany for a year. One person sadly reported that MSW students had been placed in a center by group work faculty and had to be removed after six weeks because supervision was difficult and experience meager.

Some centers did have group work as well as community organization and administration students. One center encouraged teens who grew up in the center to work there and eventually go on to graduate school in social work. Many had at one time been in the traditional role of junior counselors in the center's day camp.

There seemed to be few attempts at in-depth group work training for staff. As mentioned above, at least one opinion was that few of the trainers were trained. One organized training program was for the paraprofessional staff. One center took many teens to a resident camp for six weeks each summer to help develop, increase and reward skills. One worker experienced with such populations was skeptical about the possibilities of training many indigenous workers and stated "The old settlement workers brought a value system where it didn't exist. It is difficult to train indigenous workers to shake their roots and identify with this value system."

Most centers used volunteers to work with groups, but not all. Often they seemed to be extra hands to fill in for short resources. For some there were minimally organized programs for their use. In contrast however, were those centers who specifically involved their teen members as volunteers in the center and in camps. One center mentioned VISTA workers with street people, in night and in day shelters.

It is clear that the area of professional social work education and staff training for group work needs attention. It also appears that the disappearance of group work or its frequent transformation into a purely clinical mode in social work education has contributed to the inability of centers to find staff and support group work services.

Funding

Information was gathered about funding patterns and other sources of support. Various strategies and sources were used for funding group services. What the funding sources and other providers of resources are willing to fund is the major determinant of what centers can do. There is a wide range of options.

Obviously the major primary sources are the United Ways. In recent years United Ways, following more and more sophisticated and technocratic social planning models, have developed profiles for each funded service and prioritized these in various ways. One such priority system provides the following ratings for various services for needs which might be met by group services:

Group I   Crime Prevention
                Alcohol and Drug Prevention

Group II   Group Social Adjustment
                School Age Parents

Group III Special Care for Developmentally Disabled
                Neighborhood Organization and Development
                Communicatively Impaired
                Residential Services
                Intergroup Relations

Group IV Group Social Development
                Volunteer Services
                Adult Day Care
                Immigration and Cultural Transition Services
                Health and Physical Education

Unfortunately none were in the very low priority "Group IV." Two in "Group III" priority, but not currently funded by the local United Way, were Mental Health Services and Services for the Blind. In general it is that, with the only obvious exceptions being "Neighborhood Organization . . ." and "Intergroup Relations," these are primarily conceived of as personal and individual or family oriented social services. It would appear that group workers would have to be very creative to conceive and carry out programs which would be funded under some of these categories. In any case, to be funded a service has to fit a category, and the low priority categories tend to have funding reduced in successive years while the higher priorities have increased funding.

The ten agencies providing "Group Social Development," including two with "Youth Development Group services," were faced with the prospects of declining funding. If the services could be recast as "Group Social Adjustment," future funding might increase—if the priorities did not change in successive years. Two of the critical factors rated in the priorities system include "Significance/Importance of the Problem" and "Population at Risk/Who is Affected."

There was concern in one city that the United Way was currently planning to reduce the funds allocated for group services to one center. In another city a center was consistently receiving ten to twelve percent increases per year from the United Way.

One center was obviously very successful in developing the rationale for Mental Health Board funding for the over a half million dollars in funding for group services, with the prospects increasing every year. This center, as quoted above, says that "money is coming into group services for prevention. We knew what it was long before the term was invented."

A second center, as also mentioned above, has received a major grant from the state for work with children at high risk. It had to compete with other major agencies of family service and mental health traditions for this grant.

Another program for families and adults was developed from Title XX contracts and is now funded by the county children's services.

The executive director of one center is on city council, a position which allows the concerns of the center to be expressed in public policy decisions as well as its needs to be recognized by various funding sources.

Finally, one center is seeking foundation funding for a major development grant for group services. It should be recognized that in some large cities centers are to a great extent responsible for raising their own funds, while in others they are dependent on central fund raising and allocating organizations. Obviously the former are more free to interpret needs and services to their own supporting constituencies, while the latter must conform to the expections of the third party payors for the services. The latter are usually either directly or indirectly various Federal government agencies, with other state and local funds added in along the way.

Research and Evaluation

Related to the area of funding support is the concern about formal research and evaluation of the effectiveness of group work within centers. The lack of adequate general research support or specific program evaluation is often the stated rationale for not supporting or reducing the support for group services by United Ways, foundations, and government agencies.

Perhaps one telling fact is that very few centers reported doing any formal research or evaluation on group services. One reported "we have good output measures," and its continuing increased funding provides some evidence of the importance of this area of concern.

A search of a local United Way library did not reveal any reports on current research or evaluation projects related to group services in neighborhood centers.

Problems and Recommendations

Workers voiced a variety of specific problems encountered and recommendations to improve the support of group work in neighborhood centers.

Most significant was the paucity of documentation by the centers of the validity of group work, particularly in the academic and general presses and professional journals. A paper presented by this writer at the second Symposium (Ramey, 1986) discussed the need for evaluative procedures for group work. In general it does not appear that the situation has improved significantly in the intervening seven years.

Perhaps most pervasive was the belief that social work education was not preparing students for or encouraging them to practice group work in neighborhood centers. There seemed to be general lack of trained and sophisticated group work staff as well as a lack of graduate or undergraduate group work staff as well as a lack of graduate or undergraduate students in field placement. Some good graduate programs in group work still exist but many of the formerly strong ones are defunct or considerably weakened. The need for a training center was voiced several times.

Another group of observations included the fact that there seemed to be very few inspirational leaders in the centers. Executives are mostly careful, professional administrators. The centers seem to be very diverse, each one an island unto itself. In large cities the centers are not really of as great importance in the overall service delivery picture as they were historically. They are not on the center-stage as they were in the past. There are many other private and public programs, other community based agencies with greater access to public funding. Thus there is no core group of neighborhood residents who identify with the center and support it as in the past. One must also observe the general impermanence, physical disruption and disintegration of many of the neighborhoods served by the centers.

It appeared to one person that no real practice issues were discussed at meetings of the United Neighborhood Centers of America (UNCA). Why does a center develop groups? How do you do it? What do you do with different groups of people and different kinds of groups? How do you develop self determination? What is the philosophical basis of neighborhood center work with groups?

SUMMARY, CONCLUSIONS, QUESTIONS AND PLANS
FOR FURTHER INVESTIGATION

In general, the original hypothesis of this investigation has been confirmed. Group work is still practiced in various forms in neighborhood centers throughout the U.S. But it is just one professional intervention mode available among the various specialized services offered by centers. The centers seem to have become, as Trolander (1987) suggests, one type of agency among many. In line with Sosin's (1987) analysis, each center seems to have selected a mix of service strategies which provide for survival within its "niche" in its environment. Instead of the settlement movement, the agencies have become "multi-service centers" as Helen Harris Perlman projected many years ago. And group work in various forms and purposes is one of those services rather than part of the centerpiece of a social movement. Even so, group work is alive and we should nurture it.

One may conclude that the group work services of centers are not well documented, analyzed and evaluated in line with current professional practice. Nor, as a consequence, is information about group work services in centers written about, published or shared to any great extent. As Trolander (1987) observed, "printed primary sources . . . are quite meager since World War II," and even "secondary sources for the recent decades are almost non-existent" (243). Moreover there appears to be little academic investigation or research on the current functioning of neighborhood centers in regard to group work or any other mode of service. This lack of internal and external professional and academic communication about group work and other services of centers is debilitating. It is still true that knowledge must be certified by academic networks and published to have any real lasting or general impact. Thus, as this writer (Ramey, 1986) advocated for all group work services, research and validating strategies need to be developed. These must result in publication for the profession and for the general, supporting public.

Finally, the shift away from professional preparation for social work with groups in neighborhood centers has resulted in deficits of personnel, knowledge and skill. The lack of general theoretical perspectives or models is in part a reflection of the lack of social workers in supervisory and direct service positions and the general withdrawal of graduate and undergraduate education from considering work in neighborhood centers as a valid context for social work practice. A considerable effort needs to be made to convince graduate schools to reintroduce specific group work and neighborhood center concepts into curriculum, to do research and evaluation, to use centers for field placements, and to encourage graduates to seek professional employment in and commitment to centers.

One encouraging note is that the United Neighborhood Centers of America is in the process of bringing out a new professional periodical, "The Neighborhood Centers and Community-Based Services Journal," scheduled to begin publication in the near future. This should help fill the internal communication void. One would hope for some articles on group work in centers to appear therein. The development of a formal affiliation between UNCA and the Association for the Advancement of Social Work with Groups is also a development which should bring access to research and personnel for group work in neighborhood centers.

The investigation initiated with this paper is intended to be part of an effort to fill at least some of the void. Work is beginning to continue gathering material from the United States, to expand to include Canada and perhaps other nations, and to further document and publish on a broader scale exactly what settlements and neighborhood centers are doing at this point in history and what they project doing in the near future.

Groups are the basic units of social functioning. They are the units in which people, when they reach beyond the family, create and shape the nature of the society in which they live. We all must learn through experience how to participate most effectively in group life and to focus groups on the issues and activities which are of importance to us. People in the communities served by neighborhood centers generally have little other opportunity to develop the skills and experience necessary to fully participate in their communities through their membership in meaningful groups. Nor do they often have other opportunities to focus on and learn about issues and problems from the unique perspective and value base of the neighborhood center. One can be hopeful that social work and the centers will again work together to bring the residents of their neighborhoods into the mainstream of community life through participation in carefully developed groups in neighborhood centers throughout the United States. It is hoped as well that this exploratory study will help lead the way to this renaissance of group work.

REFERENCES

Berry, Margaret E. "One Hundred Years on Urban Frontiers: The Settlement Movement 1886-1986." Washington, D.C. 1986, United Neighborhood Centers of America.

Chambers, Clarke A. *Seedtime of Reform: American Social Service and Social Action: 1918-1933.* Minneapolis 1963, University of Minnesota Press.

Davis, Allen F. *Spearheads for Reform: The Social Settlements and the Progressive Movement: 1894-1914.* New York 1967, Oxford University Press.

Drake, St. Clair. *Race Relations in a Time of Rapid Social Change: Report of a Survey.* New York 1966, National Federation of Settlements and Neighborhood Centers.

Hall, Helen. *Unfinished Business in Neighborhood and Nation.* New York 1971, The MacMillan Company.

Hillman, Arthur. *Neighborhood Centers Today: Action Programs for a Rapidly Changing World.* New York 1960, National Federation of Settlements and Neighborhood Centers.

Ramey, John H. "Evaluation and Multi-Level Validation of Group Services: A Brief Review of Requirements, Problems, Options and a Proposal." in *Group Workers at Work; Theory and Practice in the 80's,* Paul H. Glasser and Nazneen S. Mayadas, Eds. Totowa, New Jersey 1986, Rowman & Littlefield, Publishers. Pp. 265-274.

Reid, Kenneth E. *From Character Building to Social Treatment: The History of the Use of Groups in Social Work.* Westport, Connecticut 1981, The Greenwood Press.

Sosin, Michael. "Private Social Agencies: Auspices, Sources of Funds, and Problems Covered," *Social Work Research and Abstracts,* Vol. 23, #2, Summer 1987, pp. 21-27.

Trolander, Judith Ann. *Professionalism and Social Change: From the Settlement House Movement to Neighborhood Centers.* New York 1987, Columbia University Press.

Wilson, Gertrude, and Gladys Ryland. *Social Group Work Practice.* Cambridge 1949, Houghton Mifflin Company.

Supportive Group Services in the Workplace: The Practice and the Potential

Nina Wegener

INTRODUCTION: WORK

Most employed adults spend more time at work and in work related activities than they do in any other activity, including sleeping.[1] How does this affect the individual?

Freud maintained that work has a greater effect than any other technique of living in providing the individual with a secure attachment to reality.[2] Through work, an individual is linked to a social network. The financial and emotional rewards of work provide a sense of having an impact on one's environment, and contribute to a person's self-esteem and self-worth.[3]

In contrast to such depictions of work as a positive factor in a person's life, a Health, Education and Welfare task force reported that for only a small fraction of workers does work provide the satisfaction that comes from a sense of achievement, accomplishment, and responsibility.[4] In fact, Freud notwithstanding, the report portrayed alienation as a major problem among workers, citing evidence linking such mental health problems as anxiety, worry, tension, and impaired interpersonal relationships with job dissatisfaction. And such work experiences as job insecurity, unpleasant working conditions, and hazardous tasks may lead to alcoholism, drug abuse, and suicide.[5]

At the same time, a person's life circumstances outside of work undeniably affect his or her work situation. Increased professional interest in this area has generated research which unsurprisingly reveals that developmental stages in a person's life — such as marriage, the birth and parenting

---

Nina Wegener, PhD, Teaneck, NJ.

207

of a child, caring for an elderly parent, and preparing for retirement — affect an individual's work.[6]

Whether work is the positive component in a person's life described by Freud, or a "violence — to the spirit as well as to the body" inflicting a "daily humiliation"[7] on the individual, the social work profession cannot ignore work's power to affect the individual's total life situation. Although in the 1950s and 1960s social work writers such as Bertha Reynolds and Helen Harris Perlman[8] acknowledged the influence of work on an individual's life situation (and, conversely, the impact a person's life situation can have on his or her work), it was not until recently that the social work profession recognized the workplace as a viable agency for intervention. Likewise, only recently have business, industry, and labor unions begun to concern themselves with the worker as a total person, rather than solely as a means of production.[9]

Against this background, the industrial social worker has assumed an increasingly active role as advocate, labor negotiator, clinician, educator and community liaison and organizer. Yet, despite the seemingly versatile role of the industrial social worker, the literature attests that the treatment modality, in both unions and management (with the exception of training groups or seminars and workshops which address groups in a lecture format) consistently has been individual casework.[10]

As this paper will demonstrate, through a review of related literature and through a discussion of interviews held with practitioners in the field, the needs of workers can be effectively met, and their lives enhanced, through a supportive group modality: the workplace is an appropriate (though not necessarily congenial) environment for the formation of support groups. The following delineation and examination of factors which may contribute to the success or failure of a support group serving the working population, is intended to provide industrial social workers with guideposts and encouragement for establishing supportive group services as an integral and valued part of employee or member assistance programs.

PRESENTATION OF DATA AND LITERATURE REVIEW

Literature relevant to serving the working population is plentiful. Specific topics include treating the working alcoholic, ethical dilemmas of the industrial social worker, points of intervention for the social worker, and meeting the needs of specific populations of workers. Because of the pioneering nature of industrial social work, the literature abounds with possibilities existing for the industrial worker in this burgeoning field.

It is therefore surprising that supportive group services are rarely mentioned in the literature as a feasible modality for serving the worker. A similar blind spot exists in group work literature, which seems to ignore the needs of a functional, working population.[11] The paucity of literature is not indicative of service provision in the world of work, but, in part, reflects a time lag between current literature and current practice: Industrial social workers *are* using the group modality – and using it successfully – with the working population.

The data presented in this paper consists of interviews with five practitioners in the world of work. Two of them direct Employee Assistance Programs (EAP's) in large hospitals, two work in union-based Members' Assistance Programs (MAP's), and one is the director of an EAP at a large metropolitan college. The experience of the practitioners will be discussed within the context of relevant literature.

PRE-GROUP PLANNING: INFLUENTIAL FACTORS

Providing supportive group service in an industrial setting requires extensive and careful pre-group planning. The first step in this planning should be an examination of such factors as: the attributes and needs of the working population in general; the demographics of the specific population to be served; the influence exerted by the host agency; the orientation and staffing of the program; and the group leader's interests, needs and capabilities. Following this initial planning is the next stage: determination of the group's purpose, type of group (e.g., long-term or time-limited, open or closed, etc.), outreach methodology, and the leader's role in the group. In the following section the influence of these factors will be explored in detail.

The Working Population: Needs and Attributes

A worker's most basic need is to work. Work, or the lack of it, affects all aspects of a person's life.[12] Applying Maslow's need theory to employment, a worker's needs can be categorized into two groups:[13]

1. Life maintenance needs (such as safety, freedom from hunger, etc.)
2. Human growth needs (such as achievement, responsibility, and power). These needs relate directly to the individual's opportunity to attain love, self-esteem. and self-actualization.

If the first level of needs is not met, the individual's growth toward self-actualization will be stunted. Dysfunctions at this level implicate the need for casework intervention with the provision of concrete services. In the era of Reaganomics, the ranks of the underemployed have swelled and the need for this type of service—linking the working individual with social welfare resources—is increasing.

As Martha Ozawa notes, workers are no longer satisfied with an unequal relationship with their employer. She observes that workers want to be viewed as total persons, not merely as "economic tools."[14] But workers' needs for self-esteem and self-actualization are not being fulfilled at the workplace. Schwartz refers to this as a "symbiotic diffusion."[15] Although it is not openly acknowledged, the employer needs the employee as much as the employee needs the employer (this symbiotic relationship is directly expressed through the worker's most powerful tool—the strike).

Symbiotic diffusion in the workplace may create or exacerbate mental health problems, alcoholism, or other substance abuse. And the worker suffering from mental health or substance abuse problems is generally estranged from helping systems. The working class population is largely neglected by existing social services. If individuals are able to hold a job, they are generally considered functional; it is the dysfunctional individual who is serviced by agencies. Furthermore, working class people are often caught in the bind of earning too much to be able to use public services, while being unable to afford services in the private sector. As a consequence, their mental health needs go unmet, and the worker experiencing mental problems may be forced to reach the dysfunctional stage before being able to obtain help.

Bargal depicts the worker needing help as a normal adult temporarily in need of support. He suggests that a financial or developmental crisis, such as marriage, birth, or divorce, and the stresses attached to these life events, may have a negative impact on the worker's employment.[16] Kurzman and Akabas similarly intimate that problems which do not immediately endanger job performance, such as the child-care needs of single-parent families or families in which both parents work, may ultimately jeopardize the individual's job.[17]

It is the attribute of the worker as a functional, self-sufficient individual which constitutes one of the major impediments to the development of group services. Workers have traditionally underutilized social services, not only because of their incompatibility with their life-style, but also because of the values held by workers which relate to self-sufficiency. While a worker experiencing a crisis may seek help in the form of casework services—often concrete services—from the EAP or MAP, it may be difficult for that same worker to imagine that he or she could benefit from a group experience. And society's and the social service agency's view of the worker as a functional individual and consequently outside the parameters of the "helping" system mirrors the worker's self-perception.

Another obstacle to the development of group services is the nature of the workplace as a competitive sphere. Collaborative group efforts may seem alien in this environment.

It is also important to bear in mind the changing demographics of the working population. The rapidly increasing number of women in the labor force has created numerous demands and needs. The changing role of women (and thereby men, as well) creates stresses within the family. In the dual-career family, separate jobs may cause conflict within the job situation (for example, if one spouse is transferred to another location) or within the home (who is responsible for housework; how are chores to be divided?, etc.). Upon entering the work force, married women with small children have their attention divided between work and home; changes in role and status will occur. In addition, high divorce rate and the subsequent entrance into the workplace of displaced housewives or single parents also implicates a need for supportive services. In increasing numbers, women are dissatisfied with the financial status of traditional "women's work" and are entering such non-traditional jobs as fire-fighting, auto repair, telephone line work, etc. Here, too, the changing status and changing role of women creates a stressful situation which may be played out at work or at home.

Assessing the Specific Population

After looking at the needs and attributes of the working population in general, it is necessary to focus on the specific population served by the EAP or MAP, looking at age, gender, socio-economic status, job categories and needs specific to the working population served. Each of these factors will influence the determination of purpose and type of group, and will affect the success or failure of a small group. For example, as a result of differential gender socialization, women in the workforce are more likely to recognize an existing problem, and to seek help.[18] Women will also more readily join groups and share personal experiences. In each of the five work settings served by the practitioners interviewed in the preparation of this paper, women constituted a majority of the working population and, with the exception of alcoholism recovery groups (which were male dominated), the participants in the groups were overwhelmingly female.

Socio-economic status is also a determining factor in group success.

Although the population served by hospital EAPs comprises professionals, clericals, secretaries and custodials, at the observed institution only the clericals and secretaries attended small group sessions. A similar situation existed at the college EAP; only clericals and secretaries participated in the group services of the EAP, whereas the utilization of casework services was more representative of the entire working population (professionals, clericals, secretaries, and custodians).

A partial explanation may be that blue collar workers, or workers in the lower socio-economic status are not as socialized to the group process as are middle-class workers. But probing more extensively into the work and life situation of this specific population may reveal other factors prohibiting these workers' participation in small groups. At the college EAP, for example, it was discovered that the timing of the group sessions (sessions were held from twelve o'clock to one, and from one o'clock to two—traditional lunch hours) did not coincide with the work schedule of custodians, who are allowed only a half hour lunch period from eleven o'clock to eleven-thirty. Also, outreach flyers for the groups at the college were printed only in English; a majority of the custodial workers spoke only Spanish. In order to accommodate the needs of those workers, group sessions were held after their shift ended, and were run by a bilingual social worker.

The Host Agency

One of the most influential factors contributing to the successful development of group services is the existence of a program as a part of the host agency. Sanction from the host—not just to exist, but to provide the services one chooses—is essential.

In a clinical setting such as a hospital, both management and staff are acculturated to treatment modalities which may include group treatment. Organizational resistance to innovative service provision in such a setting may be minimal. Conversely, social work practice in a union or corporate setting fundamentally involves practice in a non-human-service host setting, a setting which may be suspicious of group-work efforts.

The social worker in such a setting must always be systems-oriented, i.e., aware of the larger system into which one group or program fits. A union, for example, is inherently political and, like a corporation, has a defined power structure. Despite the seemingly hospitable setting of a labor union for group work, the power base of a union, like that of a corporation, may view the formation of small groups as threatening. Corporate management may view the social worker as tampering with industry's organizational make-up and conditions. The union may likewise be wary of the social worker's efforts to "treat" the work environment.[19]

Since the EAP or MAP exists as a tenuous and peripheral service in these host settings, the social workers in the program will need to work towards gaining institutional sanction. This may mean offering services to employees or members which will tangibly benefit the parent organization. Therefore, the social worker seeking to form groups in a union-based MAP may have to pick and choose those issues with which the union feels most comfortable. For example, groups which relate to work and work transitions (e.g., pre-retirement) may be the easiest to form, at least initially. It might also be desireable to involve union officials in the planning stage.

The Structure of the Program

Whether a program is well-established and known throughout the working population will affect the social worker's ability to form groups. For example, it may be premature to offer group services before a program is firmly settled in the host agency. Members or employees who have used the casework services of the program, and have developed trust in the program, may be more likely to join a group.

Other factors within the program to consider include: staffing (is there sufficient staff to devote the time necessary to group formation?); program policy, (for example, a program designed to provide in-house counseling may be more amenable to providing supportive group services than a program structured for needs assessment and referral).

Location especially was found to be a crucial factor both in establishing a group and maintaining it. If a group is held on the worksite, the union MAP is entering the employer's turf and may be interfering with the employer's view of its right to space; likewise, if the group is held in union space, the group leader may have to justify the use of that space to the political base of the union.

Furthermore, although a worksite location addresses a pragmatic need, it may exacerbate confidentiality concerns of workers. A "neutral" location, close to the worksite would be ideal. For example, a hospital EAP held group sessions in an office building owned by the hospital and physically very close to it. Such a location addressed both the confidentiality and practical concerns of involved workers.

Group Leader Characteristics

Finally, in the initial pre-group planning stage, the social worker who is anticipating forming and running the group will need to look at his or her own needs, interests, skills, and capabilities. Providing group work services requires a great deal of time, effort, and persistence. Time and effort are required for formulating a plan and choosing and designating an appropriate outreach. Dogged persistence is required initially, to overcome resistance to group formation both within the agency and among workers, and secondarily to sustain the group. Confronting these obstacles may tax the social worker's initiative and patience. The social worker must honestly assess his or her ability to persist despite repeated failure.

A group which develops out of the social worker's own needs or interests may help assist him or her to persist. For example, at a hospital EAP, two social workers who had recently returned to work after maternity leave formed a group for new mothers returning to work. Their personal investment and enthusiasm for this issue sustained them throughout the planning stage.

OUTREACH

The initial planning stage is essential for determining the type of outreach to be done for the group. In a union-based program, where the host may be suspicious, groups frequently form from seminars or workshops organized around issues such as working and parenting or pre-retirement. Participants in the workshop are asked if they would be interested in forming a time-limited group to discuss the issue further. The social workers in the program can then go to the union saying, "The members want this," rather than saying, "*We* want to do this." If the program is well-integrated into the host agency, social workers will be able to use the host structure for outreach. For example, a hospital-based EAP uses the hospital newspaper, which is well-read by the employees, to publicize its groups.

Another form outreach may take is case-finding. At a union, several social workers were working individually with members whose job jeopardy stemmed from the difficulty of being a single parent. Through case-finding, a time-limited group for single parents was formed.

Unless outreach is done through case-finding, it is very important not to present the group as problem-focused. Each of the interviewees cited examples of groups that were not subscribed to because of threatening or stigmatizing factors.

The flyer advertising one ill-fated group, for example, urged employees to "come and share your experiences and feelings." Groups are typically associated with therapy. The invitation to "share feelings" reinforces this perception. Consequently, workers, viewing themselves as functional individuals outside the realm of human services, may reject this invitation as not pertinent to their situation and threatening to their self-perception.

Another group designed to meet the needs of recently divorced employees likewise was not subscribed to. It was felt, in hindsight, that although divorce is common, the stigma attached to being a divorcee nevertheless remains, and workers may be reluctant to discuss the issue within the sensitive workplace setting.

RESISTANCE

Individual resistance to group formation may stem from factors other than stigmatizing factors associated with an employee's situation. One potential obstacle to group formation which must be considered in the planning stage is the issue of confidentiality. In forming groups with workers consideration of this issue is crucial. The largest threat to confidentiality comes not from professionals or management but from other workers.[20] Given the long hours spent in the company of other workers, and the ties which may develop, it is understandable — and to be expected — that casual remarks which unintentionally disclose information will be made. The professional must be prepared to confront the issue directly with group members, defining, with the members, explicit rules for group conduct.

While confidentiality concerns may pose a major hindrance to group formation, the informal alliances formed among workers may assist the social worker in overcoming this obstacle in the formative phase. For example, one of the interviewers noted that even in seminars presented in a fairly didactic style, participants raised personal issues. In this instance, it may be attributed to the population participating in the group sessions — secretarial and clerical staff comprised of middle-aged women who had been working together for a long time. Participants often brought co-workers and friends from the same department in which they worked. Since there were few secrets kept from one another, the groups were marked by open sharing of personal concerns. The social worker forming a group could draw upon the relationship developed among workers by suggesting in the outreach phase that potential group members bring friends.

Another source of individual resistance may stem from a misunderstanding about the nature of the service. In industrial social work, clarification of purpose is especially critical since the worker may not perceive a need. It is essential that the professional be clear about the function and the purpose of the group, and that he or she disarm some initial resistance by addressing this issue directly, asking members if they have questions or concerns about the group.

CATEGORIES OF GROUPS

Having considered the profile of a worker and the related elements impacting upon supportive group formation among a working population, one can begin to formulate specific types of groups which can provide a meaningful and relevant experience for the worker as well as meet some measure of success. Three categories of groups will be discussed here:

1. Groups formed to meet developmental needs.
2. Groups formed in response to work-related needs.
3. Treatment groups.

Groups Formed to Meet Developmental Needs

Groups within this category directly address the worker as a total person with personal and family needs outside the sphere of work. The value of groups in this category is that they legitimize topics which people might treat as private dilemmas not requiring or deserving of professional help.

With the exception of one hospital based EAP, each of the interviewees had attempted to form groups around such developmental issues as working parents, parenting an adolescent, adult children of the elderly, pre-retirement, and women living alone in their fifties and sixties. These groups frequently formed out of seminars or workshops and often sustained the educational component by integrating it with the supportive group modality. This was done by occasionally providing speakers for the group.

The more successful groups in this category were those which were the least problem-focused. For example, in each of the settings the most popular group proved to be one formed for working parents. By contrast, one of the more difficult groups to form and maintain was designed to meet the needs of adult children caring for their elderly parents. While working parents will experience joys from their situation which may offset the stress inherent in their dual commitment, adult children caring for their elderly parents do not share that balance.

Although an assessment of the population served may indicate a need for a support group for adults caring for elderly relatives, formation of such a group may be difficult. The social worker attempting to form such a group should be sensitive to the resistance of workers to join problem-focused groups and design outreach accordingly.

Groups Formed in Response to Work-Related Needs

If a unit in the work organization has a specific need that is work-related, the organization may contract with the EAP or MAP to provide a group service to address that particular problem. Groups in this category similarly legitimize problems of workers, but the identifiable problem is located within the work sphere rather than within the personal life of the worker. The group work service offered is not a frill or an option; it is provided on work-time for all of the workers affected by the defined problem. Two interviewees had conducted groups in this category.

At one of the hospital EAP's, the social worker was asked by the head nurse of the neo-natal unit to provide supportive services for the nursing staff assigned to that unit. The nurses worked twelve-hour shifts and encountered life and death situations daily. The accumulated stress from the nature of the work was being expressed through angry interactions and hostile silences among the staff. It was hoped that a support group would provide the staff nurses with a safe place to express the often overwhelming and intense feelings which result from caring for at-risk infants. As a result of the group sessions, staff nurses became more supportive of one another, and the mood on the unit noticeably changed from being tense and angry to caring and supportive.

The social worker's efforts in this group involved not only group skills but also collaborative work with the head nurse. Although the head nurse had initially requested the service, and appreciated the resulting change among staff nurses, at times she became concerned that she might be the topic of conversation in the sessions and consequently became suspicious of the group. To insure the continuation of the group, the group leader needed to meet individually with the head nurse, exploring her concern about the group. At the same time, it was imperative that the group leader assure group members that her meetings with the head nurse did not breach their confidentiality.

The group had met continuously for four years and has inspired the formation of support groups for staff nurses in other high-stress units.

Another group of this type was formed at the college EAP. It was composed of employees whose jobs involved frequent student contact. The group was time-limited. Its purpose was to allow the workers to express the frustration they experienced while dealing with the public, and to help them problem-solve around coping more effectively with the stress which resulted from their frequent interactions with students.

Treatment Groups

Unlike groups in the other two categories, treatment groups openly focus on an identifiable problem which is located within the individual and extensive enough to cause dysfunction in either or both the work and personal sphere. Such groups are purposefully designed to treat the individual's problem in a group modality.

An example of a group in this category is the alcoholism recovery group. In a union or corporate setting an alcoholism recovery group may be the easiest type of group to form. Frequently the alcoholism unit is not included in the union or corporation's budget, but, rather, receives separate funding through grants. Consequently, practitioners can act independently, without having to justify their services to the political base of the union or to corporate management.

Alcoholism recovery groups are most often long-term, open groups, allowing for the entrance of new members throughout the life of the group. Members frequently come to the group having used the casework services of the MAP or EAP for counseling and referral to a drug treatment program. Group attendance may be mandated by the employer for the employee whose job is in jeopardy due to alcohol abuse. As was stated earlier, these groups are male dominated.

CONCLUSION

The social worker desirous of integrating a group modality with the services offered by the program will need to carefully consider factors which may contribute to the success or failure of a group.

First, it is essential that the services offered be functionally directed and meaningful to the population. This may require a study of the work environment, collaborative contacts with union officials or management, and an examination of the demographics of the working population served by the program.

Other factors may affect the social worker's freedom to provide the services he or she deems necessary. One of the most critical factors is the existence of the EAP or MAP within a host agency. Union officials or management may be wary of groups, and the social worker will need to allay suspicion through collaborative work. Limitations may exist with the program itself: staffing may not be sufficient; or the policy of the program may be merely to assess clients' needs for referral to community agencies rather than to treat the client. The practitioner will also need to look within, assessing his or her own ability to advocate for group services and to persist despite the wide array of resistant factors.

Consideration of these factors will help determine the purpose and type of group, and the form outreach will take. Groups for workers which provide a preventive service may be formed to meet the developmental needs in a worker's personal life, or may respond to the work-related needs of a specific unit within the work organization. Alternatively, groups may also be designed to treat the already dysfunctional worker, or the worker whose job is in jeopardy.

When careful attention is given to the factors mentioned above, it is possible to provide meaningful, supportive group services despite the formidable obstacles inherent in the work setting.

IMPLICATIONS

This paper has examined the possibility for the provision of group-work services for workers within the framework of existing obstacles. Although the difficulties inherent in providing group services in the work place are many, the newness of the field suggests a potential for innovation and growth. The role of the industrial social worker is not defined so narrowly as in other fields. Also, the broad range of needs and experiences of the client population provide the industrial social worker with expansive possibilities for service provision.

In order to formulate groups in the workplace, the social worker initially will need to consider resistant factors and creatively adapt group service provision within that framework. As mentioned earlier, one of the foremost obstacles inhibiting group formation among the working population is the worker's self-perception as a functional, self-sufficient individual. Yet, this characteristic is not only a formidable obstacle, but is also a prodigious strength. For, because the client population is functional, a supportive group modality within the workplace may enable workers to consider institutional and social as well as personal problems. Institutions or social systems which are inhibitive or non-supportive of individual change indicate to the social worker modification of the system rather than of the behavior of the individual.

The group, formulated for support and mutual aid, may begin to draw from its strength to address the question of influencing the environment, i.e., the workplace, itself. Collective action to effect change may become one of the goals of the group and may be built into the structure of one group. For example, a group formulated around developmental needs such as working parents, adult children of the elderly or pre-retirement may be encouraged to look at elements within the work environment which negatively affect their situation and consider avenues for action.

If the group consists of union members within a Members' Assistance Program, a union official, such as an organizer assigned to the shop where group members work, may become an integral part of the group. With the assistance of the organizer, the group may devise contract proposals designed to specifically address their needs as working parents, adult children of the elderly, or individuals facing retirement.

Within an EAP, the supportive group seeking to effect change within the workplace may need to either open or strengthen communication channels with management before the issues affecting their situation can be addressed. In this instance, the social worker's sensitivity to the host agency is crucial. If the industrial social worker employed by an EAP is successful in mediating the needs of workers with the demands of management critical groundwork has been laid for beneficial communication between the group and management.

Supportive group services in the workplace — whether oriented toward ego-strengthening, social change, or treatment — are greatly needed. It remains for the industrial social worker to tackle the formidable obstacles of individual and organizational resistance and to tap the possibilities for creative service provision.

ENDNOTES

1. B. Googins, "Employee Assistance Programs," *Social Work* 20 (June 1975):464.

2. Sigmund Freud, *Civilization and Its Discontents*, (London: Hogarth Press, 1930), p. 24.

3. Leon W. Chestang, "Work, Personal Change and Human Development," in Akabas and Kurzman, eds, *Work, Workers and Work Organizations* (Englewood Cliffs, N.J.: Prentice Hall, 1982), p. 65.

4. *Work in America*: Report of a Special Task Force to the Secretary of Health, Education and Welfare (Cambridge, MA: MIT Press, 1973), p. 56.

5. Ibid.

6. In juxtaposition to current concerns and values reflected in recent research, one recalls Dickens' insinuating associations between work, family life, and the inseparability of the two. Charles Dickens, *A Christmas Carol, in prose: Being a Ghost Story of Christmas* (London: Chapman & Hall, 1843; reprint ed., New York: Holt, Rinehart and Winston, 1975).

7. Studs Terkel, *Working*, (New York: Random House Inc., 1972), p. 6.

8. See Bertha Reynolds, *Social Work and Social Living*, (New York: Citadel Press, 1951) and Helen Harris Perlman, *Persona*, (Chicago: University of Chicago Press, 1968).

9. David Bloomquist reports that a recent survey of upper and middle management in New York showed that ninety percent of those surveyed felt that personnel should be concerned with the total person, not just with daily output. From "Social Work in Business and Industry," *Social Casework* 60 (October 1979): 459.

10. In fact, in a review of nearly forty articles relating to either group work or industrial social work, only three mentioned supportive group services as a modality for helping workers.

11. An exception to this is an article describing a time-limited group formed around the issue of dual-career families. See Janice and James Prochanska, "Dual-Career Families are a Challenge for Spouses and Agencies," *Social Casework* 63 (February 1982).

12. Although I also firmly believe in the value of supportive group services to those lacking employment (i.e., the unemployed or retired members of the work force), I will confine my remarks here to employed members of the work force.

13. A.H. Maslow, *Motivation and Personality*, (New York: Harper and Co., 1954).

14. Martha N. Ozawa, "Development of Social Services in Industry: Why and How?" *Social Work* 25 (November 1980): 467.

15. William Schwartz, "The Social Worker in the Group," *Social Welfare Forum* (New York: National Conference on Social Welfare, 1961) p. 155.

16. David Bargal, "Professional and Ethical Issues in Providing Social Services in Work Settings," *International Journal of Sociology and Social Policy* 3 (Spring 1983):38.

17. Paul Kurzman and Sheila Akabas, "Industrial Social Work as an Arena for Practice," *Social Work* 26 (January 1981): 57.

18. "How to Get the Women's Movement Moving Again," *New York Times* 3 November 1985, sec. 6, p. 89.

19. Rosalie Bakilinsky, "People vs. Profits: Social Work in Industry," *Social Work* 25 (November 1980): 473.

20. William R. Schleicher, "Employee Assistance Programs," *Practice Digest* 5 (September 1982) p. 5.

21. Judith Nelsen, "Dealing with Resistance in Social Work Practice," *Social Casework* 56 (December 1975): 588.

BIBLIOGRAPHY

Akabas, Sheila H. and Kurzman, Paul A., eds. *Work, Workers and Work Organizations: A View from Social Work*. Englewood Cliffs, N.J.: Prentice Hall, 1982.

Bakilinsky, Rosalie. "People vs. Profits: Social Work in Industry." *Social Work* 25 (November 1980): 471-475.

Bargal, David. "Professional and Ethical Issues in Providing Social Services in Work Settings." *International Journal of Sociology and Social Policy* 3 (Spring 1983): 37-46.

Bloomquist, David C.; Gray, Daniel D.; and Smith, Larry L. "Social Work in Business and Industry." *Social Casework* 60 (October 1979): 457-462.

Dickens, Charles. *A Christmas Carol, in prose: Being a Ghost Story of Christmas.* London: Chapman and Hall, 1843; reprint ed.. New York: Holt. Rinehart and Winston. 1975.

Freud, Sigmund. *Civilization and its Discontents.* London: Hogarth Press, 1930.

Friedan, Betty. "How to Get the Women's Movement Moving Again." *New York Times* 3 November 1985, sec. 6.

Googins, B. "Employee Assistance Programs." *Social Work* 20 (June 1975): 464-467.

Kurzman, Paul A. and Akabas, Sheila H. "Industrial Social Work as an Arena for Practice." *Social Work* 26 (January 1981): 52-60.

Maslow, A.H. *Motivation and Personality.* New York: Harper and Co., 1954.

Nelsen, Judith C. "Dealing with Resistance in Social Work Practice." *Social Casework* 56 (December 1975): 587-592.

Ozawa, Martha N. "Development of Social Services in Industry: Why and How?" *Social Work* 63 (February 1982): 118-120.

Perlman, Helen Harris. *Persona.* Chicago: University of Chicago Press, 1968.

Prochanska, Janice M. and Prochanska, James O. "Dual-Career Families are a Challenge for Spouses and Agencies." *Social Casework* 63 (February 1982):118-120.

Reynolds, Bertha. *Social Work and Social Living.* New York: Citadel Press, 1951.

Schleicher, William R. "Employee Assistance Programs: Running an In-House Program." *Practice Digest* 5 (September 1982): 5-6.

Schwartz, William. "The Social Worker in the Group." *The Social Welfare Forum.* New York: National Conference on Social Welfare, 1961.

Terkel, Studs. *Working.* New York: Random House, Inc., 1972.

Work in America: A Report of a Special Task Force to the Secretary of Health, Education and Welfare. Cambridge, Mass.: MIT Press, 1973.

POWER

A Model for Social Work
with Involuntary Applicants in Groups

Cyrus S. Behroozi

Labeled "hard-to-reach," "resistant," or "unmotivated," involuntary applicants are referred to social workers by coercion and for reasons not of their own choosing (Goldstein, 1986). Although the number of involuntary applicants has been growing in recent years (Cingolani, 1984; Murdach, 1980), the literature reflects only limited attention to working with them. In spite of the special potential of the social work group for helping such applicants, scarcity of knowledge in this area is striking.

This limited attention is curious in a society that values democracy and individual freedom (Harris and Watkins, 1987:16). It is particularly serious for social work because of the profession's special concern for clients' self-determination. It has contributed to social workers' frustration and their loss of credibility in working with involuntary applicants.

This paper proposes a general model for social work with involuntary applicants in groups. The paper includes a discussion of the problem and issues, a theoretical perspective, several principles for practice, and application of the perspective and principles to social work with groups.

Cyrus S. Behroozi, PhD, is Professor at Indiana University, School of Social Work.

223

THE PROBLEM AND ISSUES

In social work, as in other professions, involuntary applicants are often designated "involuntary clients." Such a designation is self-contradictory because the term "clients" should be reserved only for persons who contract for the professional services of a social worker under mutual agreements (Perlman, 1979:14; Specht and Specht, 1986). Involuntary applicants do not become clients unless they enter into such a contract.

Involuntary applicants may or may not be in institutions. They include juvenile or adult law offenders, alcoholics or other substance abusers, child or spouse abusers, unmarried teenage mothers, runaways, and members of socially or economically disadvantaged communities. In all cases, they share a sense of reluctance that goes beyond, and complicates, the usual ambivalence toward accepting help in general (Shulman, 1979:322) and joining a group in particular (Lakin and Costanzo, 1975:209; Manor, 1986). Given a choice, they avoid any contact with the worker (Vriend and Dyer, 1973).

In social work with involuntary applicants, the foremost practice aim should be to help them transform to clienthood, e.g., voluntary membership in the social work group. The necessity of such a transformation becomes more evident as the following issues are addressed.

Ethical Issues

One of the major principles in the current (1979) Code of Ethics of the National Association of Social Workers is that "the social worker should make every effort to foster maximum self-determination on the part of clients." Other helping professions also adhere to the principle of clients' self-determination. For example, in relation to group membership, the Association for Specialists in Group Work maintains that persons should not be coerced into joining a group and that they should have the freedom to leave it (Corey, 1985:68-69).

In social work, as pointed out by Abramson (1985), self-determination is one of the most enduring ethical principles. She defines the principle as a "condition in which personal behavior emanates from a person's own wishes, choices, and decisions." Such a condition allows for the freedom to act as one wishes as well as for the freedom from coercion and interference by others. One's self-determination is limited only if one's action is harmful to oneself or others. However, particularly in such cases, Abramson cautions social workers that they should always ask themselves whether their responses are motivated by their clients' interest or by their own interest.

As Garvin (1987:255-256) points out, another ethical issue is the conflict between the principle of self-determination and the principle of respect for the worth and growth of the person, particularly in relation to those whose capability for self-determination may not have been fully developed or may have been impaired. In practice with such persons, he asserts that not only must their families be consulted regarding the social work service, but also efforts must be made to obtain their own informed consent whenever possible.

Practice Effectiveness Issue

In social work, it is generally accepted that clients' voluntary participation is essential to successful practice outcomes. In related professions, too, predominant practice models are based on the same principle. For example, as cited by Paradise and Wilder (1979) and Vriend and Dyer (1973), this is the case in the counseling models developed by such theorists as Carkhuff; Combs, Alvia, and Purkey; Eisenberg and Delaney; and Rogers. This principle is central also in the insight-oriented psychotherapy (Berman and Segel, 1982) and, at least implicitly, in the behavioral counseling model (Vriend and Dyer, 1973). In fact, citing a study of practice in juvenile institutions, Harris and Watkins (1987:11) report that forced treatment can be harmful. Supporting the same position in relation to forced group counseling, Corey and Corey (1987:289) have concluded that such counseling would entrench negative attitudes. This conclusion is consistent with the findings of several studies, indicating that forced group experience not only is ineffective (Mitchell and Piatkowska, 1974; Romano and Young, 1981) but also can have negative consequences for its participants (Cornbleth, Freedman, and Baskett, 1974).

As implied by the designation "members," voluntary participation is even more crucial in practice with groups. Corey (1985:68-69) reports that voluntary membership is considered an important factor in varied approaches to practice with groups, including those developed by Lakin, Schutz, and Yalom. In the "mainstream" model of social work with groups, voluntary participation is a primary feature of group membership (Papell and Rothman, 1980).

Professional Double Bind Issue

Another issue with significant implications for working with involuntary applicants is how practitioners can reconcile their professional obligations to such applicants with the requirements of their employing institution (Ritchie, 1986). A serious consequence of ignoring this issue is that it may lead to misrepresentations of the professional role (Riordan, Matheny, and Harris, 1978). In social work, Alcabes and Jones (1985) argue that the profession must differentiate between the problems that it can resolve and those that it cannot in order to resist the pressure to accept responsibility for the latter. This issue is considered by Garvin (1987:254-255) in relation to social work with groups in "social control" situations. He views such services as complementing the institution's social control function by helping group members to meet their own needs in socially acceptable ways. However, he asserts that the services should be in the interest of clients and, as such, should not be controlled solely by the mission of the institution.

THEORETICAL PERSPECTIVE

How can involuntary applicants be helped to become voluntary members of the social work group? In order to address this question, it is first necessary to discuss significant dynamics of involuntariness, a social work practice orientation responsive to such dynamics, and practice principles consistent with the orientation.

Dynamics of Involuntariness

All involuntary applicants are not alike in every respect. However, in spite of their differences, they may share certain attributes. The universally common attribute is their reluctance. Such reluctance is a natural and, indeed, healthy sign that they are grasping for a share in the control of their destiny (Riordan et al., 1978). It also represents their demands to understand the meaning of their referral for the service and their response to having been manipulated by others (Vriend and Dyer, 1973). Furthermore, it is a way of maintaining personal integrity against threats to self-image. As such, it is a valid position (Larrabee, 1982) and a coping state (Goldstein, 1986).

Involuntary applicants perceive themselves as having been coerced to submit to undesired judgment and conditions set by others (Perlman, 1979:116). Thus, they may be immobilized by feelings of failure, uncertainty, and incompetence (Oxley, 1981:290). They may be embarrassed and angry because they have been judged incapable of handling their own problems (Ritchie, 1986). They may experience a loss of control, self-respect, human dignity, and freedom (Harris and Watkins, 1987:45). They may be unfamiliar with the purpose and expectations of the professional service. They may be suspicious of authority figures and reject the worker as a representative of the system that has been their adversary (Riordan et al., 1978).

Besides their response to the coercion, the involuntary applicants' reluctance stems from two other sources: perception of the problems and perceptions of the need for change and of the attainability of change (Goldstein, 1986; Harris and Watkins, 1987:88; Ritchie, 1986; Vriend and Dyer, 1973). The intensity of their reluctance can be understood in terms of these sources along a continuum. Accordingly, the most reluctant involuntary applicants are those who deny their problems as defined by others. Next are those who admit their problems and want to change, but are unable to change because they do not know how and do not believe that the helping experience will benefit them. The least reluctant involuntary applicants are those who are aware of their problems, of their need for change, and of the attainability of change.

Practice Orientation

The general profile that emerges from the dynamics just considered is that of persons who experience powerlessness, incompetence, and inability to make and implement decisions for managing themselves and their situations. In response to such a profile, the practice orientation proposed here combines ideas from three interrelated processes: empowerment, competence-promotion, and choice-making.

Empowerment is a process of assisting persons from a stigmatized social category to develop an ability to perform valued social roles (Solomon, 1976:6). As such, empowerment helps people develop a capability for formulating self-determined goals, identifying alternatives for goal attainment, and using resources of their own and those of others for achieving such goals (Solomon, 1976:342).

Related to empowerment, the competence-promotion process attempts to improve the person-environment transaction as part of helping the person to change (Maluccio, 1981:11). It maximizes participation of the person in the helping process and emphasizes the person's strengths and potentialities (Maluccio, 1979:14). The key personal manifestations of competence are self-confidence, trusting one's own judgment, and the ability to make decisions (White as cited in Maluccio, 1981:4).

Inherent in the development of such competence is the awareness that, at any given time, one has available alternative courses of action, that any action represents a choice, and that one should accept responsibility for the choices that one makes. The necessity of this awareness does not negate the effect of circumstances beyond one's control. Rather, it assumes that, in spite of those circumstances, there is always the possibility of a variety of responses at any point in time (McEvoy, 1967). It also assumes that any person is potentially capable of making choices. However, making a "free choice" requires one's heightened awareness of reality, particularly recognition of available alternatives and their consequences (McEvoy, 1967). Thus, in social work practice, the central purpose is to help people become aware of their power of choice-making through developing competence to select and implement meaningful and informed alternatives. In fact, Harris and Watkins (1987:50) suggest that the nature of almost all counseling is "helping clients to accept appropriate responsibility for choosing alternatives from among available options." It is particularly important for involuntary applicants to learn how to make choices among positive alternatives in order to deal with their sense of powerlessness. For this purpose, the "affirmation approach" developed by Rios and Ofman (Larrabee, 1982) begins with helping involuntary applicants to face the reality of their lives in order to see that they have chosen the way they lead their lives for understandable reasons.

PRACTICE PRINCIPLES

Several basic principles for practice can be identified as consistent with the foregoing theoretical perspective. It is assumed that these principles are relevant to working with various involuntary applicants. However, their relevance may be limited for practice with some institutionalized involuntary applicants, particularly those who have strong antisocial tendencies or those whose social functioning has been severely impaired because of mental illness or other problems. In practice with such persons, approaches other than social work may be more appropriate, such as the "correctional model" reported by Harris and Watkins (1987:74-76) for working with prison inmates.

Aims of Practice and Types of Applicants

1. In social work with involuntary applicants, the foremost and primary aim should be to help them transform to clienthood by developing a service contract. In social work with groups, such a contract signifies their membership in the social work group.
2. In developing the membership contract, the focus should be on helping involuntary applicants to deal with the sources of their reluctance. Thus, a beginning task in working with them is to assess such sources.
3. On the basis of the assessment of the sources of their reluctance, three types of involuntary applicants can be identified. The first type of applicants bring their response to the coercion, but are aware of their problems, accept their need for change, and believe that change is attainable. The second type of applicants also bring their response to the coercion, are aware of their problems and of their need for change, but do not believe change is attainable. The third type of applicants bring not only

their response to the coercion but also their denial of their problems and, consequently, of their need for change. Practice with each type calls for particular foci and processes responsive to the particular sources of reluctance.

Dealing with Response to the Coercion

1. In the beginning, the reluctance of involuntary applicants should be recognized and accepted (Perlman, 1979:121). This recognition and acceptance should involve empathizing with feelings associated with the coercion, such as anger and embarrassment. Furthermore, involuntary applicants should be helped to understand the meaning of such feelings (Vriend and Dyer, 1973).

2. Premature confrontation of involuntary applicants forcing them to accept others' interpretation of their problems or to confess guilt should be avoided (Ritchie, 1986). Rather, their perceptions and even evasions should be heard and accepted for the moment, and confrontation about these can come later (Perlman, 1979:119). As Larrabee (1982) suggests, involuntary applicants should be helped to explore their reluctance in terms of its positive and negative aspects as a choice made by them rather than as something to be overcome through confrontation. Accordingly, they should be helped to see that each position taken in life, including reluctance, has both positive and negative aspects. However, he also suggests that affirmation of their rights to believe differently from others (e.g., their referral source) should not be a sanction for continuing self-defeating behaviors.

3. The worker should differentiate himself or herself from the referral source by clarifying their different functions; however, criticism of the referral source should be avoided (Harris and Watkins, 1987:38). In spite of such a differentiation, the worker should not take personally the possible expression of hostility and rejection by involuntary applicants, nor should the worker be immobilized by being unappreciated (Corey and Corey, 1987:289).

4. From the beginning, involuntary applicants should be provided opportunities to make choices and to experience success. For example, they should be allowed to choose appointment times and to comply with a minor request before a major one (Ritchie, 1986).

Dealing with Perceptions of Problems and of the Need for Change

1. A central practice principle well-known in social work is to "start where the client is." In working with involuntary applicants, observance

of this principle calls for understanding their perceptions of their problems and their expectations, which may be different from those of their referral source and others.

2. Involuntary applicants should not be considered "unmotivated." They do bring to the helping situation their needs and interests, which should be explored, understood, and reconciled with the expectations of others. In the beginning, it should be expected that some involuntary applicants are primarily concerned with their basic survival needs rather than higher order needs (Harris and Watkins, 1987:46). In any case, they should be understood as being motivated by what will give them most gratification and least discomfort (Harris and Watkins, 1987:134-35).

3. Involuntary applicants should be understood in the context of their environment; thus, the definition of their problems and the focus of change should include such a context (Oxley, 1981:315). In practice with institutionalized involuntary applicants, assessment of the problem should include their institutional conditions so that they can look also within themselves for sources of the problem (Garvin, 1987:261).

4. Available services should be explained to involuntary applicants in a way that is understandable and unambiguous, promising tangible and demonstrable usefulness to them (Oxley, 1981:312-313). Use of professional jargon (e.g., "therapy") or labeling (e.g., "resistant") that may be threatening to them should be avoided (Harris and Watkins, 1987:62).

5. In the end, involuntary applicants' perceptions of the problem and of the need for change may be considerably different from those of the worker or others (Perlman, 1979:134). Such perceptions, including their decision not to seek help, should be respected once they become aware of their alternatives and of the consequences of their choices (Oxley, 1981:312). After a discussion of the advantages and disadvantages of alternatives available to them, the choice is theirs. However, as Corey and Corey (1987:289) suggest, the process of choice-making should include finding alternatives to the service refused.

PRACTICE WITH GROUPS

In addition to its universal significance for human development and change, group experience has special potential for working with involuntary applicants. As reported by Levine and Gallogly (1985:15-21), such an experience can reduce applicants' denial, facilitate their acceptance of the existence of their problems, increase their motivation for change, and facilitate their development of more acceptable ways of dealing with their problems. It has been reported also that group experience can be the strongest force for reconsideration of norms that require change (Garvin, 1987:259). Furthermore, particularly because of the issues of authority and trust, confrontation of involuntary applicants by their peers in the group is more effective than by the worker on a one-to-one basis (Harris and Watkins, 1987:55-56). Thus, with some exceptions, it is assumed that practice with groups is the method of choice for helping involuntary applicants. The exceptions may include acting-out individuals, those who are extremely anxious, and those who lack minimal capability for constructive relationship and interaction with others.

Three Phases of Practice

The general model presented here for practice with groups consists of three phases: pre-group, group, and post-group. The pre-group phase includes group formation, preparation of members, and contracting. In the group phase, the group matures as a social unit through several stages of development. The post-group phase is concerned with members' experience following the termination of their membership in the group.

In this model, the group phase is based on the developmental stages theorized by Lacoursiere (1980:29-41). Accordingly, at different points in the life of the group, members manifest different predominant social-emotional and task-related behaviors. These points or stages of group development are called orientation, dissatisfaction, resolution, production, and termination. Unlike other theories, Lacoursiere's theory differentiates between the beginning stage of group development for voluntary participants (i.e., the orientation stage) and the beginning stage for involuntary participants (i.e., the negative orientation stage). Such a differentiation makes his theory particularly applicable to practice with involuntary applicants.

The orientation stage is characterized by participants' mild to moderate eagerness and positive expectations. At the same time, they experience a certain degree of anxiety generated primarily by their ambivalence and lack of full knowledge about the new experience. Furthermore, they are quite dependent on the group leader, and the amount of work accomplished is moderate since much energy and time are spent dealing with the developmental issues. Major issues for members include their concern with having the competence necessary for satisfactory use of the group experience.

In the dissatisfaction stage, participants become aware of differences between what they want from the group experience and their perceptions of what is actually happening in the group. This perceived discrepancy leads to feelings of frustration and even anger in relation to the purpose, the authority figure, and members of the group. Other negative feelings, such as discouragement and rivalry, may also be experienced. These feelings lead to decreased morale and productivity in the group.

The resolution stage occurs between the period of maximum dissatisfaction and the beginning of the production stage. During the resolution stage, members' expectations and realities are reconciled, and their competence to participate in the group successfully is achieved and recognized. Consequently, there is increased self-esteem and decreased animosity among members and between them and the leader. These feelings are generated partly by implicit or explicit agreement about the group norms. Manifested in this stage are stronger group cohesion and gradual increase in work, which continues into the production stage.

In the production stage, positive feelings about the experience characterize members' relationships and performance. These feelings lead to more efficient use of time for accomplishing the group purpose. However, the actual production stage reflecting a high level of work and positive feelings may be a relatively small part of the group experience.

Finally, in the termination stage, members concern themselves with a review of their accomplishments in the group and with its impending dissolution, leading often to a sense of loss. During this stage, the work related to the group objectives considerably decreases.

In Lacoursiere's developmental stages, when participation in the group is involuntary, participants begin their group experience with hostility, suspicion, and other feelings stemming from their reluctance about being in the group. These feelings are manifested by a lack of cooperation and even by rebellion. Such a beginning is called the negative orientation stage. Depending on the degree of participants' reluctance, this kind of beginning usually blends into the dissatisfaction stage. Thus, the resolution stage should address not only the usual dissatisfaction but also the participants' reluctance. If such a resolution is achieved, the group continues into the production and termination stages successfully.

In practice with involuntary applicants, this paper proposes that the special attention be given to the pre-group phase and the beginning of the group phase. During these periods, the membership contract is developed for their voluntary participation in the social work group. As Alcabes and Jones (1985) suggest, contracting should be understood primarily as a process of socialization into the role of a client. In such a process, individuals remain in the role of an applicant until they agree to the expectations of clienthood (i.e., group membership).

Three Types of Involuntary Applicants

This paper has identified three types of involuntary applicants in terms of the sources of their reluctance. Furthermore, the paper has suggested that, for the development of the membership contract, involuntary applicants should be helped to deal with the sources of their reluctance. As shown by Figure 1, the development of the membership contract with each type of involuntary applicants calls for special practice foci and processes appropriate for the particular sources of their reluctance.

FIGURE 1

Types of Applicants	Pre-Group Phase	Group Phase
Type I	PROCESS: Worker-applicant interaction SPECIAL FOCUS: Dealing with response to the coercion CONTRACT: Membership in the social work group	STAGES OF GROUP DEVELOPMENT: [Negative Orientation] – Orientation-Dissatisfaction/Resolution–...
Type II	PROCESS: Worker-applicant interaction SPECIAL FOCUS: Dealing with response to the coercion CONTRACT 1: Trial participation in the social work group	STAGES OF GROUP DEVELOPMENT: Negative Orientation – Resolution–... SPECIAL FOCUS: Dealing with perceptions of the problem and of change CONTRACT 2: Membership in the social work group
Type III	PROCESS 1: Worker-applicant interaction SPECIAL FOCUS: Dealing with response to the coercion CONTRACT 1: Participation in the exploratory group PROCESS 2: Exploratory group experience SPECIAL FOCUS: Dealing with perceptions of the problem and of change CONTRACT 2: Membership in the social work group	STAGES OF GROUP DEVELOPMENT: [Negative Orientation]- Orientation-Dissatisfaction/Resolution–...

Type I

These involuntary applicants bring their negative response to the coercion, but are aware of their problems, accept their need for change, and believe that change is attainable. Therefore, the special focus of practice with these applicants should be to help them deal with their response to the coercion and with the universal issues related to the ambivalence towards accepting help and group membership.

These responses and issues can be addressed primarily through working with such involuntary applicants individually during the pre-group phase, and the membership contract can be developed by the end of this phase. However, it is possible that some of their issues, particularly those related to the coercion, may not be adequately resolved during the pre-group phase. In those cases, members take their unresolved issues to the beginning stage of the group phase, manifesting a brief negative orientation stage. However, the negative orientation stage will soon change into the orientation stage followed by the other stages. Implications of the negative orientation stage will be discussed later.

In working with such involuntary applicants during the pre-group phase, the practice principles for dealing with their response to the coercion can best be incorporated into the framework developed by Oded Manor (1986) for dealing with the ambivalence of prospective members when they meet individually with the worker. To negotiate the membership contract with them, he proposes a sequence for dealing with their personal and social issues (i.e., anxieties and goals). The sequence begins with addressing personal issues (e.g., am I understood?) and continues through responding to personal goals (e.g., to be comforted), social goals (e.g., concern with concrete, basic needs), and social anxieties (e.g., will I be put down?).

Type II

These involuntary applicants also bring their negative response to the coercion, are aware of their problems and of their need for change, but do not believe change is attainable. Thus, the special focus of practice with these applicants should be to help them deal with their response to the coercion, to help them explicate what needs to change, and to help them accept the social work group experience as an effective means for change.

Dealing with the applicants' response to the coercion and explicating the problem and focus of change can be accomplished through working with them individually during the pre-group phase. However, it is unlikely that these applicants will accept membership in the social work group. The major reason for this is that their interpersonal experience with authority figures and others have usually been characterized by distrust, pessimism, and disappointment. Worker's assurances may not diminish the effect of those experiences for them to want to join the group, particularly because they cannot anticipate with much accuracy the nature of what McEvoy (1967) calls "experiences not yet." Therefore, the focus of the contract during the pre-group phase may have to be only getting a commitment from them to try the usefulness of the social work group by participating in it for, as Manor (1986) suggests, at least four meetings. This trial experience serves as an opportunity for increasing their choices and for providing a basis for choice-making (Corey and Corey, 1987:289). After the period of trial, their pre-group contract should be reviewed and should be advanced to the membership contract, if they agree to become members of the group.

Because of participants' unresolved issues about joining the group, their trial group experience may resemble the negative orientation stage, replacing the orientation stage and blending with the dissatisfaction stage. As Lacoursiere (1982:240) suggests, in addition to dealing with the issues inherent in the usual beginning, the negative orientation stage requires helping participants to examine the reasons for their reluctance and to consider what would happen if they would not join the group. It requires also helping participants to appreciate the usefulness of the group experience.

Type III

These involuntary applicants bring not only their response to the coercion but also their denial of their problems and, consequently, of their need for change.

During the pre-group phase, individual work with such applicants can help them deal with their response to the coercion. However, they would not probably agree to participate in the social work group even on a trial basis because they deny their problems and their need for change. The process proposed in this paper for working with such involuntary applicants is similar to what Garvin (1987:259) calls "a planned sequence of groups." As such, the pre-group phase includes a two-part membership contract. The first part, negotiated with applicants individually, seeks their agreement to participate in an open-ended, exploratory group to examine whether they have a problem needing resolution. The second part, negotiated as a possible result of the exploratory group experience, seeks their agreement to join the social work group.

Reported by Levine and Gallogly (1985:73-81, 134-135) as groups for motivation and acceptance, these exploratory groups are effective particularly in working with denying alcoholics. The authors suggest that, in such groups, participants should receive initial support to express their denials in order to lessen their defensiveness. The exploratory group should also help them to examine possible reasons for their behavior and for their reluctance to change. In the initiation of group services for reluctant persons from socially and economically disadvantaged communities, Christmas (1972:768) has reported another kind of exploratory group called "intake group screening." The primary purpose of such a group is to prepare individuals for membership in rehabilitative groups, particularly by helping them to deal with feelings of threat and by providing the reassurance that they will be with others having similar backgrounds and problems.

Participants in an exploratory group agreeing to join the social work group may still enter the latter group with some degree of reluctance. While such reluctance may lead to the negative orientation stage for them, that stage is expected to change shortly into the orientation stage followed by the other stages.

SUMMARY AND CONCLUSION

This paper has proposed a general model for social work with involuntary applicants in groups. In developing the model, the paper has analyzed the problem of working with such applicants in relation to the ethical, practice effectiveness, and professional double bind issues. It has also presented a theoretical perspective that includes the dynamics of involuntariness, an orientation for practice, and several practice principles.

The theoretical perspective and principles have been considered for practice with three types of involuntary applicants differentiated in terms of the sources of their reluctance, i.e., their response to the coercion, their perception of their problems, and their perceptions of the need for change and the attainability of change. Emphasizing the pre-group phase and the beginning stages of the group phase, the paper has proposed that the special aim of practice with involuntary applicants should be to help them deal with the sources of their reluctance. The intended outcome is the membership contract, reflecting their transformation from involuntary applicants to voluntary participants in the social work group.

This paper is only a beginning effort to develop a model that may be generalized to practice with various types of involuntary applicants. Clearly, it needs testing and further development, particularly through its application in working with involuntary applicants representing different problems, characteristics, and situations.

REFERENCES

Abramson, M. (1985). The Autonomy-Paternalism Dilemma in Social Work Practice. *Social Casework, 66,* 387-393.
Alcabes, A., & Jones, J. (1985). Structural Determinants of "Clienthood." *Social Work, 30,* 49-53.
Berman, E., & Segel, R. (1982). The Captive Client: Dilemmas of Psychotherapy in the Psychiatric Hospital. *Psychotherapy: Theory, Research and Practice, 19,* 31-42.
Christmas, J. (1972). Group Rehabilitative Approaches in Socially and Economically Disadvantaged Communities. In C. Sager & H. Kaplan (Eds.), *Progress in Group and Family Therapy* (pp. 764-773). New York: Brunner-Mazel Publishers.
Cingolani, J. (1984). Social Conflict Perspective on Work with Involuntary Clients. *Social Work, 29,* 442-446.
Corey, G. (1985). *Theory and Practice of Group Counseling* (2nd Edition). Monterey: Brooks/Cole Publishing Co.
Corey, M., & Corey, G. (1987). *Groups: Process and Practice* (3rd Edition). Monterey: Brooks/Cole Publishing Co.
Cornbleth, T., Freedman, A., & Baskett, G. (1974). Comparison of Self-Acceptance of Conscripted and Voluntary Participants in a Microlab Human Relations Training Experience. *Journal of Community Psychology, 2,* 58-59.
Garvin, C. (1987). *Contemporary Group Work* (2nd Edition). Englewood Cliffs, N.J.: Prentice-Hall.
Goldstein, H. (1986). A Cognitive-Humanistic Approach to the Hard-to-Reach Client. *Social Casework, 67,* 27-36.
Harris, G., & Watkins, D. (1987). *Counseling the Involuntary and Resistant Client.* College Park, MD: American Correctional Association.
Lacoursiere, R. (1980). *The Life Cycle of Groups: Group Developmental Stage Theory.* New York: Human Sciences Press.
Lakin, M., & Costanzo, P. (1975). The Leader and the Experiential Group. In C. Cooper (Ed.), *Theories of Group Process* (pp. 205-219). New York: John Wiley.
Larrabee, M. (1982). Working with Reluctant Clients through Affirmation Techniques. *The Personnel and Guidance Journal, 61,* 105-109.
Levine, B., & Gallogly, V. (1985). *Group Therapy with Alcoholics: Outpatient and Inpatient Approaches.* Beverly Hills: Sage Publications.

Maluccio, A. (1979). *Leaning from Clients: Interpersonal Helping as Viewed by Clients and Social Workers*. New York: The Free Press.

Maluccio, A. (1981). Competence-oriented Social Work Practice: An Ecological Approach. In A. Maluccio (Ed.), *Promoting Competence in Clients: A New/ Old Approach to Social Work Practice* (pp. 1-24). New York: The Free Press.

Manor, O. (1986). The Preliminary Interview in Social Groupwork: Finding the Spiral Steps. *Social Work with Groups, 9,* 21-39.

McEvoy, T. (1967). The Existential Dynamics of Free Choice. *Journal of Existentialism, 8,* 1-17.

Mitchell, K., & Piatkowska, O. (1974). Effects of Group Treatment for College Underachievers and Bright Failing Underachievers. *Journal of Counseling Psychology, 21,* 494-501.

Murdach, A. (1980). Bargaining and Persuasion with Involuntary Clients. *Social Work, 25,* 458-461.

Oxley, G. (1981). Promoting Competence in Involuntary Clients. In A. Maluccio (Ed.), *Promoting Competence in Clients: A New/Old Approach to Social Work Practice* (pp. 290-316). New York: The Free Press.

Pappel, C., & Rothman, B. (1980). Relating the Mainstream Model of Social Work with Groups to Group Psychotherapy and the Structured Group Approach. *Social Work with Groups, 3,* 5-21.

Paradise, L., & Wilder, P. (1979). The Relationship between Client Reluctance and Counseling Effectiveness. *Counselor Education and Supervision, 19,* 35-41.

Perlman, H. (1979). *Relationship: The Heart of Helping People*. Chicago: The University of Chicago Press.

Riordan, R., Matheny, K., & Harris, C. (1978). Helping Counselors Minimize Client Reluctance. *Counselor Education and Supervision, 18,* 7-13.

Ritchie, M. (1986). Counseling the Involuntary Client. *Journal of Counseling and Development, 64,* 516-518.

Romano, J., & Young, H. (1981). Required Group Counseling/Study Skills for Academic Improvement: How Effective Are They? *Journal of College Personnel, 22,* 492-496.

Shulman, L. (1979). *The Skills of Helping Individuals and Groups*. Itasca, IL: F. E. Peacock Publishers.

Solomon, B. (1976). *Black Empowerment: Social Work in Oppressed Communities*. New York: Columbia University Press.

Specht, H., & Specht, R. (1986). Social Work Assessment: Route to Clienthood — Part I. *Social Casework, 67,* 525-532.

Vriend, J., & Dyer, W. (1973). Counseling the Reluctant Client. *Journal of Counseling Psychology, 20,* 240-246.

Empowering Groups
Through Understanding Stages
of Group Development

Toby Berman-Rossi

Most of us have belonged to groups throughout our lifetimes. Groups have been organized for us, and others we have organized ourselves. Some have been formal, some informal. Some have been productive, while others have not. We have been part of family groups, friendship groups, school groups, work groups, professional groups, therapy groups, tenant groups, and educational groups, to name just a few. The range within these groups has been wide: those with clear problem solving foci, others with vague purposes to be established by members. We have all known workers, leaders, teachers, and therapists who contributed to our sense of satisfaction and we have also known those whose behavior stifled us as individuals and stifled the development of the group as a whole. How our groups have developed as working units has also been part of our experience. Mutual aid known in one group may not exist in another. We have known groups to be: cohesive/fragmented, polarized/united, productive/unproductive. Productivity stands out as a critical group component. We join groups in the hope that we will accomplish a purpose or goal. Despite the vagueness or certitude of our initial motivation, we experience the hope that we will gain something in particular from joining groups, something which will make our expenditure of energy and affect worthwhile. Once in groups, we notice that they feel different as time passes. Middles seem different from beginnings and beginnings certainly different

Toby Berman-Rossi, DSW, is Assistant Professor at The School of Social Work, Columbia University, New York, NY 10025.

The author gratefully acknowledges the helpful comments of Alex Gitterman and Peter Rossi.

239

from ends. Be we members or workers, we sense that groups as a whole and relationships among members develop over time.

As practitioners we feel pleasure when our groups develop into strong working units. Our sense of satisfaction is shared by members. We also notice the times our groups get stuck, mutual aid is weak and productivity is lessened. We are challenged to understand obstacles to development and to skillfully find ways to help the group move on.

Development of the group as a whole is predicated upon the character of two internal group processes, that of member to authority and member to member relationships. As the group evolves, these two sets of relationships can change dramatically. A once feared worker can become viewed as a source of help. Participants can move from isolation and alienation to engagement expressed through mutual aid. Progress in the development of the group as a whole parallels progress in the development of these two sets of relationships. Strong worker to member and member to member relationships are not present at the beginning of the group. In a manner similar to the development of the group as a whole, they develop over time.

While we hope that these two sets of relationships will evolve positively, such growth is not automatically a necessary outcome of group association. Potential obstacles to group development, to the development of a strong working relationship between worker and members and to the development of a process of mutual aid among members are ever present. Our clients often come suspicious of us as institutional authorities. Mistrust of peers seems understandable in light of the fragmentary interpersonal relationships many members have experienced. The reality that our groups develop as well as they do is living testimony to their healing and strengthening power. It also points to our skill as practitioners, to help set such a process in motion, against great odds.

This paper concerns itself with a discussion of stages of group development and how a working knowledge of this core concept is helpful to group practioners. As a necessary accompaniment to presentation of this concept, we will highlight a discussion of member to authority and member to member relationships. Our orienting question will be: what is happening to the internal workings of the group as the group as a whole develops. These components are interactional, reciprocal and interdependent. Each exists in the context of the other and gives rise to the character of the whole.

The method of analyzing a group suggested in this paper provides a tool for assessing where the group is in its development and how it is progressing. The appropriateness of a worker's activity can therefore be related to more objective correlates. As part of this assessment we will be able to look at the interrelationship between the development of the group as a whole and the development of member to authority and member to member relationships.

Our interest in group development is instrumental. The more fully developed a group is, the greater is the likelihood that member to member relationships will strengthen. The greater the degree of mutual aid, the greater the development of the group as a whole. Less dependent upon the worker, the group becomes inherently more powerful. Groups are empowered when they can fully use their energy to address and satisfy members' needs which brought them together. Therefore our practice strategy is directed toward the development of the group as a whole as well as toward the development of member to authority and member to member relationships. When this core interactive process is understood, practitioners can act with a high degree of consciousness with regard to central group tasks and can concentrate upon the development of attendant social work skills necessary to assist the group in its progress.

STAGES OF GROUP DEVELOPMENT

The concept of "group development" is one which concerns itself with the growth process groups experience over time.[1] While the literature reflects varied philosophical and psychological traditions, and offers differing explanations for why groups develop as they do, there is a high degree of consensus that groups do develop as time passes. Even attempts to examine the negative evidence end with the conclusion that the evidence is not persuasive. Rather, it is suggested, that counterarguments should be thought of as a call for refinement of the concept, rather than elimination of it.[2]

The concept of "the group as a whole" or "it" is at the heart of the well developed literature on stages of group development. When we use the word "it," as in the case of "it" develops, we are referring to a consideration of an entity which has an identity separate from and beyond the individual participant within the group. This "it" concept is an artificial construct. We cannot see "it," or touch "it" but we can describe "it" and when we do, as in the case of "it is fragmented," or "it is productive," we are speaking about something beyond the individual group members.

Writers use stages, phases, or trends interchangeably when speaking of group development.[3] These terms identify distinct periods when different dominative group behavior is demonstrated and the character of the group, as a whole, changes through an evolving process.

There are many striking aspects of this process.[4] *First*, is the aspect of predictability. The stages themselves are not arbitrary. We can look from group to group and find an orderly progression more similar than dissimilar. For example, in the initial stage of group development, all groups will engage in orientation activity in which they will be unsure of how their relationship with the worker and with each other will evolve. *Second*, is the concept of developmental tasks. Each stage sets developmental challenges which must be successfully addressed if future stages are to be effectively experienced. This is not to suggest that all developmental issues associated with a particular stage are resolved before the group progresses to the next stage, but rather that the issues must be sufficiently worked through if the group's energy is to be freed for its succeeding work. Suggestions of former stages can always be found in a present stage, while the present portends the future. Take for example challenges to our authority within the group. Just when we thought the issue was put aside, a new challenge arises only to remind us that such issues are never fully resolved, but rather they appear through the life of the group. Recognizing the stage of development in which the challenge occurs will enable us to better understand the meaning of the challenge and the collective strength of the group in addressing the issue before it. This aspect of group development is especially crucial for practitioners who are always struggling with the question of when the issue has been discussed enough. *Third*, we note how the group develops over time. We can look inside our groups and see how "it" is developing. Is it fragmented? polarized? productive? Has the group progressed in its development? How does it move — with much movement backwards and forwards or in a rather even, steady manner? And *fourth*, and finally, is the idea of value associated with movement to the next stage. Each progressive stage signifies movement towards greater maturity on the part of the group as a whole. We believe our groups are progressing positively when they move to the next stage. Therefore, we direct our energy to assisting the group in its development towards the next stage, a stage which by definition signifies greater maturity on the part of the group as a whole. While we can all recall the pleasure of the initial "honeymoon" stage, we recognize that unless our groups wrestle with our authority, in a satisfactory manner, they will not be able to move on to using each other fully. Defining where the group is in its development, and how it is progressing provides a tool for assessment and thereby helps inform practice strategies.

TYPES OF DEVELOPMENTAL MODELS

There are three types of developmental models described in the literature: linear-progressive, life-cycle, and pendular.[5] Each model attempts to capture elements thought to be neglected by the others and offers practitioners a useful range in which to attempt to place their groups. The first model, with which most of us are probably familiar is linear-progressive. Benis and Shephard's (1956) model would fall into this category. Briefly, linear-progressive models are models where linearity is derived from movement "onwards and upwards" and progression is derived from the group's movement towards resolution of two distinct critical issues: dependence upon the worker and interdependence among the members, with dependence preceding interdependence. Critical here is the belief that the members cannot move on to the development of their relationships with each other unless in some significant manner their relationship with the authority is sufficiently resolved. This "power and control" stage represents the high point of the empowerment struggle. While the "authority theme" is never really resolved, these models state, it must be dealt with sufficiently so that members can lessen their preoccupation with the power of the leader and can move on more securely towards the task for which they came together. Only in this way can the members and the group as a whole realize their power. Drawbacks of linear thinking are minimized through the understanding that these stages are not discrete, but rather that elements of former stages are found in latter stages. Dominative group patterns, rather than exclusivity of characteristics, are described by this model.[6] This model most typically would apply to formed, open or closed-ended groups which were not time limited. Tuckman's (1965) formulation of: forming, storming, norming and performing follows these lines. Members join together, gain initial familiarity, engage in and resolve a struggle with the authority, establish norms of work and conduct, and move forward in performance.

Our own practice with groups would suggest that while offering a major contribution to our understanding of group development, the linear-progressive model fails to appreciate the terminal aspect of group development. Who among us has not struggled with the power of ending a meaningful group and who among us has not viewed successful termination as a central group task? Addressing the final stage of a time limited group, with feeling, cognizant of the process of loss becomes particularly important to our members who must find a way to dissolve their ties, without dissolving what the group has meant and provided. That which the members worked so hard to create will be no more. The life-cycle model addresses this gap by adding an end stage of development. This model largely constitutes a linear-progressive model with a terminal stage as a final stage of group development and is applicable to all time limited groups.[7] Tuckman and Jensen's (1977) later formulation of forming, storming, norming, performing, and adjourning attends to the ending stage of groups.

In the main, our profession has utilized knowledge developed by social scientists about stages of group development and applied that knowledge to practice and its analysis. For example, Seitz (1985) utilized the stage developmental and social work practice literature to analyze change within a group of women post-mastectomy who moved from concern with themselves to concern for others. A seminal exception from our own profession has been the work of Garland, Jones, and Kolodney (1973), who developed a life-cycle model. Based upon extensive content analysis of process records, they defined stages of group development as: (1) Pre-Affiliation, (2) Power and Control, (3) Intimacy, (4) Differentiation, and (5) Separation. While essentially similar to other life-cycle models, within Garland, Jones, and Kolodney's schema, stage 2, Power and Control, refers to power and control issues among members, i.e, status, ranking, the development of norms, while in other paradigms this stage specifically refers to the authority relationship between the worker and the members. For Garland, Jones, and Kolodney (1973) the worker remains the most crucial influence in resolving these interpersonal and structural tensions, but is not the focus of the tension itself. Glassman and Kates (1983), based upon an affinity for the work of both Bennis and Shephard (1956) and Garland, Jones, and Kolodney (1973) offer a merger of these two sets of ideas by demonstrating how the "authority theme" could be included within the work of Garland, Jones, and Kolodney (1973).

Those theorists who provide syntheses of linear-progressive and life-cycle models, despite their different emphases, are essentially in agreement that the stages of group development are: orientation, dissatisfaction, resolution, production, and termination.[8] Member to member relationships, worker to member relationships, and an overall characterization of the group as a whole, are highlighted as key aspects of this process of development.

The third model, the pendular or recurring cycle model, suggests that groups do not progress in linear fashion, but rather experience a pendular movement back and forth which ultimately takes on a cyclical nature because of the persistence of issues rather than their resolution.[9] There is the sense of enduring difficulties which continue to need to be addressed. These issues are never "resolved" but rather achieve different positions of ascendence at different points in the life of a group. My own experience suggests that groups experiencing pendularity, i.e., open-ended groups particularly of long term nature, develop linearly but utilize an internal process of a cyclical nature. In these groups the introduction of new members continuously reawakens earlier developmental issues. I recall two experiences, with the same open-ended, long term care floor group, which suggested that similar issues are resolved differently at different stages of group development. In the first instance, Mr. Dixon joined four months after the group was formed. At his first meeting he suggested I, rather than the group, handle a conflictual matter with the medical department. He reasoned that I, being more influential than they, would be listened to more. The group debated the suggestion for two sessions before deciding that, while they weren't totally confident, they thought they might be strong enough to initiate contact on the matter. Six years later, with the same group, a similar incident occurred. Mr. Barbero, also a new member, suggested that I take their complaints to the Dietary Department. This time the group was quick to answer that they didn't need me to do that. They only used me that way, they said, when they were convinced that they could not be influential. The point at which new members join open-ended groups as well as the character of the group, at that particular time, become important variables in determining how their presence affects group development.

As we consider the "goodness of fit" between these three models and our own groups, we are immediately confronted with the reality that placing groups within this typology is even more complex than we anticipated. Our groups do not always involve pure types. The groups with which we work utilize a broad range of structures. Even with similar types, differences are significant. For example, how would a seven week open-ended girls baking group, compare with my seven year open-ended floor group in a long term care facility in terms of group development? Our own practice literature has yet to fully consider the influence of structure upon stages of group development. Schopler and Galinsky (1984), in their writing on development within open-ended groups where the worker is the constant, have made an important beginning.

In sum, these stages form a predictable order. Each stage sets developmental challenges which must be successfully addressed so that future stages can be effectively experienced. Such successful attention does not demand resolution of issues. Elements of previous stages can always be found in the present. Such a progression is vitally important to groups if they are to devote the majority of available energy to the tasks at hand, rather than towards the resolution of tensions within their development. Not all groups will go through all of these stages but failure to achieve the work of one stage will either prevent movement to the next stage or will significantly affect the way in which that next stage develops.

Having described the overall development of groups, let us now look inside the group to the two critical sets of relationships which ultimately define the character of the group as a whole: member to authority and member to member.

MEMBER TO AUTHORITY AND MEMBER TO MEMBER RELATIONSHIPS

Our developmental literature informs us that members must reconcile the power and authority of the worker, in some kind of significant way, before they can fully develop their relationships with each other. While we recognize that the worker-member relationship is a dominant concern during initial stages of group development, it is not the group's only concern. The relationship between the worker and members does not develop in isolation of the members growing relationship with each other. While the members are working on their relationship with the practitioner, they are simultaneously developing their relationships with each other. They watch, and listen. While they are, as yet, unable to make substantial claims upon each other, they notice what each does. Though sorely underdeveloped at initial stages of group development, it is this set of peer relationships, which contributes to how the group as a whole "takes on the leader."

From our vantage point of practitioners, three critical variables particularly influence our behavior during the initial stage of group development: (1) our definition of function within the group, (2) our view of members, and (3) our understanding of the group as a collective enterprise.

As group workers, we learned early that we would always have a unique relationship with our groups. Our movement into settlements, the streets and neighborhoods, defined the very nature of our contacts. Once in members' milieu, ownership of the experience was shared. The group experience itself taught us that members were both part of their own solution as well as instrumental in contributing to the solutions of others.

"Truth" could not be transmitted from worker to members, but would become created via member action, via members helping each other. Participants would always be key to their own salvation. Ours would be a relationship of doing with, not doing to. We would ". . . act to help others act."[10] Our practice strategies would be directed away from a dependent, paternalistic relationship between worker and members and directed towards a partnership relationship through which the group could be strengthened to increasingly command its own fate. This strategy itself would influence the "resolution" of the "authority issue."

The definition of our role would become inextricably tied to our understanding of the group experience and the ways in which members contributed to each other. We would enter the group believing that mutual aid among members was central. While all who worked with people in groups instinctively understood this process of mutual aid among members, it was Schwartz (1961) who developed the concept and brought it center stage for all to use. Our practice literature is filled with the ways in which the concept of mutual aid has been useful to practitioners in shaping their thinking and practice.[11]

Conceiving of the group as an enterprise in which there are a multiplicity of helping relationships carries with it accompanying ideas about the relationship between the worker and the group and has direct bearing upon the way in which the initial stage of group development is experienced. An interactional focus, with worker and members influencing each other, shaping the meaning and character of the other within the group, has a profound effect upon the role relationship between worker and members within the group. Germain and Gitterman[12] state "In this view, client and worker roles shift from those of subordinate recipient and superordinate expert, often assumed to be characteristic of a 'professional' relationship." The worker is only the source of help; his/her vision and ideas part of multiple visions within the group. The worker's continual faith in the symbiotic connection between the group and its social institutions deemphasizes the centrality of the worker as *the* source of help. The worker's contribution is instrumental. Within this configuration the worker is taken out of the position of sage and moved into the position of working partner, though a partner with an interdependent function, different from that of the members. Each time the worker holds his/her view up for scrutiny there is movement towards more egalitarian relationships within the group. This posture on the part of the worker is particularly powerful when the group is beginning. It is through action that the worker demonstrates the kind of authority he/she will be. The creation of egalitarian relationships directly influence the way in which the authority theme is addressed and how the group ultimately develops. This is not to suggest that the power and control stage is ever easy for us, but rather, that the "resolution" of the conflicts integral to that stage proceed differently when the worker is part of a network of helping relationships than when the worker is viewed as the source of help and power and control remains located within him or her.

Once the members move beyond their concern with the worker, they can move frontally towards the development of their relationships with each other. While mutual aid always has the potential for development, obstacles to its maturation are ever present. Obstacles to the development of mutual aid among members[13] have the power to interfere with development of the group as a whole. The members must be free to use the worker and to help each other.[14] The development of social work skill in dealing with these obstacles becomes paramount. If the group does not progress in its development to a stage where members can actively be of help to each other, members are denied the strength and power of what should be theirs as a result of group association.

STAGES OF GROUP DEVELOPMENT AND THE TASKS AND SKILLS OF THE SOCIAL WORKER

We now turn to the tasks and skills of the social worker in using knowledge of stages of group development to assist the group in its growth. Defining the worker's role as helping members help each other do their work points to a strategy for action. The social worker remains at all times a centripetal force.

Knowledge of stages of group development within groups is insufficient as a guide to action. Only when this body of knowledge is combined with a definition of the task of the group can the practitioner bridge the gap between knowledge and action. Since action cannot be directly deduced from knowledge, the worker must use his/her vision of desired ends, namely, what the group is working on, as a bridging concept.[15] This point is brought home clearly when we compare Bennis and Shepard's (1956) and Garland, Jones, and Kolodney's (1973) views on how the trainer/worker should respond during the power and control stage of group development. Because the task of Bennis and Shepard's T-group members was to understand its own group process, the trainer felt no obligation to influence the development of that process in any particular direction. In contrast, Garland, Jones, and Kolodney (1973) were concerned that full catharsis would have too great a regressive potential for children whose task it was to develop social skills and have fun together. As a result, they urged social workers to limit cathartic expression before such powerful negatives could influence the group.

As practitioners face their groups, their knowledge base and understanding of the groups' tasks provide guideposts for the development of helping strategies. An articulation of helping strategies assists social workers in defining their professional tasks and the skills to be utilized in pursuit of those tasks. Five independent and reciprocal components define the interactional field of the social worker. They are: (1) character of group system, (2) character of member behavior, (3) member and collective tasks, (4) tasks of the social worker, and (5) skills of the social worker. As with all organic systems, these elements are continuously in motion, interacting with each other. The character of the group, at any point in time, is a function of this movement. While we separate our five components for analytic purposes, the group as a whole can only be known when these elements are considered together.

Discussion of Stage Integrated Components[16]

Knowledge of stages of group development inform an understanding of the tasks and skills of the social worker in helping the group accomplish its tasks. Since time does not permit a full discussion of all stages of group development, only the first stage in a group's development will be used for illustration.

Stage I: Pre-affiliation

Character of group system. At this initial stage, the group qua group is nonexistent and therefore is a source of stress rather than support to members. The work of the group is unknown and the focus ambiguous. The group is without structure or norms. A climate of trust has yet to be developed. Rules of behavior are individually rather than collectively determined. There are individual rather than collective relationships.

Character of member behavior. Members are unable to see a strong connection between their troubles and the troubles of others thereby increasing a sense of uniqueness and isolation. They have little connectedness and mistrust each other as well as the worker. Mistrust of the worker is based upon previous relationships with authorities. Indirect communication with an approach-avoidance pattern predominates. Strong social taboos and norms mitigate against intimacy and sensitive areas of work. Members are uncertain about their ability to handle the demands they imagine will be made upon them. The worker is tested before the members. Members display a visible need for acceptance and support from the worker as well as a desire to be directed. A familiar structure is desired as a means of diminishing anxiety.

Member and collective tasks. In this initial phase there is a need to develop a collective, specific idea of the work of the group based upon the connection between their need and agency service, whereby individual stakes can be located within the collective agreement. Members must establish an initial division of labor between the worker and themselves so potential benefits and obligations may be more clearly understood. The development of an initial structure for work and a culture in which authenticity and honest communication is the norm becomes important.

Tasks of the social worker. The primary task of the social worker in the initial stage is to clarify purpose and to arrive at a contract with the members as to the terms of their relationship and the focus of work. As components of this primary task, the worker is called upon to tune in and develop a preliminary understanding of what the members may be bringing to the experience. S/he is expected to help define the division of labor between the worker and the members in which respective roles are portrayed. S/he is further expected to contribute to the development of a working understanding among the members as to the terms of the contract highlighting the relationship between members' individual stakes and the stage of the group as a whole. Finally, the worker must draw from members their understanding of why they are there and get feedback on the contractual offer, all the time trying to establish a match between agency and member stakes.

Skills of the social worker. (1) To offer a clear uncomplicated statement about the mutual stake between agency and clients incoming together. (2) To generalize client need in an effort to establish connections among group members. (3) To partialize client need, making concerns understood in their specific meaning. (4) To develop receptivity to veiled client communication by responding to non-verbal and oblique expression. (5) To reach for feedback. (6) To encourage specificity in discussion and call attention to cloudiness of expression. (7) To translate covert messages.

If there were time we could apply the same schema to the other four stages of group development, to illustrate the necessary tasks and skills of the social worker over the life span of the group.

CONCLUSION

Stages of group development has been chosen as a critical concept, which when understood and utilized by the social worker, becomes a powerful tool in assessing groups and empowering them in pursuit of their tasks. The concept of stages of group development allows us to focus on the group as a whole at a particular moment and over time. Within this concept we have highlighted the importance of understanding member to authority and member to member relationships.

The following ideas are central to this proposition: (1) understanding stages of group development and the related tasks of the group enables social workers to closely link their helping efforts to the developmental needs of the group and its members; (2) the knowledge that group members must "resolve" the "authority theme" before developing intimacy among themselves, encourages the worker to not personalize challenges but rather to make his/her power open for examination and scrutiny; (3) knowledge of stages of group development when combined with an understanding of mutual aid among members directs the worker's activity to supporting connections among members and addressing obstacles to mutual aid; (4) aiding the group in its development empowers the group to become a mature helping system, capable of satisfying members' needs; (5) work with those dealing with environmental or interpersonal stressors demands a helping strategy designed to increase members' experiences of mastery, competence, power and influence. Strengthening the group as a whole is an accompaniment to such a strategy.

Within the concept of stages of group development, we have noted five commonly accepted stages: (1) Pre-Affiliation, (2) Power and Control, (3) Intimacy, (4) Differentiation, and (5) Separation. Each stage sets developmental challenges which must be successfully addressed so that subsequent stages can be mastered. Successful handling of Stage 2, Power and Control, (the authority theme) must occur if the group is to devote most of its energy to the tasks for which it has come together, rather than towards the resolution of tensions with the worker. Lack of control and hope, and loss of power, lead to an increase in alienation and feelings of impotence when members cannot adequately confront the worker's power. These feelings are already present for the vulnerable populations with which we work, i.e., the homeless, the elderly, psychiatric patients, children and adolescents. Successful handling of Stage 2 allows the group to move to the challenge of the next stage which is the creation of intimacy and mutual aid among the members. Assisting the group in helping members deal with his/her power and influence is a significant challenge for the social worker, a challenge for which a high level of skill is required.

Our discussion of stages of group development is rooted in a definition of the group as an entity in which people need each other to work on what has brought them together. Members' need for each other gives rise to an inherent multiplicity of helping relationships. The worker's helping efforts, while of a different order, are part of a system of collective helping activity. The practitioner becomes a working partner, directing his/her activity towards helping others to act. In this network of partners, hierarchical power decreases as egalitarian relationships and collective strength increases. Help is not passed from worker to members, but rather is created by members through their activity together. Only through their own efforts can members attain their goals. The worker's role is to help members work, providing skillful assistance in the process.

Knowledge of stage of group development and the internal member to authority and member to member processes becomes an assessment tool having the power to inform the practice of workers, supervisors and educators. Assessment of the group as a whole, as well as member to authority and member to member processes becomes possible. By identifying normative member and group stage related characteristics, practitioners can learn to spot departures from the norm. These departures become significant cues pinpointing specific targets towards which practitioners can direct their activity. This tool assists in determining whether the worker's activity is appropriate for the group's stage of development. Practice options relevant to each stage are increased, as well as more apparent.

As a tool for assessment, these ideas are deeply aligned with what the worker does to assist the group in its development. The social worker's tasks and skills in the group are intimately tied to the stage related, developmental tasks of the group. The same behavior at different stages of group development can have different meaning. The worker gets cues for action based on the stage of development. Similarly, we can determine when groups are not progressing in their development, locate some of the obstacles and address them with the group. And, by understanding the group's stage related capabilities, the worker can balance his/her demands to avoid overtaxing the group and increasing a sense of incompetence, or underdemanding and patronizing members.

The skill of the social worker is paramount in aiding the growth of the group as a whole. Some developmental literature suggests that cohesiveness is greatly aided by an inactive worker whom members can strongly rise against.[17] While these studies are useful in understanding group process they are inappropriate as guides for social work practice. Our function requires an active partnership with clients, not a practitioner outside the process manipulating members for their own good. Such manipulation stresses clients who are already environmentally and interpersonally stressed. Social workers, informed by an understanding of stages of group development are obligated and equipped to use that knowledge positively, by forming an alliance with group members on behalf of satisfying the needs which brought them together. These times demand no less.

ENDNOTES

1. See for example, Hare (1976), Lacoursiere (1980), Tuckman (1965), and Tuckman and Jensen (1977).
2. See Cissna's (1984) effort to examine the negative evidence.
3. Among other places, definitions can be found in Lacoursiere (1980, p. 25) and Bales and Strodbeck (1951, p. 485).
4. See Chin (1969) for a useful description of aspects of this process.
5. Gibbard, Hartman, and Mann (1974) provide a useful comparative discussion of these three types of models.
6. Most models reviewed by Gibbard, Hartman, Mann (1974), Hare (1976), and Tuckman (1965) are of this type.
7. This model can apply to all time limited groups. Mills (1964) and Mann et al. (1967) describe how these stages are revealed within the college classroom.
8. In addition to Tuckman (1965) and Tuckman and Jensen (1977) see also Anderson (1979), Babed and Amir (1978), Caple (1978), Lacoursiere (1980) and Lewis (1979) for classifications of the stages of group development.
9. Bion's (1959) work would be an example of this model.
10. Schwartz (1961) p. 159.
11. See for example, Shulman (1984), Lee and Swenson (1986), Gitterman and Shulman (1985, 1986).
12. Germain and Gitterman (1980) p. 14.
13. Gitterman and Shulman (1986), chapter 1, provide a discussion of obstacles to the development of mutual aid.
14. Gitterman (1983) suggests that interpersonal obstacles between workers and clients have additional roots, all of which make the worker less usable to the group and the group preoccupied with impasses to its work.
15. Millikan (1959) provides an important discussion of the relationship between knowledge and action.
16. The works of Caple (1978), Garland, Jones and Kolodney (1973), Gitterman and Shulman (1986), Lee and Swenson (1986), Shulman (1984) and Schwartz (1961) have informed the following discussion.
17. Lundgren (1971) makes this suggestion.

BIBLIOGRAPHY

Anderson, J. "Social Work with Groups in the Generic Base of Social Work Practice." Social Work with Groups. 2:4(1979):281-293.

Babed, E. and L. Amir. "Bennis and Shepard's Theory of Group Development: An Empirical Examination." Small Group Behavior. 9:4(1978):477-492.

Bales, R. and F. Strodbeck. "Phases in Group Problem Solving." Journal of Abnormal Social Psychology. XLVI(1951):485-95.

Bennis, W. and H. Shephard. "A Theory of Group Development." Human Relations. 9(1956):415-57.

Bion, W. R. Experiences in Groups. New York: Ballantine Books, 1961.

Caple, R. "The Sequential Stages of Group Development." Small Group Behavior. 9:4(1978):470-476.

Chin, R. "The Utility of Systems Models and Developmental Models for Practitioners." In W. Bennis, K. Benne, and R. Chin (eds.) The Planning of Change. (2nd ed.), New York: Holt, Rinehart and Winston, 1969.

Cissna, K. "Phases in Group Development: The Negative Evidence." Small Group Behavior. 15:1(1984):3-32.

Garland, J., H. Jones, and R. Kolodney. "A Model for Stages of Development in Social Work Groups." In S. Bernstein (ed.) Explorations in Group Work: Essays in Theory and Practice. Boston: Boston University School of Social Work, 1965.

Germain, C. and A. Gitterman. The Life Model of Social Work Practice. New York: Columbia University Press, 1980.

Gibbard, G., J. Hartman and R. Mann. "Group Process and Development." in G. Gibbard, J. Hartman, and R. Mann (eds.) Analysis in Groups. San Francisco: Jossey-Bass, 1974.

Gitterman, A. "Uses of Resistance: A Transactional View." Social Work. March/April(1983):127-131.

Gitterman, A. and L. Shulman. (eds.) "The Legacy of William Schwartz: Group Practice as Shared Interaction." Social Work with Groups. 8:4(1985/86).

Gitterman, A. and L. Shulman. (eds.) Mutual Aid Groups and the Life Cycle. Itasca, Il: F.E. Peacock Publishers, Inc., 1986.

Glassman, U. and L. Kates. "Authority Themes and Worker-Group Transactions: Additional Dimensions to the Stages of Group Development." Social Work with Groups. 6:2(1983):33-52.

Hare, A. P. Handbook of Small Group Research. (2nd ed.) New York: The Free Press, 1976.

Lacoursiere, R. The Life Cycle of Groups. New York: Human Sciences Press, 1980.

Lee, J. and C. Swenson. "The Concept of Mutual Aid." In A. Gitterman and L. Shulman (eds.) Mutual Aid Groups and the Life Cycle. Itasca, Il.: F.E. Peacock Publishers, Inc., 1986.

Lewis, B. "An Examination of the Final Phase of a Group Developmental Theory." Small Group Behavior. 9:4(1978):507-517.

Lundgren, D. "Trainer Style and Patterns of Group Development." Journal of Applied Behavioral Science. 7:6(1971):689-709.

Mann, R., S. Graham, and J. Hartman. Interpersonal Styles and Group Development. New York: John Wiley & Sons, Inc., 1967.

Millikan, M. "Inquiry and Policy: The Relation of Knowledge to Action." In D. Lerner (ed.) The Human Meaning of the Social Sciences. New York: Meridan Books, 1959.

Mills, T. Group Transformation. New Jersey: Prentice-Hall, Inc., 1964.

Schopler, J. and M. Galinsky. "Meeting Practice Needs: Conceptualizing the Open-Ended Groups." Social Work with Groups. 7:2(1984):3-19.

Schwartz, W. "The Social Worker in the Group." In The Social Welfare Forum, 1961, Proceedings on the National Conference on Social Welfare. New York: Columbia University Press, 1961.

Schwartz, W. "On the Use of Groups in Social Work Practice." In W. Schwartz and S. Zalba (eds.) The Practice of Group Work. New York: Columbia University Press, 1971.

Seitz, M. "A Group's History: From Mutual Aid to Helping Others." Social Work with Groups. 8:1(1985):41-54.

Shulman, L. The Skills of Helping Individuals and Groups. Itasca, Il.: F.E. Peacock Publishers, Inc. 1984.

Shulman, L. "The Dynamics of Mutual Aid." In A. Gitterman, and L. Shulman. (eds.) "The Legacy of William Schwartz: Group Practice as Shared Interaction." Social Work with Groups. 8:4(1985/86):51-60.

Shulman, L. "Group Work Method." In A. Gitterman and L. Shulman (eds.) Mutual Aid Groups and the Life Cycle. Itasca, Il.: F.E. Peacock Publishers, Inc., 1986.

Tuckman, B. "Developmental Sequence in Small Groups." Psychological Bulletin. 63(1965):384-399.

Tuckman, B. and M. Jensen. "Stages of Small-Group Development Revisited." Group and Organizational Studies. 2:4(1977):419-427.

Liberation Theology, Group Work, and the Right of the Poor and Oppressed to Participate in the Life of the Community

Margot Breton

The idea of social workers "reaching out" implies that they venture away from their traditional "turfs" and that they engage with different people than their traditional "clients" or group members. In and of itself, this process of reaching out could be construed as a straightforward extension of existing "turf" and clientele: an extension of professional and institutional power. However, this Symposium explicitly interprets reaching out as involving a challenge to the status quo, and issues a call to question existing professional and organizational power relationships.

This introduces the political factor at the center of the debate on reaching out. No longer can we be satisfied with the challenge to adjust to or create new environments in which to serve people, nor can we be satisfied with the challenge to adapt our skills or develop new ones to help new populations. If reaching out is to involve more than a pure extension of our professional "dominion," then we have to rethink our objectives in political terms, i.e., we have to question what power we are willing to forego and to what extent we are willing to redefine roles and functions.

In this paper I assume that among the people we want to reach are the poor and oppressed who have become involuntarily disenfranchised. I further assume that reaching out to them does not mean "plucking" them out of their environments and bringing them into our benevolent "arms"— agencies, institutions, services, whether these have been renewed or not. I see reaching out as a process of "re-enfranchising" whereby the poor and oppressed reclaim their right to be truly participating members of their communities.

When the Latin American liberation theologians made their radical

---

Margot Breton, MSW, is Associate Professor with the Faculty of Social Work, University of Toronto.

"Option for the Poor," they emphasized the right of the poor and oppressed to participate and share in the life of the community, and they
recognized that this meant using the "mighty weapon" of politics (Boff,
1986). It is in the noblest social group work tradition to prepare individuals to activate their right as citizens (or as franchised people) to participate in the life of the community and to engage in social action. However,
I think it is fair to say that this preparation has been perceived mainly as an
educational process of teaching individuals now to become good citizens
of a democracy. This, I submit, will not do when dealing with marginalized and involuntarily disenfranchised populations. These populations, as
liberation theologians (and people engaged in liberation movements in
general) point out, are not only needy, they are oppressed. Thus they are
not only in need of learning how to exercise their rights as members of
communities; as oppressed people who are denied these rights, their first
line of action is to have their rights reinstated.

If we acknowledge the reality of oppression, the root causes of non-
participation in the life of the community can no longer be seen to rest
primarily with the non-participating individuals. There must be a percep-
tual shift toward the causes residing in the existing socio-economic structures, which means moving from a primarily educational perception of
problems of participation to a primarily political perception. This paper is
a search for what is involved in a political perception of the problems of
the participation of the poor and oppressed in the life of the community.

In the first section, I look at how the liberation theologians of Latin
America come to the conclusion that political commitment is essential to a
theology which seeks liberative change. Then I identify some of the challenges with which the "comunidades eclesiales de base" (the small basic
ecclesial communities) confront the traditional power structures of the Roman Catholic church.

In the second section, I discuss how a number of issues raised by liberation theologians relate to our need to challenge the vested interests in the
status-quo of social group work practice. In conclusion, I deal with the
price we as professionals must pay, if we are to effectively reclaim our
own historical "Option for the Poor."

PART I: LIBERATION THEOLOGY

I am conscious of the warning from liberation theologians not to fall
into the rhetoric of liberation, or be caught in what Boff (1984, p. 74)
calls the metaphorizing mania whereby words like poverty or oppression
aren't given their real material meaning anymore but are "kidnapped"
and forced to speak in a metaphorical key, thus distracting attention from

concrete reality. Liberation theologians stress that the word liberation must be taken for what it is: "the concept of a historical reality, the reality of the social emancipation of the oppressed" (Boff and Boff, 1984, p. 81). The significance of this grounding in reality is crucial to understanding liberation theology and its impact. Segundo (1976, p. 41) points out that: "From its very inception liberation theology was a theology rising out of the urgent problems of real life." Boff (1984, p. 24) uses similar language: "There is only one, single theology of liberation. There is only one point of departure — a reality of social misery — and one goal — the liberation of the oppressed." This radical stance is reflected in the following conclusion: "For the kernel and core of liberation theology is not theology but liberation. It is not the theologian but the poor who count in this theology" (Boff and Boff, 1986, p. 1). Thus liberation theology starts not with the reading and interpretation of the scriptures but with a commitment to the liberation of the poor and oppressed.

Political Commitment

"Commitment is the First Step" (Segundo, 1976, p. 81); only after this "personal commitment to the oppressed" (ibid.) which arises out of a knowledge of the "concrete life of the people" (Boff and Boff, 1986, p. 8), does the liberation theologian turn to the (theological) "task of interpreting the word of God as it is addressed to us here and now" (Segundo, ibid., p. 8). This approach to theology assumes that "the major problems of man are definitely not tackled on a plane of certain knowledge," but that: "We live and struggle in the midst of decisive contextual conflicts without science being able to provide any ready-made option in advance" (Segundo, ibid., p. 76). Theology is no exception to this universal law and "it retains meaning only insofar as it remains in touch with the real-life context" (ibid.). It is in this context that human beings make options, including that of accepting theology and divine revelation itself. Therefore "the alleged problem of deciding whether we should or should not remain on the level of theological certitudes deduced from revelation is really no problem at all and hence can never be resolved. That is what Gustavo Gutierrez had in mind when he said that "theology comes after" (ibid.).

An exegetical analysis also brings Segundo to the same conclusion: "to place theology and its certitudes in the service of human beings who are scanning the complex signs of the times and trying to use them to find out how to love more and more, how to love better and better, and how to make a commitment to that sort of love" (ibid., p. 80). To conclude that commitment is the first step is to conclude that there can be no liberation theology without a liberation praxis, that is without taking actions that lead to the liberation of the poor and oppressed. And actions directed at liberative change presuppose a political commitment, as liberation theologians stress repeatedly, from Gutierrez in his seminal 1971 work *A Theology of Liberation* onwards.

The Basic Ecclesial Communities

It is in the light of political commitment that I look at the basic ecclesial communities and at the challenges they pose to the traditional power structures and 'modus operandi' within the Roman Catholic Church. The seriousness and extent of these challenges are captured in the title Boff (1986) gives to one of his works: "Ecclesiogenesis: the Base Communities Reinvent the Church."

The emergence of the basic church communities in Brazil began in 1956 (see Boff, 1986, for a detailed history). In a first stage, the members deepen their faith; then they begin to help each other. As they organize and think more thoroughly about their condition, they come to realize that their problems have a structural character. "Thus, the question of politics arises and the desire for liberation is set in a concrete and historical context" (Boff, 1985, p. 8). Though "The base ecclesial community does not become a political entity," it is "also the place where a true democracy of the people is practiced" . . . "For a people who have been oppressed for centuries, whose "say" has always been denied, the simple fact of *having a say* is the first stage in taking control and shaping their own destiny. The 'comunidad eclesial de base' thus transcends its religious meaning and takes on a highly political one" (Boff, ibid., p. 9).

Boff (1986) also documents the Inter-Church Meetings of the Basic Communities of Brazil, and notes that by the third meeting in 1978 "The unheard-of was happening, after 480 years of silence, a religious, oppressed people had the floor, and the monopoly of the corpus of church experts on speech was over." The fourth meeting (1981) was "a veritable celebration of the power of participation and organization lodging at the grassroots"; there Xoco Indians presented the struggles of their people in "playlets improvised on the spot," telling the story of how, armed with slingshots and facing police with rifles and machine-guns, they defended their lands.

Challenges to Professional and Institutional Power

The experiences of the basic ecclesial communities, as well as the theological reflections which conclude that commitment is the first step, have brought profound challenges to the status quo in the Roman Catholic

Church. Four challenges are particularly relevant to the theme of "Reaching out: People, Places and Power."

First, the challenge to the power of the clerics (or professionals) as representing a special class of people, the class of experts and specialists either on the theological or pastoral levels (i.e., either on the levels of theory or of practice). On the theological level, liberation theology holds that only after coming down from their ivory towers or academic 'places,' only after learning from the historical reality of the present life situations of a people, and only within the real life context of a political commitment to the liberation of the oppressed, will the theologian, along with other members of the faith community, attempt to understand and interpret the Scriptures. On the pastoral level, the vitality and concrete achievement of the basic ecclesial communities are such that Boff (1986, p. 2) would declare that the laity are "the vehicles of ecclesial reality, even on the level of direction and decision-making." In Latin America, as in many other parts of the world, the poor and oppressed form the overwhelming majority of the laity. Thus the challenge is clear: to learn from the poor and oppressed, to learn from their poverty and their oppression.

The second challenge is related both to the declericalization process and to the perception of the poor not only as needy but as oppressed. It is a challenge to abandon paternalistic concerns and practices (doing for the poor), and to adopt a conscientization or consciousness-raising model (doing with the poor). Leonardo and Clodovis Boff (1984, p. 3) capture the essential differences between the two approaches, as they explain that: "In times gone by, the Church was bound to the dominant classes, and it was through their mediation that the church reached out to the poor to whom the dominant classes were giving 'assistance.' The presence of the church was 'assistentialistic,' paternalistic. The church came to the aid of the poor, it is true, *but made no use of the resources of the poor in instituting a process of change*. Now the church goes directly to the poor . . ." (Emphasis added)

Going directly to the poor reflects the Church's "preferential option for solidarity with the poor (which) implies that it is the poor themselves, 'conscientized and organized' who must become the primary agents and operators of their own liberation" (Boff and Boff, 1986, p. 55). Latin American liberation theologians acknowledge the debt they owe to the Brazilian educator Paulo Friere "who taught us all about a 'pedagogy *of* the oppressed' (not *for* the oppressed), and about 'education as the practice of freedom' (not as a 'taming' process to facilitate the assimilation of the oppressed into the prevailing system)" (ibid.).

Indeed, the third challenge posed by liberation theologians is that of working not towards reform of the prevailing system, but towards basic structural changes or transformation of the system. This challenge stems from an analysis of the root causes of poverty and oppression in the countries of the South American continent. As Gutierrez notes (1986, p. 26): "The poor countries are becoming ever more clearly aware that their underdevelopment is only the by-product of the development of other countries because of the kind of relationship which exists between the rich and poor countries." This awareness is accompanied with a realization that "reformism . . . is synonymous with timid measures, really ineffective in the long-run and counterproductive to achieving a real transformation" (ibid.).

Liberation theology has opted for nothing less than this real transformation, that is for "structural changes which will reach the very bases of society, indeed which call for a new society" (*Puebla Final Document*, in Boff and Boff, 1984, p. 38). Let us not be mistaken, however. This new society is not one that will be "necessarily richer but rather more just and fraternal . . . more participatory" (Boff, 1985, p. 20).

The fourth and last challenge is to accept that conscientization, without which building a new society is not possible, involves a life-long struggle. As Segundo (1976, p. 210) points out, the processes of literacy-training and consciousness-training are essentially different. Unlike the former, the latter does not involve

a skill or mechanism that is 'possessed' once and for all. Instead we are dealing with an indefinite process . . . The person involved [in conscientization] becomes an active subject rather than merely a passive subject in history, life becomes more complicated, the resistance of society grows, and one must face more threats and sanctions from the social system that seeks to perpetuate itself and to reify its members. Moreover, the exercise of this new capability does not become easier with use, as a habit usually does . . . The more 'consciousness' one acquires, the more difficult it becomes to translate its growing demands into the complex and objectified social reality around one.

The people in the base communities are aware of the difficulties of translating these demands into effective political action. "A word that comes up again and again in the communities is *caminhada*: 'journey.' The people are indeed aware of the burdensome nature of their journey, a journey of resistance and struggle, not of facile enthusiasm." (Boff, 1986, p. 43).

Hopefully, this first section of the paper does not reflect a "facile enthusiasm" about liberation theology. Nor does it imply that the situations of oppression in Latin and North America are identical, or that the avowedly marxist theories used by liberation theologians to analyze socio-economic problems are the only possible theories to analyze these problems in the North American context. The premises and theses of liberation theology are presented to enrich our own thinking, as social group workers, of what it means to reach out to the poor and oppressed. To this task I now turn.

PART II: SOCIAL GROUP WORK AND THE POLITICAL COMMITMENT TO THE POOR AND OPPRESSED

Reaching out implies a challenge to professional social workers, to models for practice and to delivery systems. I look briefly at each of these challenges.

A Challenge to Models for Practice

It seems axiomatic that if social workers are to reach out effectively to the poor and oppressed, they have to question what they have learned from the "social action" and "reciprocal" models of practice. This is so because the assumptions on which these models are based do not hold for work with oppressed populations, i.e., with populations that are marginalized and involuntarily disenfranchised.

The "social action" model assumes that if individuals do not participate in the life of the community, it is because they are either unmotivated or unskilled in the art of citizenship participation. In other words it assumes that the opportunity to participate is always available to willing and able individuals in a system defined as an effectively-running, democratic and egalitarian society. Social group work contributes to that society, wrote Grace Coyle (1959, p. 100) through developing "habits and skills in democratic participation and the social attitudes and concerns which make for a healthy community life." From this point of view, it is the individual who, having learned how to be a good member of society, becomes responsible for the quality of community life. This educational approach must be recognized as an elitist approach which addresses itself to individuals who have benefitted to some extent from society and have a responsibility to give back to the community. It does not address itself, and Coyle (ibid., p. 97) admits this, to "the economically distressed." A fortiori, it does not address itself to those who are on the margin of society. People without a home, without a job, unable to feed their children or to access proper medical care because of existing social and economic conditions are not only poor, they are oppressed. And alienation is the quasi-inevitable consequence of poverty and oppression. When individuals have little control over their lives, when they have no "say" in what happens to them or around them, they become alienated and effectively disenfranchised. A model which focuses on individual responsibility cannot deal with problems of oppression and disenfranchisement.

Nor can a model such as the reciprocal model, which presupposes, between the individual and society, a symbiotic interdependence "of basic urgency to both" (Papell and Rothman, 1966, p. 74). The reality of oppression is that the oppressed are totally dependant on a society that exploits, oppresses and marginalizes them. Oppression presupposes not an interdependence but a breakdown between the individual and society: society expects nothing from the oppressed (save cheap labor when needed, or bodies to feed war machines), and the oppressed, alienated, expect nothing of society. In that situation, social workers have to conceptualize their functions as involving something different than mediation between two parties assumed to need each other and to be willing to reach out to each other. That "something" starts with political awareness of the implications of oppression and a political commitment to the oppressed, and leads to defending the interests of the oppressed against those of the oppressors. As Gutierrez (1984, p. 48) argues in *The Power of the Poor in History*: "Politics today involves confrontation . . ."

The Need for a Political Action Model: A Challenge to Workers

The need to take political action and to face the accompanying confrontation is recognized by social workers (Weiner, 1964; Germain and Gitterman, 1980; Lee, 1987); indeed Lee (ibid.) recently urged us "to break into the oppressive power system and disturb its equilibrium." But this involves more than a question of "political acumen" (Germain and Gitterman, 1980) and "political skills" (Lee, 1987), though group workers need to develop these. Acquiring acumen and skills is the easy part: the difficult part is to give up some of our power as professionals. I think this is why the calls to exercise political influence go largely unheeded and why we do not have a "political action" model—for a political action model is a power-sharing model. Perhaps we would have such a model in place had we not shunted Bertha Capen Reynolds' work aside during the McCarthy era. It is high time we restored her thinking at the core of social group work (I am indebted to Ruth Middleman for pointing this out to me).

As I reflect on Latin American liberation theology, I suspect that we group workers want to join with the oppressed but not let go of our self-appointed right to determine what is good for them; and that we are reluctant to learn from the poor and oppressed because that means giving up our claim to be the experts. I suspect that our tendency is to interpret the challenge to develop a "reaching-out" model of practice as meaning that we the professionals will find the right way of helping the oppressed and then will go and apply our new-found wisdom. In other words I suspect that if we are not reaching the oppressed and working effectively with them at this point in time, it is not especially because we lack political techniques nor because we have abandoned our social conscience: I suspect it is because we will not let go of some of our power as professionals and experts.

There may appear to be a paradox here, for workers often feel powerless vis-à-vis the enormous task of reaching and working with the oppressed. However, that feeling may simply mask a sense of frustration that *we* the professionals, *we* the educators, *we* the mediators, should have the power to change things for the better. Our challenge is to recognize the power of the poor and oppressed, and to help them recognize and harness that power — help them to become "conscientized" — so that *they* can be "the primary agents of their own liberation" (Boff and Boff, 1986, p. 31).

An example of this power took place at *Sistering*, a Toronto drop-in centre for isolated/homeless women. When the Board, because of funding cut-backs, reluctantly closed the week-end drop-in, Evelyn, the 74-year-old president of SUGI (the user group) had a petition signed up by about sixty women. She presented the petition at the annual meeting, and later at City Hall, before the Mayor and the Metro Social Services and Housing Committee. She was successful in getting the Committee (1) to vote funds to keep the drop-in open on week-ends for three months, and (2) to look into the issue of the responsibility of various levels of government for funding Toronto drop-ins (Sistering Newsletter, Summer 1988).

Group workers are familiar with conscientization at least as it applies to intra-group, interpersonal phenomena: after all, mutual aid, the process whereby group members become conscious of their power to influence one another and exercise that power, is a cornerstone of practice with groups (not only social work groups but, significantly, most psychotherapeutic ones). It is the extra-group, political dimension of conscientization that we are less familiar with or less inclined to digest. This dimension requires that individuals identify not only with a small group in which they feel they belong and in which their direct influence attempts result in a sense of greater personal well-being. The political dimension requires that individuals identify with those people outside the group who share their situation; it requires that they interact with the community of which they and the group are a part, attempting, often indirectly, to influence its institutions in order to bring about social change and greater social justice and well-being. This is why conscientization efforts should involve fostering a sense of group and *community* membership simultaneously.

Groups Open to the Community

Group workers should question why this does not happen on a regular basis: could it be that paternalism in group work takes the form of focusing on what takes place inside the group, thus "protecting" the group against the influence of the community and the demands of participation in the life of the community? We assume that members need to become attached to a small group *before* making moves toward the community: is this way of thinking a remnant of our original group practice, which was largely with children and youth? If we accept that for adults, achieving socially important goals is personally satisfying and nourishing, we need to rethink the assumption of a linear progression from personal goals to social goals.

I agree that "human connection is a prerequisite of social action" as Lee (1987, p. 1) has argued, but this should not imply that we define people only as "needy," when we should be defining them simultaneously as needy *and* oppressed. Too many groups never get close to social action of any kind, so deeply are they involved in meeting their members' needs. This happens even in groups formally designed as consciousness-raising groups: as Home (1981, p. 159) notes in her research on women's consciousness-raising groups, their tendency is "to remain on a personal level despite their avowed sociopolitical goals." It would appear, therefore, that there are different ways of "connecting" people, some leading to social action and some not, and I suggest that connections leading to social action emphasize simultaneous, dual membership in a group and in a community, or if not dual membership, dual "belongingness" to a group and to a community.

This implies that group workers search for more productive boundaries between the small group and the community — that they look at an "open-to-the-community" group concept (Breton, 1986), wherein the group is seen as constantly exchanging with the community of which it is a part. To this day, we are hindered in this kind of thinking by the fact that "we have learned to specialize by numbers'' (Schwartz, 1971, p. 19), and therefore our tendency is to leave everything that has to do with ''community'' to ''community'' workers, but one cannot conceive of politically effective groups, of groups which will help create a more just society, which are not open to the community.

Use of Networks

A greater openness to the community would lead group workers to network-building. We recognize the value of networks, yet how often do we help group members to create or use their own natural support networks? More pointedly, how many group workers convene people ''specifically with the expectation of creating 'weak' ties as opposed to 'strong' ties [even though this means] affording them access to a much wider range of resources'' (Shapiro, 1986, p. 118)? As we challenge our traditional ways of delivering services, we must ask why we neglect network-building. I submit this is partly because the more closed or insulated the group and the more the ties are strong, the more the professional group worker controls the process, including the one of mutual-aid which has come to be identified as a purely intra-group process. Last but not least, the more the resources available to people are those accessed through agency connections (i.e., through institutional networks), the more the social work agency, or the institutional system, controls both worker and group.

Challenge to Delivery Systems

If the above analysis is correct, effective reaching out to the poor and oppressed will involve more than individual group workers giving up some of their professional control and power and more than the development of new practice models; it will involve social work agencies giving up some of their institutional control and power, and accommodating to new models. In other words, change at the professional level must be backed by change at the institutional level. The experience of liberation theology in Latin America indicates that it could not have flourished without the backing of at least a part of the Latin American Roman Catholic Church hierarchy. The ''Bishops' Conferences,'' the direct involvement of a number of bishops with basic communities and their active defense of theologians against onslaughts from the Vatican testify to this support, and should encourage social workers to believe that it is possible to mount a successful challenge to the authority, power and vested interests of institutions.

CONCLUSION

This paper addresses a number of challenges, which can be resumed in the following question: Are we social group workers going to reach out to the poor and oppressed in an imperialist fashion, seeking to "colonize" people over whom, at this point, we have no influence, or are we going to join with them and accept to learn from them? If we choose the second option, we will pay less attention to what we have and what we know, and more attention to what they have and know. We will look at empowerment not as a gift that we powerful professionals make to those we identify as powerless; empowerment will mean that we recognize and accept the power that lies dormant in the poor and oppressed, and that we provide channels through which they themselves can activate that power, thus letting them be "the agents of their own destiny" (Gutierrez, 1986, p. 8). In other words, we will make use of their resources, instead of offering them no other option than to become dependent on us and our resources.

As a corollary of this liberative approach, we will not reduce competence to a set of abilities we experts teach the poor and oppressed, but we will recognize the competence which they already exercise to survive, and we will help them to use this competence to forge a more just and participatory society, a society (to paraphrase Boff, 1986) in which people are builders of services instead of merely clients or customers. A commitment to the liberation of the poor and oppressed demands this, for as liberation theologians insist: "a real sharing of power implies a real sharing of responsibility" (Boff, 1986, p. 25). Ultimately, that is the price social workers will have to pay to reach the poor and oppressed.

Leonardo and Clodovis Boff (1986, pp. 53-54) wrote that "'Good ideas' do not work *ex opere operato*. Liberation . . . is an action . . . Liberation activity can receive illumination and support from the 'thematics' of liberation, but they cannot replace it." Thematics of liberation are discussed in this paper; the real challenge at this point is for social group workers to engage in liberation activity.

REFERENCES

Boff, Leonardo. *Ecclesiogenesis: The Base Communities Reinvent the Church.* Translated by Robert R. Barr. Maryknoll, N.Y.: Orbis Books, 1977/1986.

Boff, Leonardo. *Church: Charism and Power.* Translated by John W. Diercksmeir. New York, N.Y.: The Crossroad Publishing Company, 1981/1985.

Boff, Leonardo and Boff, Clodovis. *Salvation and Liberation: In Search of a Balance Between Faith and Politics.* Translated by Robert R. Barr. Maryknoll, N.Y.: Orbis Books, 1979/1984.

Breton, Margot. "Professional Group Work Practice with the 'Hard-to-Reach' in Para-Professional/Community-Based Settings." Mimeograph, 1986.

Coyle, Grace L. "Some Basic Assumptions About Social Group Work" in Albert S. Alissi, *Perspectives on Social Group Work Practice: A Book of Readings.* The University of Connecticut School of Social Work, 1977, pp. 5-22.

Germain, Carel B. and Gitterman, Alex. *The Life Model of Social Work Practice.* New York: Columbia University Press, 1980.

Gutierrez, Gustavo. *A Theology of Liberation.* Translated and by Sister Caridad Inda and John Eagleson. Maryknoll, N.Y.: Orbis Books, 1971/1973.

Gutierrez, Gustavo. *The Power of the Poor in History.* Translated by Robert R. Barr. Maryknoll, N.Y.: Orbis Books, 1979/1984.

Home, Alice. "Towards a Model of Change in Consciousness-Raising Groups," *Social Work with Groups* 4: (1/2) (Spring/Summer 1981, pp. 155-168).

Lee, Judith, A. B. "Social Work with Oppressed Populations: Jane Adams Won't You Please Come Home?" *Social Group Work: Competence and Values in Practice*, Joseph Lassner, Kathleen Powell, and Elaine Finnegan, (eds.), Monographic Supplement #2, Vol. 10, (1987): 1-16.

Schwartz, William. "On the Use of Groups in Social Work Practice" in W. Schwartz and S. R. Zalba (eds.) *The Practice of Group Work.* New York: Columbia University Press, 1971, pp. 3-24.

Segundo, Juan Luis, S. J. *The Liberation of Theology.* Translated by John Drury. Maryknoll, N.Y.: Orbis Books, 1975/1976.

Shapiro, Ben Zion. "The Weak-Tie Collectivity: A Network Perspective" *Social Work with Groups* 9:4 (Winter 1986), pp. 113-125.

Wiener, Hyman J. "Social Change and Social Group Work Practice" *Social Work* 9:3 (July 1964), pp. 106-112.

Regaining Promise:
Feminist Perspectives
for Social Group Work Practice

Elizabeth Lewis

> The objective situation can only be modified by first changing the subjective consciousness.
>
> —Madonna Kolbenschlag

This paper explores several facets of feminist theory for its power to focus social group work practice with vulnerable populations more precisely. Through its examination of male-female relationships feminism has forced us to develop our subjective consciousness of the minute and massive ways in which one vulnerable population has been marginalized over time and in all cultures. Given this "dawning of insight" about women we may be in a better position to utilize the skills of social group work to change ourselves and the contexts of our lives.

Feminist theory should be useful to social group workers for several reasons:

1. It has current and well developed perspectives which have relevance for practitioners, three fourths of whom are women,
2. It deals specifically with a universally and historically vulnerable population, women, in whatever magnificent and confusing diversity of life stage, culture, class, race, religion, gender preference we claim,
3. It is rooted and grounded in a value,
4. Women have advanced the research knowledge about details of socio-psychological and structural vulnerability and their inter-penetration, and thus helped us to draw a more clear and practical map

Elizabeth Lewis, PhD, is affiliated with the Department of Social Service, Cleveland State University, Cleveland, OH.

for interventive strategies at the personal and interpersonal as well as the organizational level,

5. Perhaps the major reason for pursuing this analysis and seeking to draw parallels and points of relevance for social group work practice is the fact that feminist scholarship has undertaken the formidable task of analyzing major institutional structures which perpetuate disadvantage and inequality, namely

   a. the role of institutional religions, which build and maintain belief systems and laws of moral behavior,

   b. political institutions which regulate access to and participation in the development, management, and modification of the polity at all levels including national and international,

   c. economic institutions which control access to, and availability of resources that make possible not only the material necessities of life but confer the capacity to enter into cultural and intellectual creativity.

While feminist theory has focused on the structures and processes of women's victimization, this methodology of analysis can be applied with equal relevance to other vulnerable, victimized populations. There are particular parallels with conditions of minorities of color.

While this paper posits that feminist theory is preeminently applicable, it is clear that analyses of racism have preceded and oftentimes been entwined with analyses of sexism. There are differences, however. We have come to appreciate the different tasks of black women in the context of relationships with black men and their position in a racist society.

In its inception, social group work appeared to have the qualities of a social movement, based on values of equality, participation and self and societal fulfillment. It was critiqued as having little basis in theory but much in philosophy. Its technologies were pragmatic, action oriented and geared to being and doing. Its visions were of helping participants, members, to engage with one another and with some facets of their social world in an integrated and realistic effort. Its participants were socially vulnerable people.

From the perspective of a particular [any] vulnerable population a social movement is a critique of society, and projects a vision of what that society ought to be. Numbers of the population come to know the conditions of their oppression and disadvantagement in a conscious way through sharing and talking, primarily in small face to face groups. These experiences and insights represent the unravelling of one tapestry of life with its flaws and imperfections. Feminists have called it the process of "de-construction," the Chinese call it "speaking bitter" and Friere (and others) in South America called it "conscientization"; or, to return to the analogy, find and reveal the other side of the tapestry of life.

My recent, and late, explorations of the feminist movement resulted in a sense of familiarity. In an ambiguous way many ideas seemed familiar; much of the pain of discrimination and marginality expressed by women resonated to concerns about racism, equity in the work place and economic justice, which focused efforts of members, workers and agency on social issues and goals of social reconstruction in the early days of practice.

In some ways it seems to me that the practice of social group work has succumbed to the pressures for containment and management of symptoms and to the definition of participants (clients) not as equal partners and members in a common endeavor but as somehow damaged and defective beings. "Clients" by nature and endowment become less than capable of exercising their power, less than capable of exploring and naming the conditions of their vulnerability, and consequently being left with no choice but to act out the script which was written by others, whether inadvertently by worker, more instrumentally by agency, and by social definition and evaluation, by the wider society.

Feminist perspectives contribute to the regaining of the promise of social work practice in a number of ways. Through group experiences, we may develop:

1. A *common consciousness* of the embedded details of victimization
2. The systematic *de-construction* of negative and disadvantaging definitions of reality
3. The process of *naming*, of identifying the consequences of established structures and patterns
4. Trust in the *processes within the group* to reconstruct a new reality and to provide the context within which to test and practice new language, behaviors, expectations and aspirations
5. A belief in the *power of the group*, united to bring about desired changes in the context, however small these may be
6. A *sense of community* through the experience of reaching out and discovering allies and "same-thinkers and doers" in the wider social context.

Social group work (and social work) directs our attention to the importance of both identity and a sense of competence, both autonomy and relatedness of persons, to the paradox of a unique yet social person. Our own theorists of practice have helped us to conceptualize holistic, ecological, life space definitions of persons in society. Feminist theorists have advanced our knowledge of the process of "being and becoming," a term which Gertrude Wilson used to described social group work objectives.

CONSCIOUSNESS

Ruether (1983 p. 184) (Sexism and God Talk) speaking of the importance of connectedness says: "Consciousness is much more of a collective social product than modern individualism realizes. No one can affirm an idea against the dominant culture unless there is a sub-cultural group that gives people both the idea and social support for an alternative position." Modern feminism affirms in specific terms the philosophical and value positions of social group work, adds a complex analysis of historical and researched data about the inseparable nature of social humanity, yet needs the technical expertise of workers with groups to accomplish the consciousness and competence within members and groups to redefine identity and to develop alternative patterns of relating.

IDENTITY: DE-CONSTRUCTION

Early feminists did not necessarily challenge the "social construction" (Berger & Luckman, 1963) of female identity as spiritual, nurturing and tenderly emotional, but sought to enter the public arena through causes and associations most legitimate to "womanly" concerns. History identifies a concern for praxis over theory, for example, the cause of abolition of slavery—a public and highly political issue, but one in which "women's nature" could legitimately be involved; the issues of child labor, of care of mentally ill, of child health, all fall within the realm of appropriate "womanly" concerns. Social work itself was/and is a properly "woman's profession" by that definition.

It is interesting to note that the major contexts for early social group work practice were settlements and the Y.W.C.A.* Each had close ties to

---

*I would like to acknowledge the considerable help I have received from Margaret Berry, retired Executive Director, National Federation of Settlements, for insights on the Social Gospel and its importance to the development of church sponsored neighborhood settlements and centers, and for the Y.W.C.A. history of work with employed girls and women; to Dr. Ruby B. Pernell for insights into the historical efforts of Blacks to redress racial discrimination during and after the Civil War as well as in the 1960s; and to Ms. Evelyn Hunt for providing guidance to the formidable resources of feminist theory and theology.

religious institutions and gave opportunity to exercise the "social gospel" of Protestant denominations for men and especially for women. Think of the settlement house as a "home" within which women of education and means could create a "family" of concern. This was often with other women in a close and supportive community of affection and ideals; an opportunity to live in a neighborhood with neighbors, and gather a secular community of women (primarily within the Protestant tradition) so as to legitimate a single and presumably celibate, rather than married state. Women were able to enter the public or political realm through the concerns of neighborhood, within the context of family life and care and concern for children, for family health and safety, for the proper education of girls and young women in womanly arts, for reduction of poverty and of child labor, and for causes of peace (Porterfield, 1980, pp. 162-170).

Although remaining within a patriarchal church, nuns in holy orders were able to sidestep the challenge to feminine identity and definitions represented by celibacy, an unmarried state, through the idea of "marriage with Christ," and at the same time to achieve many of the advantages of maleness: advanced education, management of the organization and the often considerable resources of land and buildings, and selected industry, as well as to exercise professional responsibilities such as nursing and teaching and social service. These all are safely within the definition of femininity: spirituality, the vows of poverty, chastity and obedience to authority, are all reassuring commitments to a male defined identity and social order. The revolutionary and unintended subversions result from their demonstrated competence as women to reason and argue, to think creatively and to demand mastery and competence of themselves and of their students; to manage complex organizations, to acquire and manage property and to be role models of the whole woman.

While the Y was generally concerned with social justice for all, the Industrial Girls Department was concerned with programs for young working girls, factory girls, and with legislative efforts aimed at safe working conditions, protection from hazards, improved pay, and union organizing, a radical attempt to develop power to change systemic conditions. The Y residences provided safe and inexpensive housing, a home away from home, for young women without the protections of family or husband. If one were a bit cynical, the lack of support for the Y.W.C.A., even the efforts to combine YM's and YW's might be viewed as attempts to reduce options for young women to remain single and employed, since wages would hardly permit an independent life-style. Again, the women leaders staffed and managed organizations that provided an acceptable context within which to exercise women's capacities within the public as contrasted with the private/family domain.

Current and recent feminist theory challenges the biological and social definition of women, casting out the exclusivity of nurturance, spiritual purity, and emotionality as *peculiarly* feminine. The efforts to change thus move beyond either the political or economic to the theological and social/cultural, and thus challenge all institutional realms within which a delimited female identity is maintained. There is a difference in thrust. Biology no longer is destiny. There are clearly differing biological capabilities of reproduction, lactation, menstruation. These manifestly different functions are now accessible to greater control by women. While women will carry a child to term, there is an opportunity for choice rather than an inevitable acceptance of pregnancy. This element of choice in sexual matters is ultimately the major arena of battle between men and women.

While it is perhaps a human weakness to subsume another's identity within one's own familiar and valued self-picture, perhaps this process is more starkly visible when there are but two sexes, male and female. Over time and history, cultures and classes, races and religions, geographical locations and principalities and powers, women's identities have been subsumed in men's identities. Perhaps the universality of this oppression is what makes the feminist movement both most revolutionary and dangerous to the existing order and at the same time most promising as a vehicle for achieving a more just and human society. Feminism has a history of emergence and re-emergence over time and place, and a history of co-optation and containment not only by men, but by women who fear the danger of a lost feminine identity, circumscribed as it may be.

Group workers are familiar with the anxiety and conflict resulting from challenges to identify which result from the normal development in a new group. One is anxious in a new group when one's identity, competence and personal definition of desires and aspirations, to be achieved within the limited relationships with others may be, usually is, challenged. If the group is to become what it has the capability to become, each member must be willing to risk, and undergo the pain of a changing self-identity and discover and incorporate new and expanding capacities, knowledge and skills which come about with emergence of community. Daly (1973 p. 2) makes reference to the need for "existential courage to see and be in the face of the nameless anxieties that surface when a woman begins to see through the masks of a sexist society . . ." So too, new definitions of self and others in group formation and development are part and parcel of member/worker responsibilities in social group work.

At one time role theory provided important insights for social group workers. Feminists have explored in much detail the process of socialization to sex role. It is a conditioning process beginning at birth, within the family and reinforced by most institutions and social forms, especially the small face-to-face group. Both persons and mass media, clothes, toys, and professionals, such as teachers, doctors, social workers, all contribute to the process. "This happens through dynamics that are largely uncalculated and unconscious, yet which reinforce the assumptions, attitudes, stereotypes, customs and arrangements of sexually hierarchial society" (Daly, 1973, p. 5).

It should be apparent that the small social group, whether focused on consciousness-raising or on tasks in the surrounding environment, gives promise of developing the full range of human potential, not discarding spirituality, nurturance or emotion, but adding capacities for assertiveness, conflict resolution, decision making, cooperation and accomplishment of important social [public] tasks.

DE-CONSTRUCTION

Recalling our analogy of the tapestry, "de-construction" calls into question the image of the world largely woven by men. We are charged to see another side into which is woven the vast subtle and gross manifestations of power, and thus of systematic, patterned vulnerability. De-construction brings into question the idea of natural or inherent differences between the sexes beyond the genital, upon which most consequent definitions and expectations are constructed.

Research in other arenas, maternal-neonatal interactions, object relations theory, (Mahler, 1975, Gertrude and Rubin Blank, 1987) for example, demonstrate the impact of nurture and interaction rather than nature in this regard. Feminist researchers have attended to the inherent capacity of humans to construct language and to impart symbolism, i.e., meaning and worth through the spoken and written word, and to the patterning of thought and ultimately of behavior which comes about. The human organism seems capable of almost infinite varieties of language and thus of infinite ways of constructing meaning and interactive responses.

Daly (1963, 1978, 1984) is, without a doubt, the most radical of feminist writers in de-constructing words, language, meaning. "The-rapist," "gyn-ecology," "man-ipulated," "pre-history" rather than "his-tory" or "her-story" illustrate the fun we can have with this process! We are sensitized to the need to examine not only verbal but non-verbal cues which convey meanings, expectations, and the impact on self and others' identity.

The exploration of the behavioral, non-verbal has not limited feminist theorists in their attempts to move from the experiential to the more cognitive, conceptual realm of knowing, to affirm the affective, emotional knowing, to give it validity because it is real even if it cannot easily be measured or quantified. In other words, feminist theorists have pursued rigorous research on the human condition which is as valid as the more popular (masculine) model of rational, positive, quantifiable research. Perhaps if we were to use more familiar terminology we would speak of moving from the un- or pre-conscious to the conscious knowing, or as we used to say jokingly, "aha, the dawning of insight."

Feminist theorists speak of de-constructing essentially other-dominated (male) definitions and explanations, proscriptions and prescriptions with their built-in assumptions of power and privilege by developing essentially woman-constructed definitions, explanations and rules, built out of women's experiences. As Blacks and other minorities of color have come to reclaim and reconstruct their own histories, contributions and leaders, so women are emulating that process of exploring and identifying and including their own leaders, ideas and contributions to human history to make a more complete, holistic conception of human life.

Feminist theorists have concerned themselves with relationships, of self to self, to others, to family, friends, groups and associations and to the wider circles of belonging and participation. They have been concerned not only with access, but also with participation and with a quality of participation which is non-hierarchical, which seeks to respect diversity in the pursuit of community (unity). The pursuit of inclusiveness, which is difficult, is essential. Does this resonate to social group work goals? The promise within our practice should be quite apparent.

Social group work process, interpersonal interactions, become both medium and message, the opportunity for de-construction and re-construction at the most basic and perhaps intimate level. This can happen only when worker and members have learned to think in a critical mode, examining built-in assumptions and subtle consequences. From beginnings — with choices of members in the process of formation — through struggles to clarify purposes and objectives, develop norms of cooperation — through work/activity which is not confined within the boundaries of the group but extends in the surround of agency and community — skillful practice of social group work has the promise of freeing participants to discover and practice liberating modes of human endeavor.

THEORETICAL PERSPECTIVES

While there are numerous parallels between feminist perspectives and social group work practice perspectives, there are also some critical differences. As we are aware, the theoretical frames for practice cause us to attend to some factors and overlook others. Each has consequences for our interventions. Certainly, feminist perspectives incorporate a holistic view of the interlocking and inter-penetrating effects of material, social, intellectual and spiritual facets of human existence—what we have simplistically distilled into "system perspectives" or "ecological perspectives." This orientation closely parallels current social work and particularly group work perspectives, and enhances the congruence of these two realms. However, one critique of "systems" is its implication of naturally adaptive processes wherein the person and the social context arrive at a "goodness of fit." Goodness for whom? This appears to be an evolutionary, generally conservative time frame for change. Feminist perspectives, on the other hand, require the capacity to critique the system, to de-construct it in its essentially discriminatory aspects and to call by name those attitudes and expectations, terms of language, behaviors and social arrangements which cumulatively have a disadvantaging, marginalizing effect. A differently defined situation promotes alternative interventions and plans of action, within group between members, between group and context, or both. Actors may address a situation in radically different ways and results may be more profound than in the processes of gradual evolutionary change. We speak here of radical in the sense of getting at root causes, as compared with more cosmetic or symbolic changes which may leave the basic outcomes little improved. Mary E. Hunt (speech, Women-church conference, October 1987) highlights the place of emotion in this process of change, calling us to the holy use of rage, the commitment to structural, societal reconstruction which comes through the felt reaction to institutionalized marginalization, dehumanization and exclusion from full human participation.

In the realm of psychological theory the deterministic formulations of Freud and Erikson, Skinner, among others, receive critical analysis. Each is sexist, being designed in the male mode, and each has deficits in the limitation of human potential for personal and social "becoming." Daly (1973, p. 40) identifies "the need for knowledge which is subjective, affective, intentive and con-natural"; that which is available to worker and members within the immediate and experienced "now" of the group. She suggests that it is this knowledge, intuitive and as immediate apprehension of first purposes which provides direction and meaning for technical knowledge. Daly critiques severely what she identifies as purely technical or theoretical knowledge. The separation of theory from purpose makes theory insular, dogmatic and destructive and thus inherently damaging to the psychological and social sciences and to the professions which draw upon them.

In the philosophical realm much feminist writing is built on existentialism. This perspective had its advocates in the social work field, particularly as it stressed the "here and now" of life, self-actualization and indeterminacy. As with any other philosophical stance, extremes may have negative consequences. To me, the great emphasis on *self*-actualization, and a morality which is self-centered, is potentially hedonistic and counter-productive to the sense of community for which we strive. While this can be understood as an attempt to correct the sex-biased definition of women as self-sacrificing, self-abnegating, other-oriented, it represents the opposite side of the coin, and runs the risk of promoting merely a change from male domination to female domination. Individualistic and self-aggrandizing activity, male or female is counter-productive whether within a group or in the wider society.

Even the Roman church, persistently patriarchical, and certainly not existential has some flexibility, permitting an evaluation of an act within the particulars of context, i.e., self-responsibility and freedom of choice. It does not absolve one from the social consequences nor the necessity of weighing the personal and the social good and making decisions which have both proximate and long term outcomes, and which in most cases are made within ambiguous circumstances.

If I understand it correctly, existentialism does focus on the here and now, the nature of the moment, and on the potential for choice and the idea of "being and becoming." In this way it serves to counteract the fixety of a rational, positivist, essentially masculine definition of the world in which the games, rules, positions of the players, and the rewards are pretty much defined so that one team always wins. Feminist perspectives not only illuminate the idea of a win-win situation but suggest equity of positions and rewards, and most important, a different game and different rules.

Feminist perspectives draw our attention to the constructed world, language, words and names, behaviors, looks, actions, the unconscious absorption of norms and expectations, i.e., to the minute, the every-dayness of actions, interactions, thought and behavior patterns which perpetuate the social structures of discrimination and disadvantagement—which make vulnerable all members of a population which has either ascribed or achieved (or not achieved) attributes. For the population "women," feminist perspectives diagram in methodological detail how biology converts gender to inferior status which is then reinforced by language, by the construction of norms of behavior, social roles, and by designations of proper or natural relations between the sexes. It has sensitized us to the impact of historical recall or neglect of female contributions, the use of theological precepts in organized religions to reinforce essentially male prerogatives over women's bodies, minds, and life activities and expectations. In the United States these essentially social constructions of women's reality are included in all systems, economic and political, social, educational, theological, and familial. The potency of feminist perspectives lies exactly in that they have drawn attention to the subtle, unconscious and daily exercise of attitudes, beliefs, and behaviors which define and reinforce a despised status.

TRUSTING GROUP PROCESS

The relevance of feminist perspectives for social work practice with groups lies in the place of the small group including informal networks and collectivities as the major context and arena for experiencing social influence, for practicing and experimenting with different, even divergent behaviors, and for evaluating the outcomes of these social inventions. Next to familial interactions, small group interactions have both the potential for flexible performances, and for critique and reinforcement of behaviors which produce equity, harmony and personal development, or for structuring impetus for growth. Members/participants in small groups experience a range of difference or divergence over short periods of time, with a worker who brings her/his own perspectives on what is "good." They provide a safe arena for experimentation and analysis, and perhaps most important, for discovery of action-consequence connections. It is not surprising that the women's movement has utilized the small, relatively informal "club" type of group, with relatively homogeneous membership and female leadership (indigenous or otherwise) to enter the experimental and analytic world.

In social group work it is perhaps the danger inherent in empowerment, the potential loss of control represented by the developing consciousness and "we-ness" of the group entity, the members' capacity to name and define the inequities of the wider social context—which restrains workers and agency from pursuing goals of change beyond the members personally, beyond the confines of the group. It appears risky to deal with social structural change.

COMMUNITY

The feminist vision embraces community, the idea of unity in diversity, transcendence beyond either male or female, encompassing humanity. John L. McKnight (*Social Policy*, Winter 1987, pp. 54-58) in "Regenerating Community" sharpens our awareness of American society as bipolar, not in terms of male or female, but as individuals and institutions. The weakness inherent in such bi-polarity is that institutions may produce the opposite of what they are intended for: "crime-producing corrections systems, sickness-making health systems, stupid-making school systems" (p. 56). Institutions are designed to control people. McKnight makes the case for community as the large middle ground within which life is lived. He says "community is the social place used by family, friends, neighbors, local enterprises, associations as the major social domain." The structure of associations is the result of people acting through consent (p. 56). Associations are in his words the informal small groups which form the networks of support for every-day life. Summing the community of associations, he says they "provide a social tool where consent is the primary motivation, interdependence creates holistic environments, people of all capacities and fallibilities are incorporated, quick responses are possible, creativity is multiplied rather than channeled, individual responses are characteristic, care is able to replace service, and citizenship is possible" (p. 57).

McKnight offers three visions of community: the "*therapeutic*, requiring professionals and their services; the *advocacy*, in which labelled people will be protected by advocates, legal, support, locators, facilitators, a defensive wall of helpers; and finally, *community*, where people are enabled to contribute their gifts — the right of labelled people to be free."

Familiar threads are woven into this tapestry of community:

> *capacity* the fullness of each member to contribute; *collective effort* shared work that requires many talents; *informality* a critical element of the informal economy, authentic, unmanaged relationships, care, not service; *stories* reaching back into common histories and individual experiences for knowledge about truth and direction for the future; *celebration* associations in community celebrate because they operate by consent and have the luxury of allowing joyfulness to join them in their endeavors; *tragedy* the explicit common knowledge of tragedy, death, suffering. To be in community is to be part of ritual, lamentation and celebration of our fallibility. (p. 58)

This juxtaposition of universal community with feminist perspectives poses an ongoing tension for the social group work practitioner, operating within the institution, (the social agency) with its socially defined and circumscribed purposes and hierarchies. While these may serve as supports and functional parameters at some points, they may also represent the stereotypical definitions and expectations of a discriminating society, providing service to individuals who come as labelled, oppressed and victimized persons. The tasks for worker and members is to lose "no single thread" (Lewis, Beavers, et al., 1986) in the reweaving of the tapestry of life, to include all of the multi-colored threads of human capability, to help the members to own their group and to help this promise of community to be achieved.

REFERENCES

Berger, Peter and Luckman, Thomas, *The Social Construction of Reality*, Garden City, N.Y., Doubleday, 1966.

Blank, Gertrude, *The Subtle Seductions: How to be a Good Enough Parent*, Jason Aronson, Northvale, N.J., 1987.

Daly, Mary, *Beyond God The Father: Toward a Philosophy of Women's Liberation*, Boston, Beacon Press, 1973.

Friere, Paolo, *Pedagogy of the Oppressed*, New York, Seabury Press, 1970.

Hunt, Mary E., Speech, Women-Church Conference, Cincinnati, Ohio, October, 1987.

Kolbenschlag, Madonna, *Kiss Sleeping Beauty Goodbye*, N.Y. Doubleday, 1979.

Lewis, Jerry, Beavers, W. Robert, Gosseth, John T., Phillips, Virginia, Austin, *No Single Thread*, N.Y., Brunner/Mazel, 1976.

Mahler, Margaret, *On Human Symbiosis and Vicissitudes of Individuation*, International University Press, 1968.

McKnight, John L., "Regenerating Community," *Social Policy*, Vol. 17, #3, Winter 1987, pp. 54-58.

Porterfield, Amanda, *Feminine Spirituality in America*, Philadelphia, Temple University Press, 1980.

Ruether, Rosemary Radford, *Sexism and Godtalk: Toward a Feminist Theology* Boston, Beacon Press, 1983.

ADDITIONAL READINGS

Affilia: Journal of Women and Social Work, Feminist Press, N.Y.

Chambers, Clark A., "Women in the Profession of Social Work," *Social Service Review*, March 1986.

Freeman, Jo, "The Origins of the Women's Liberation Movement," *American Journal of Sociology*, Vol. 78, #4, January 1973, pp. 792-811.

Miller, Casey and Kate Swife, *Words and Women*, Garden City, N.Y., 1976.

Signs: Journal of Women in Culture and Society, University of Chicago Press, from 1976.

Social Work With Groups, Special Issue on Group Work With Women/Group Work With Men, eds. Beth Glover Reed and Charles Garvin, Vol. 6, #3/4, The Haworth Press, Inc., N.Y., Fall/Winter 1983; see esp. Guest Editorial: "Gender Issues in Social Group Work."

Van den Bergh, Nan and Lynn B. Cooper, eds., *Feminist Visions for Social Work*, Silver Springs, MD., N.A.S.W., 1986.

Consumer Control of Social Agencies: Case Study of a Black Mothers' Group

Betty Reid Mandell
Phil Postel

The clinical model of social work assumes that a treatment plan must be done cooperatively with the client, and must take into account the client's willingness to enter into the kind of treatment that the clinician is prepared to give. It also assumes that, if there is a diagnostic label to be given to the client, the clinician, as the expert, will give it. In order to engage the client in treatment, mutual expectations need to be clarified and, as Timms and Mayer say,[1] the client may need to be educated in the kind of treatment that the agency is prepared to give.

This model may work fairly well for people socialized into the culture and expectations of those who run agencies, predominantly white, middle-class people. It seems to work less well for people of a different social class/or race than agency personnel. Timms, for example, showed how baffled many white working-class clients were with therapeutic expectations of a family service agency in England.[2]

The civil rights movement, the War on Poverty, and the women's movement gave voice to a great deal of criticism of white, patriarchally structured, middle-class agencies and their treatment of women, minorities, and the poor.[3] Those groups often saw social agencies as part of the problem, rather than part of the solution. One of the most militant spokespersons for this point of view was Malcolm X, who, in his autobiography, cried out in rage and anguish against the state's social agencies that had broken up his family and put him and his siblings into foster care:

Betty Reid Mandell, MSW, is Professor of Social Welfare at Bridgewater State College, Bridgewater, MA. Phil Postel, MSW, is associated with the Massacuhusettes Department of Social Services, Plymouth, MA 02360.

Soon the state people were making plans to take over all of my mothers' children. . . . A Judge McClellan in Lansing had authority over me and all of my brothers and sisters. We were "state children," court wards; he had the full say-so over us. A white man in charge of a black man's children! Nothing but legal, modern slavery—however kindly intentioned. I truly believe that if ever a state social agency destroyed a family, it destroyed ours. We wanted and tried to stay together. Our home didn't have to be destroyed. But the Welfare, the courts, and their doctor, gave us the one-two-three punch.[4]

We believe that an important step toward empowering clients is to give them an *organized* and *institutionalized* part in shaping policies of the agency, in defining treatment, and in challenging labels and other expert views of the professionals. Many services that grew out of social movements, such as the civil rights and the women's movement, did just that.[5] Most professionalized social agencies did not. We suggest that their treatment effectiveness could be improved if they took this crucial, and difficult, step. As one contribution to a dialogue on how this might be done, we present here a case study of group work in a highly professionalized residential treatment institution that moved in that direction. We make no claim to scientific objectivity in this case study. It is one person's story, and others who were involved in the story may well tell it in a different way. Nevertheless, we believe that it contains a true message for social workers.

This is a story told by Phil Postel, a black social worker who several years ago worked in a private residential treatment institution. The story was told to a class of BSW students taught by Betty Reid Mandell, who taped it and now writes it down for the benefit of the social work community. Except for some editing for the sake of brevity, it is told in Phil's own words. Also included is some of the class discussion, which brought out some valuable points. Finally, we discuss the story from a theoretical point of view.

THE STORY

I was a very young, naive social worker entering a new agency, a private agency in a suburb about 10 miles from Boston—nice, lily-white suburb. I was hired as what they called a clinical associate, to see children and their parents once a week for counseling. Before I came to the agency, unbeknownst to me, they had this master plan about what I was going to do.

This was a place I wanted to go to because I had read about its philosophy in *The Other Twenty-Three-Hours*.[6] The thing I found attractive about it was that there was less emphasis on the one hour in therapy. The emphasis in this philosophy is on the hours outside the therapy session — a holistic look at people — and I was very impressed with that.

Let me tell you a little about the place. The suburb where it was located was a very white-oriented environment, and the institution very much reflected its environment. It was by and large white. I felt very isolated in terms of what that was about, very uncomfortable, and in moving into this place and trying to get situated in work with a lot of these people, I'm feeling just a bit uneasy about my own blackness. As it turns out, the plan was for me to serve the black clientele exclusively. I didn't know it was going to be that way, but that's the way it was. So they gave me my caseload and in reviewing it I found out that all the consumers who are assigned to me are black. My feeling is, "Well, this seems right. I feel comfortable with this. I think I can deal with this." So I kind of launched into it.

Well, it turns out that I was into one of the biggest surprises of my life. What they thought about me was that I was the Uncle Tom, the white spy, the one who kind of defected and went with *them*. So, in a sense, I might as well have been white. That threw me right off.

These women were described to me as "character disordered." Again, in my naivete, I didn't quite understand the far-reaching meaning of "character disorder." To me they appeared like most black people appeared, you know what I mean? They were all black ladies, they were all single mothers, they all had sons (obviously, since this institution served only boys). They all had been married at least once, and all their marriages had failed. The amazing thing about these 8 women was that, even though their sons had been at this institution for at least 2, and some going on 3, years, *none of them knew each other*. In fact, some of these mothers had never even *seen* each other, which I thought was pretty profound — that they had this kind of thing in common, but they didn't know it. Now part of that is geography. These mothers all came from the inner city of Boston — Roxbury, Dorchester, Jamaica Plain. So there were all kinds of issues that I began to discover in working with these people. One was the old classic problem that these people didn't have any wish to come to therapy, whoever the therapist was, so that was interpreted as some form of resistance, or non-caring on their part, that they couldn't get these mothers to come out and do their one hour of therapy, or whatever it was supposed to be at the time. They did not see the very logical issue of transportation being a problem, that these mothers had no transportation, that there was no public transportation to this facility. They were poor. Somehow that never got to be a concern for the agency. Anyway, I decided that my approach would be a little different, that I would not ask them to come out to this institution.

I was trying to get a co-leader for the group, and was unsuccessful. None of the employees wanted to touch it. In fact, it was clear that these mothers' sentiments about this agency were *felt* by the agency, because a lot of these employees were intimidated by these mothers, and really didn't want to be involved with them. In fact, at all costs they tried to avoid them. They were afraid of these women. So I didn't get a co-leader.

However, at some point this young woman comes to do an internship at the agency. The director kind of guided her my way. I don't know what she was into, but she said, "You ought to go check with Phil because he seems to be into some real interesting things this year. He's talking about doing a group of mothers. Go check with him." This lady comes into my office and there she stood—blond hair, blue eyes, I mean a picture of— you know—the ideal suburban white intellectual, explaining to me what she's about and how she's working on her doctorate and this and that, and the director says that you're doing this and I am kind of interested in that and I'd like to do something with you."

I told her, "Absolutely not, there is no way that I would go to face you with these black ladies. *No way.* I would get tarred and feathered by them, and so would you." To make a long story short—this lady was real persistent. She came back the next day: "I think this, and I think that. I think you should do that. . . ." I smiled and said, "I don't care what you think. You don't know what I've been through over the last year. You don't know what I'm dealing with. So I can appreciate your persistence about wanting to do something but it ain't here, it ain't with me. It's gotta be with somebody else out there."

In any case, this woman *was* persistent, boy, I'll tell you. She was back again on my back, and finally I relented. I said, "I will do this. I will think about entertaining you as a general observer, student observer. You'll have no authority whatsoever, in terms of the planning, you'll have no part of that, and I will at least try to sell that. Because the other thing that I recognized about this young lady was that she was a very bright young woman who had really developed some good skills. I was impressed with her insightfulness about me. As a matter of fact, she read me like a book, and I was impressed by that. And there was something about her throwing a hook in me that made me think, "There is something very good about this lady. She's very insightful." She was a really caring, sensitive, warm person who had a strong commitment to this field. And that put a hook in me. I wouldn't let her know that that was what was going into my feelings about her, but it was there, and that's why I entertained the possibility of her being with the group.

We went through a lot of planning. We decided that we would meet in the city at some local community place very familiar to them in the black community. And I was able to acquire some space in a building for free. It was very accessible by public transportation. I was *their* turf, known turf. That was attractive to them, that they didn't have to trek way out to . . . with no transportation.

We started out to introduce the group. We introduced the group's purpose as a discussion group around issues that they had about the institution and working with children and families at this institution. It was real safe, it was real broad, and that kind of was the stage of our first meeting.

I must tell you about my introduction of this young lady, who was with me at the first meeting. I obviously was fumbling and I was very awkward in trying to introduce this lady, and there she sat . . . I mean, she looked like a model, she was a very pretty lady. If she didn't look like white city, nothing did. And they had been giving me that business all year long. . . . You know you're an Uncle Tom, and you know you sold out to whitey, and blah, blah, blah, blah, on and on all year, so here I come with the evidence, right? Anyway, awkwardly I try to introduce her . . . and I quickly make the point about how she has no authority, and this and that, and I'm running this and this and that . . . at least try it at least once. . . . So we went through that whole ritual and tried to set a tone which was very safe and I was able to stimulate a really good dialogue with them and it kind of went well.

The second session I decided that I would try to get a film, to try to get away from my doing a lot of dialogue. I found this film. I thought it was a great film which seemed to reflect a lot of what their real world's about. The focus of the film was around a single mother, black, who's struggling. It seemed to fit all of what I was seeing in their personal experience. So I decided, " This is great stuff! I'll just show this film and this will be the *big* break-through. They really will finally kind of get at what I've been trying to tell them all along."

Showed the film. Put on the lights. What'd you think of the film? Silence. Nothing. Come on, get out some opinion about that. Turns out that these women were *extremely* angry about this film. Went on to tell me it had *nothing* to do with their lives—that they felt offended and indignant. They didn't need no help and they're tired, goddam it, of people telling them how to cope and what to do, and that's all that film was doing again. And you know, this was crapola, and you should have never brought it. And I felt about that high, because I thought I had a big winner and I just didn't know what to do with it. Frustrated, feeling real helpless. It was an amazing thing, because after their blast—believe me, they got worked up, they blasted me, all of them, some of them in harmony. They blasted me about that whole thing for the rest of the night.

It must be obvious to you by now that I was an inexperienced group worker. I had not lead a group before, and I had read very little about group process and group dynamics. If I had known then what I know now, I would have expected this "storming" behavior[7] and it wouldn't have thrown me as it did then. Now I understand better the mistrust that clients have toward institutions and "helping people" and the rage this creates. I understand better how group members need to challenge the leader's authority, and that this "authority theme" is never completely resolved, but is a continual interactive process between the worker and the group members. I know that the worker continually strives to deemphasize the centrality of the worker as *the* source of help, and becomes instead a working partner in an egalitarian relationship.[8] I know too that groups go through predictable stages of development. Now I recognize that the group members lashing out at me was part of what Garland, Jones, and Kolodny describe as the "power and control" stage of the life-cycle of the group.[9]

Now I am a more sophisticated group worker. Yet, despite my inexperience in group process at the time I led this group, I think that my basic honesty, empathy, and commitment to the democratic process, along with the skills that my co-worker brought to the process, somehow saw us through to a successful conclusion of the group.

At the next meeting I went to them, and I laid out my feelings. I laid out how frustrated I was, how helpless I was feeling, that I really did want to address what they thought were legitimate concerns, but I was throwing up my hands at this point and saying, "I don't know what you people want. In fact, do you want this group or not?" What came out of that was a major significant turnaround which I did not anticipate. They began to say that they thought the group was of some value. I said, "Oh, really? Well, what do you want to do with it?" What came out of that was they began to bring their concerns, their agenda, their issues, all to me. Which was what I was trying to get about all the time. In effect, they had kind of humbled me and said, "You are not going to tell us how to deal with our lives and dictate to us." What I kind of told them, "Hey, I've had it." It was sort of a humbling process. Then they were able to bring the things that did concern them. And it's amazing, because even I, who thought I had some very clear insight about what might be their priorities, was missing the point. There were some very common sense kinds of things, like their frustration and anxiety about the environments they live in, meaning "what I'm feeling helpless about is when my kids go out in the streets, I have no control. I mean, it's the kids in the streets who influence my child, dictate a lot of what that child's about, be it delinquent or crime or whatever."

They were very worried about their boys getting caught up in that whole scheme of things. Most mothers who live in those environments are *very* concerned about it, but they feel very helpless because they don't have any sense of control over it. It's nothing more than "I have to trust this child that he'll do the right thing when he's out there."

Another concern—one or two of these mothers had daughters—was the fear about their daughters becoming pregnant. With the age group that we're concerned about, young adolescents, it was a problem that was very pronounced in the black community . . . and they were feeling very helpless to do anything about it.

A significant thing that came out of that discussion was their perception of men. They were all *very, very* angry at men, and you can see how I could be a nice whipping boy for them. But they obviously had all had very painful experiences in their relationships with men. All of their marriages had failed. They felt that the men in their lives had contributed to the failure, the pain. They felt that they had been abused by men, both emotionally and physically, and were able to say how they were very angry at being deserted. They were left with these children, and those were things that had been festering with these women for a good number of years, a long number of years. It was interesting that one of the women was even able to say how, after having failed with a number of men, she realized that she was setting up a pattern for herself that was destined to fail by the way she approached men. Her expectations of them were the same all the time, so every time she went to another man, it always seemed to fall through. She was able to discover some of that herself and report that to the group.

Do you understand how rich, how significant that kind of dialogue amongst themselves was? Don't you understand that in that kind of dialogue, they were doing the best therapy that could be given? And the significant thing in all that was they began to resolve the feeling of feeling absolutely alone. In other words, "I'm the only mother who has to cope with this problem, this damned kid. No one else has to cope with this problem or this damned kid. No one else has to deal with that." And when they heard each other—"Wow! I'm not alone. I must not be such a bad person after all." It was an amazing session, and it began to set the tone for a lot of the remaining meetings.

Now let me come back again to this young lady who I started out talking about. As the sessions went along, she eventually became a much more involved person in the process, in terms of the planning and all of it. It was very important to me in terms of what she was able to contribute. She was able ultimately to win the trust of these mothers beyond what I had ever known with them. Now, I would attribute that to the attitude of caring that they were able to feel from her. She would go out of her way to pick up people at their home in her car, and drive them to the meeting place and drive them back home and she was also a woman.

More and more I kind of was on the outside, kind of looking in. I thought, "I'm the leader of this group; this woman is really *in* it." After a point I began to sit back and I looked at it. It was amazing, phenomenal, what had actually transpired in all of this time. And I began to really have a real appreciation of what was happening here, and I felt really good that these changes had come around.

We accomplished a lot that year, a tremendous amount. Because of the way things were structured, much of that they were able to do for themselves. That's the significant thing that I learned from all of that, that people need to have control of their own destiny. People need to feel empowered to overcome their own problems. That's significant, if you really want to be effective. And that's what was going on. And it was the first time that it had ever happened for them in their lives, around an institution.

We were coming to our last planned session, and a very touching thing happened. They decided that at the last session they were going to treat the leaders of the group to dinner, at one of the mother's house. They all decided they were going to get this meal together for us because they felt that ultimately we were of some importance, particularly the young lady. That was their way of showing us their appreciation for what that year had been about. And it happened, and it was tremendous. It was a wonderful, wonderful experience, that last session. And at that dinner, we talked about how we could close out the year. And they came up with the idea of addressing the people at this institution. They were a lot clearer with themselves now, and they wanted to bring out their concerns about what this institution ought to be about in dealing with minorities. And they wanted to offer them, as well as some suggestions about some of what they thought the agency ought to be about. So they put it together, the whole agenda. They requested that the director of this agency be the moderator of this meeting. They wanted to address the entire staff, and that was arranged.

I remember the director saying to me (I think he was kind of cautioning me), "Well, Phil, let me tell you this, that it's a possibility that the turnout for this session with your mothers might not be as great as you think it's going to be. In other words, it's likely that a lot of the staff won't show." All right. That's some of that old stuff that was still lingering and festering there—their perception of them. As it turned out, the majority of staff did show, although there was a good number that didn't—just were so afraid to go in there because they thought that they would probably be the subject of attack, or of chastisement of some sort. Because these mothers really were quite angry at one point and very verbal about expressing it. But the presentation itself went extremely well.

What are we looking at here? What you're looking at here is that the consumers, in fact, in taking on this task, began to run the agency. And I'm one who always believed that if that element is not in there somewhere strong you're not doing the right thing, and the agency is not doing the right thing. Ultimately, ideally, what *should* happen is that the consumers should in fact be running the entire scheme, because they know how to help themselves better than we do, actually. All right—systems are not really set up to accommodate that as easily, but you can still get at it. And, more important, you can always leave a person with a sense of control of her own destiny. *You* can do that as an individual, in any system. And it's *significant*.

That is the way that session got closed out. It was the most rewarding experience I've ever had in my life. I learned many, many things. It really isn't all that significant what color you are. You see that through all this? It really doesn't make any difference. The more significant thing is whether you really care about them or not. They have an acute sense of awareness, and they know when you approach them and how you approach them, how you talk to them, whether you really care about them or not. Their view is, "Somebody's coming to intrude in my life some more, to take some more of my intimate personal self away, to exploit whatever way they want." And believe me, that's a real reality out there. It happens all the time. And the difference was that that wasn't there.

At the last dinner, I remember we were talking a little bit about those issues when they first started, and this young lady whom I introduced, and they began to reveal some of their private thoughts about what they were thinking at the time I was introducing her. I mean, it was a fun session, because we were very close and the trust issues had been established and the bonding had been established. It was hilarious some of the things that they said to me that they thought that I was about, introducing this lady. And they kind of capped it by saying, "Well, in this room here, we're all black, and particularly this particular white lady." And if that isn't the essence of what I'm trying to show you here, then I can't show it to you any other way. If there's an issue around race, color, or any of those things, by and large it lies with you and how you carry yourself. It gets back to a sense of your own awareness and the world around you. Yeah, you and where you came from is very important, but also who you're dealing with and that world as well. In approaching any minority, if you have a wish to learn more about the culture, it's because it will enable you to demonstrate or illustrate the effectiveness of dealing with those people and caring about those people more proficiently. That's what it's really about.

CLASS DISCUSSION

Students made several astute comments, which we shall summarize here. One student asked Phil if he felt set up by the agency, and Phil agreed that he was set up to fail. Although he was not the only black the agency had ever hired, he had heard that the few other blacks who had worked there were people who were incompetent, so he had a bad track record to overcome. This put more pressure on him.

A student wondered if the fact of his co-worker being a woman was perhaps more important than the fact of her being white, in that she could relate better to the other women. Phil agreed that that was important, and also agreed that some of their hostility toward him was due to his being a man.

A student asked what his supervision was like. Did he get any help with these issues? Phil said that he was supervised by a psychologist who headed up the clinical department. He was seemingly very warm and nurturing, a caring person. Clinically he was quite astute, and was able to give a lot in this area. However, he was very naive about the issues involved with these women. His perceptions were stereotyped. In terms of these women's concerns, he was way out of touch. Phil had to discover most of the things he learned on his own.

A student asked if Phil thought the label of "character disorder" which had been given these women had something to do with the problem. Phil agreed that it did, and said, "I think there was a lot of what I would call cultural behavior, that other people would call 'black behavior,' that gets labeled. And I think it gets labeled with all kinds of things. One of their main issues, and one they were very angry about, was before they even got to this private agency, their kids had failed in the public school system. See what I'm saying? It was all before they got to this agency. They got labeled 'emotionally disturbed.' They were angry as hell about that, this labeling process, and they were very in touch with that. That's part of what I think contributed to their resentment about the agency, because as they viewed it — myopic as it is — it was 'white people doing this to me.'"

A student asked what follow-up has been done. Now that issues have been raised and brought out into the open, is the agency responding more to the needs of those women? Are they working better with the staff? Phil said he doesn't know as he has not been in touch with the agency for several years. However, that was the first time at this agency that parents had come to address the staff in the fashion that they did. It was done so constructively and so positively that there was a rash of groups that came up the next year. Everybody wanted to be in a group and there were groups all over the place. It was the glamorous thing to be about. So it did have some positive impact on the agency. At least minimally, it gave all parents and families — white, black, whatever — a sense of being empowered, a sense of being able to choose their own destiny.

Phil continued, "I left shortly after that year with the group. In fact, in terms of continuing to work with these mothers, it was phenomenal, because they were their own support group, their own network. They spent a lot of time with each other on a friendship level, such as baby sitting — 'Come on, bring your kids over here.' There were all those things that made their life pleasant. They were able to use themselves, and they felt empowered."

DISCUSSION

This story contains a thickly woven tapestry of meanings. We shall spin out a few of the most important threads to look at their theoretical implications, and their implications for social work practice. First, let us consider the location of the agency — 10 miles away from the community of the clientele, and inaccessible by public transportation. Does it raise again the question of community-based, community-controlled agencies? This proposition has been on the agenda since at least the 1960s in this country, and although some progress has been made since then, much remains to be done. In foster care and institutional care for children, it is a known fact that a child's ties to his or her family are strengthened when the placement is easy to visit. When children are placed far from home and visiting is difficult, they are less likely to ever return to their families than are children who have frequent contact with their families.

But, leaving aside the question of community-based services, let us look at the agency's lack of sensitivity to issues of social class. They seemed to have had no clue as to what it means to be poor, in practical, day-to-day terms. They probably did not live with, or near, the poor, and perhaps never did. If they were once poor, they had evidently forgotten what it was like. Their education apparently had not exposed them to the real life issues of poverty. Their professional education seemed to have dealt mainly with intra-psychic clinical issues, with little or no attention to sociology, anthropology, or political economy. When they worked with poor people as clients, they emphasized clinical pathology (the medical model) rather than social and environmental systems (the sociological model). This made them insensitive to some of the most powerful determinants of behavior — social class, race, gender, and culture.

Next, let us look at the intake policy of this agency. Why were only eight Blacks accepted as clients? In the Boston area, there is a great need for good placements, and there are never enough of them. Keeping the number of Blacks low guarantees their marginal status within the institution, making both the dominant culture and the minority culture forever aware of their *minority* status. It diffuses the potential impact that the minority could have. From her study of men and women in corporations, Rosabeth Moss Kanter[10] developed a slide-tape presentation called "The Story of O" to illustrate the problems of minority status in an institution. Her study focused particularly on women in corporations, but "The Story of O" applies to any minority in any institution. When there are 1 or 2 Os among many Xs (the dominant group), O's are assumed to be inferior, different, odd, not as knowledgeable, potentially dangerous because their very presence challenges the dominant culture. Similarly, a foreigner in a country is assumed to be at least a little dumb, and often quite laughable, simply because she or he does not understand the language and culture. This is reflected in popular humor and literature.

Now, using these insights, let us consider the agency's hiring policies. What did it do to black staff members to be the "token" black? Is it possible that those allegedly incompetent blacks who preceded Phil were no more incompetent than some of the white staff, but because they stood out as the "odd O" in a mass of Xs, they were perceived as inferior, different, odd? Flo Kennedy once said, "I am looking forward to the day when incompetent women and minorities can get the same jobs that incompetent men have held all along." In the case of a social agency, we would have to say "the jobs that incompetent women have held," since social workers are predominantly female.

At any rate, whether or not they actually *were* incompetent, they were perceived that way by the agency staff and this perception probably lent some support to their feeling that "Os are incompetent; therefore this new O who has just come is also likely to be incompetent." As the student commented so perceptively during the class discussion, it was a set-up. The new black social worker was handed a caseload that the other workers had found too hot to handle. Having done this, the staff probably felt a sense of relief that this problem was taken care of—the "uppity" black women had been given to the black man to take care of, and nobody else needed to worry about them any more. The staff was certainly not interested in co-leading a group with Phil—they had finished with *that* problem! It was fortunate that the new intern arrived without any stereotypes about Os and Xs and could see this particular task as an exciting challenge.

Now let's consider the implications of giving Phil an all-black caseload. First, the agency did it without telling him that this was their plan. He was not consulted about his wishes any more than the black mothers had been consulted about theirs. Possibly the agency's thinking went something like this: "Obviously a black person will understand black people better than do white people, because he belongs to the same culture." While this is more often true than not, it nevertheless did not take into account social class and gender differences, and it showed no awareness of the sociological implications of this decision. The clientele did not perceive it as a favor; they perceived it as the agency trying to "cool the mark": by giving them a black 'Uncle Tom" to act as a buffer between them and the agency. Fortunately, Phil was no Uncle Tom, and rather than "cooling the mark," he helped the women articulate and channel their anger to bring about constructive change.

And what was the medium used to bring about this change? A group. Individual therapy had only alienated these women and made them feel more manipulated. But in a group they overcame their isolation, developed a social perspective on their problems, formed strong bonds of community together, and moved on from there to try to change their environment (the agency). If they are structured well, groups are powerful instruments for bringing about both individual and social change. Why don't agencies use them more? Sometimes it is out of fear. One welfare worker, for example, when asked why he didn't organize AFDC mothers into groups, said that he was afraid of what they might say and do if they were organized—he was afraid they would *turn on him*! He knew how much anger they felt against the system, and possibly against him, and he could control them better when he dealt with them individually.

Groups could help combat the terrifying and debilitating isolation that is so pervasive among people today. It is this isolation that is at the root of many problems that social agencies deal with. The incidence of child abuse, for example, is highly correlated with isolation and poverty. Social workers often say that politics has nothing to do with their clinical work; that good clinical practice is a-political. Politics must wait until after work. Yet the very choice of a treatment modality can be a political choice. In choosing to do individual therapy rather than to organize a self-help group, a worker is often making a political as well as a clinical choice. In her study, *The Origins of Totalitarianism*, the political philosopher Hannah Arendt talked of the methods that totalitarian rulers use to control people. The most central of these methods is to isolate people, and the most important way to combat totalitarianism is to help people come out of their isolation.

> ... terror can rule absolutely only over men who are isolated against each other ... therefore, one of the primary concerns of all tyrannical governments is to bring this isolation about. Isolation may be the beginning of terror, it certainly is its most fertile ground; it always is its result ... power always comes from men (sic) acting together ... isolated men are powerless by definition.[11]

One of our most critical tasks is to help people form bonds of community together. Phil and his co-leader did this with 8 mothers. The pleasure and security which they found in the community that they formed undoubtedly radiated out to their children and helped to form stronger family bonds. It most certainly radiated throughout the agency. We hope that, through this article, it will radiate through the social work community.

REFERENCE NOTES

1. N. Timms and J. Mayer. *The Client Speaks*. London: Routledge & Kegan Paul, 1971.

2. *Ibid*.

3. One of the most notable studies of how Black children were treated in child welfare agencies is Andrew Billingsley and Jeanne M. Giovannoni, *Chil-*

dren of the Storm. New York: Harcourt Brace Jovanovich, 1971. A valuable study of 54 social agencies nationwide that serve predominantly minority clientele is Shirley Jenkins, *The Ethnic Dilemma in Social Services*. New York: The Free Press, 1981.

4. Alex Haley and Malcolm X, *The Autobiography of Malcolm X*. New York: Grove Press, 1965, pp. 20-21.

5. For a unique and valuable study of social services that grew out of social movements, see Ann Withorn, *Serving the People*. New York: Columbia University Press, 1985.

6. Albert E. Trieschman, *The Other Twenty-Three Hours: Child Care Work with Emotionally Disturbed Children in a Therapeutic Milieu*. Chicago: Aldine Publishing Co., 1969.

7. "Storming" is taken from Tuckman's formulation of the stages of group development: forming, storming, and performing. Tuckman, B. "Developmental Sequence in Small Groups," *Psychological Bulletin*, 63 (1965);384-399. Tuckman and Jensen later added another stage to this formulation, "adjourning": Tuckman, B. and M. Jensen, "Stages of Small-Group Development Revisited." *Group and Organizational Studies*. 2:4(1977):419-427.

8. This formulation of the worker's role is taken from Toby Berman-Rossi, "Empowering Groups Through Understanding Stages of Group Development."

9. Garland, J., H. Jones, and R. Kolodney, "A Model for Stages of Development in Social Work Groups." In S. Bernstein (ed.), *Explorations in Group Work: Essays in Theory and Practice*. Boston: Milford House, Inc., 1973.

10. *Men and Women in the Corporation*. New York: Basic Books, 1977.

11. Hannah Arendt, *The Origins of Totalitarianism*. Cleveland: World Publishing Co., Meridian Books, 1958, p. 474.

What Difference
Could a Revolution Make?
Group Work in the New Nicaragua

Maureen G. Wilson

Following the July 1979 victory of the *sandinista* forces, social work entered a period of crisis in Nicaragua. A view was held by some within the revolutionary alliance that the essential function of social work had been to contribute to the perpetuation of the old regime and that thus, with the revolution, this profession was no longer necessary. This idea initially prevailed, and in 1980 Nicaragua's only school of social work was closed to new admissions. The country's social work community quickly mobilized itself in response to this and was successful in persuading authorities of the need for social workers in the implementation of the nation's new social policy.

During the years prior to the victory of the popular insurrection, social workers in Nicaragua were already engaged in a reexamination of their roles and perspectives on practice. The usefulness of the functionalist perspective of the mainstream of North American thought which had dominated Nicaraguan social work practice until the early 1970s was thrown into question, and a search began for models more appropriate to the Nicaraguan reality. This paper examines the nature of group work in the context of the emerging models of social work practice in Nicaragua, as social workers redefine their roles in relation to the society's new social and political realities.[1]

Nicaragua was run virtually as a private estate of the Somoza family from 1933, when the U.S. military left the country with a U.S. trained and equipped National Guard under the command of Anastasio Somoza, until 1979 when this group was driven from power by the *sandinistas*. When the Somoza dynasty fell in 1979, Nicaragua's annual GNP per cap-

Maureen G. Wilson, PhD, is Associate Professor, Faculty of Social Welfare, University of Calgary, Calgary, Alberta.

301

ita was a very poorly distributed $800 U.S. Most people had annual incomes of $200 to $300 U.S., while the cost of living was almost as high as that in the U.S. Life expectancy was 53 years, ten years less than that for Central America as a whole and eighteen years shorter than that for Cuba.

A social service bureaucracy was first created in Nicaragua in the early 1960s in order to take advantage of U.S. foreign aid programs introduced as part of John F. Kennedy's "Alliance for Progress" initiatives. Few benefits, however, trickled down to the mass of the people. The new programs served largely as a way of providing employment and opportunities for the personal enrichment of the Somoza elite and its middle-class allies.[2] There was a growing international demand for cotton during this period, and peasants were once again driven from their land.[3] The social service bureaucracy which might have helped address the problems of the rural dislocation and rapid urbanization resulting from this was so hopelessly corrupt and inept that the problems of the poor were largely neglected.[4]

In spite of tremendous economic problems,[5] the Nicaraguan revolution ". . . achieved more social reform in five years than most prerevolutionary Latin American countries had accomplished in decades."[6] "Despite the hardships, war, poverty, and errors, the revolution has provided the majority of Nicaraguans with access to education, health care, and land — three primary desires of the once dispossessed."[7] A massive literacy campaign quickly reduced the illiteracy rate from approximately half the population to about ten percent. Health care, which had previously been available largely only to the urban and the wealthy, was extended to the entire population, and measles, polio, and diphtheria were virtually eliminate. These advances have been acknowledged by both the World Health Organization and UNICEF in granting Nicaragua their awards for best health achievement in the third world, and in UNESCO's unanimous choice of Nicaragua for its Grand Prize in recognition of the national literacy crusade.[8]

EMERGING MODELS OF SOCIAL WORK:
NICARAGUA IN THE LATIN AMERICAN CONTEXT

It is against this background that Nicaraguan social workers have engaged in the process of reconceptualizing their practice. It is interesting to note that, in contrast with a number of other professional groups, there appears to have been little division among social workers with respect to their support of the 1979 insurrection.[9] It would be a separate project of considerable interest in intellectual history/sociology of knowledge to analyze the dynamics of the various influences and experiences within the Nicaraguan social work community which would account for this, and for the relationship of this phenomenon to the emergence of the currently prevailing model of the professional social worker in Nicaragua. The scope of our task here, however, will be limited to the identification of some of these influences, an examination of the elements of this model, and an exploration of the implications of these for social work practice in general, and social work with groups in particular.

The emerging views of many Latin American social workers on the role of their profession in relation to the social formation are reflected in María del Carmen Mendoza Rangel's work, *Una opción metodológica para los trabajadores sociales.*[10] As Mendoza points out, the professional attitudes and methods of intervention of social workers in Latin America have been closely related to the historical moments in which the social workers have found themselves. Thus, in the early stages of capitalist development the emphasis has been on "social assistance," with "traditional" social work methods being applied, in the traditional forms of case work, group work, and community work. Corresponding to the stage of advanced capitalism, the emphasis has been on "social security," with the expansion of social programs to cover a larger proportion of the population, and attempts at unification and integration of these programs. Associated with this stage is an emphasis in social work methods on administration, supervision, and research.

In the historical conjuncture of a social transformation to a new society, the emphasis in social work is on the promotion of social change. That is to say, social workers recognize the need to work for a change in the structure of the society. Here, a dialectical method is employed by social workers, based on a "scientific method/theory of knowledge." This is described as a "collective" method, incorporating the knowledge of the social sciences and employing Freire's model of "popular education." Thus social workers, working now more directly with the poor, facilitate groups in analyzing their own positions in the historical moments in which they live, and in determining courses of action for themselves. In this model, social workers do not see themselves as politically neutral, but rather as actively taking the side of the poor.[11]

How is this thinking reflected in the practice of social work in Nicaragua? Some sense of this would be expected to be found in the view of social work practice represented in the design of the program of professional social work education: its declared goals, and the methods for attaining these goals.

Social work education began in Nicaragua in 1961 with the establishing of a program by the Nicaraguan Institute of Social Security (INSS), in response to a need for interviewers to handle applicants for pensions and other social benefits. In 1964 the first thirteen social workers completed this training. The following year the School of Social work moved to the National Autonomous University of Nicaragua (UNAN).[12] The curriculum of the School of Social Work until 1974 was greatly influenced by North American thought: its perspective was functionalist. Social workers during this period were engaged largely in palliative programs, charged with distributing eyeglasses, clothing, and food through INSS, the National Social Assistance Council (JNAPS) or religious organizations, or acting as functionaries in the administration of the corrupt and restrictive system of social security benefits.[13] In the field of community development social workers worked within poor communities, with the support of international organizations supported by the U.S. government, to promote the idea that these groups could work without violence to achieve a better life.[14]

While the above-described reconceptualization of social work was developing elsewhere in Latin America, and against the background of the growing Sandinista popular movement, dissatisfaction had begun to manifest itself among Nicaraguan students and professors with respect to their program of social work education. In 1973, some professors who insisted upon a traditional "social assistance" conception of social work were asked to resign and new professors, mostly sociologists, were hired who were to have an important influence in the search for a redefinition of social work which would be appropriate to Nicaraguan society.

Together, professors and students embarked on the task of a complete review of the program of social work education. After a semester of intensive work, a new plan of studies had been produced based upon a vastly altered conception of the profession. In 1974, this new program received the approval of university authorities. It reflected a marked shift away from the *tecnicismo* which had characterized the School's curriculum throughout its thirteen years of existence, and toward an emphasis on theoretical development. In the concern with overcoming this blind *tecnicismo* and producing social workers capable of the social analysis necessary for the promotion of social transformation, however, some imbalance now developed in the School's program. During this transitional period, the high level of theoretical content was not well articulated with concrete practice methods.[15]

In 1980, following the defeat of the Somoza regime, Nicaraguans entered into a process of review and transformation of their system of higher education as a whole. Included in this review was the country's only School of Social Work. As a result of this process, the decision was taken to admit no more new students, only allowing those already registered to complete their programs. The explanation given for this closing was that the function of the program and of the profession had effectively been to contribute to the perpetuation of the old regime and its gross injustices, and that for that reason it was no longer necessary.[16]

This decision impacted not only on the School and its approximately 150 students, but also on the roughly 200 practicing social workers. These groups united in a campaign to persuade university authorities and the Council of Higher Education of the need for social workers for the implementation of the country's new social policy.

Following these efforts, the decision of the Council of Higher Education was revoked, and in 1984 the program was reopened. It reopened, however, with new plans and new programs of study. Fifty students were admitted, on a regional basis, to daytime classes in a four-year program.[17] The curriculum is now said to be "based in a scientific conception of the world informed by the disciplines of philosophy, sociology, research and social planning, political economy, theory and methodology of social work, and social policy."[18]

What is the nature of this new program of social work education? According to a current mission statement of the School, the goals of the School of Social Work are consistent with "the political project of the *sandinista* popular revolution, based on [the following principles]:

- the revolutionary principles guiding the structural changes the country requires to achieve a more just and egalitarian society, suppressing all forms of oppression, domination, and exploitation of man by man [sic];
- the democratic principles which rest on a view of men [sic] as protagonists in their own history, free and conscious [political] subjects, architects of their own destiny;
- the principles which conceive of workers and peasants as the central propelling force of the revolutionary changes in our society, to which the rest of the social strata and popular sectors are articulated; [and]
- the antiimperialist principles that struggle to make our society free, autonomous, and capable of self-determination and of freely deciding its own future.[19]

It declares that, among other things, its graduates should be prepared to facilitate the democratic process of popular participation in the structural changes required to achieve a more just and egalitarian society. In defining the social work profession, it is noted that social work, notwithstanding the function it had served under the previous regime, has always been unique in its close contact with the social base — the popular majority.

> No profession in our country, no matter how old and traditional it may be, can define itself outside the revolutionary process in which we are living. Social Work, as all the other professions, assumed from its inception the sphere and the function assigned to it by the dominant class. Under this conception it developed as an instrument of reproduction of the existing conditions of domination — subjecting the great popular majority in our country. Nevertheless, this profession from its beginnings was characterized by its close contact with the social base, through its use of techniques of direct intervention in the social reality at different levels: community, group, family, and individual. This particular characteristic of social work, maintained and enlarged today as a necessity for the construction of the new Nicaragua, differentiates [social work] from other related professions.[20]

Interventions at the microsocial level, then, along with the contribution of the social sciences, help to provide bases for interpretations of the macrosocial reality. As a new definition of social work must base itself on the need of service to the process of social transformation, it follows that intervention at the microsocial level must serve the interests of the popular sectors. Social work thus

> . . . can be operationally defined as the profession which is characterized by its direct action with the popular sectors with the purpose of investigating and diagnosing their social needs in order to implement programs and projects directed toward the meeting of these needs. This work implies sharing of an objective knowledge of reality . . . [to facilitate] the carrying out of a systematic process of planning, execution, and evaluation of specific social projects . . . [These social projects] are not conceived without . . . the sensitization and organization of these popular sectors, [which] allows them to make themselves subjects of their own transformation.[21]

To the surprise of many Latin American social workers who look to the Nicaraguans for a model of future social work practice, this new program design has not involved an abandoning of either the traditional 'case work/ group work/community work' forms identified earlier as approaches to intervention appropriate to early stages of capitalist development, nor of the emphasis on administration, supervision, and research which emerge with the stage of advanced capitalism.[22] Rather, it would seem that these forms or categories of practice have been retained, but with methodology which is "rooted, generated, and developed in the context of the reality of [the Nicaraguan] people."[22]

Methods of case work, group work, and community work are taught in integrated methodology classes. Within each of the identified fields of practice (mass organizations, health, housing, social security, social welfare, labor, and education), the functions of the social worker are seen as including

- . . . the *design and implementation of social research* . . . for the implementation of social programs and projects directed at individuals, groups, and communities, as a result of needs [identified] by the popular sectors and [within] guidelines set by the state institutions;
- to *plan*, to *administer*, to *execute*, to *supervise*, and to *evaluate* . . . *social programs and projects* directed toward satisfying needs of a social and economic nature, with the purpose of treatment and/or prevention of the exacerbation of a specific social problematic: Housing, health, work, education, social welfare, etc.;
- to promote and consult on *community development* projects which encourage the conscious participation of the popular sectors in the meeting of concrete needs;
- to plan, coordinate, execute, and evaluate *training* of the work force of (both productive and service) enterprises or institutions;
- to organize *groups* at institutional and community levels for the treatment and prevention of problems or needs specifically of the group;
- to carry out studies, diagnoses, and treatments of social cases, including the *family* and the *community*, to the end of solving *individual problems*; and
- to determine, through socioeconomic studies of individuals and families, the possibility of obtaining *social benefits* given by different institutions.[24]

There is a strong emphasis on research, beginning with the first year of the program. While there is no intention to discontinue the teaching of conventional research methods and statistics, the major developmental concern in this area is in the area of methods of participatory research, which is seen to be more compatible with the popular education model.[25]

GROUP WORK
IN NICARAGUA'S NEW SOCIAL REALITY

Taking course materials related to group work methods as an illustration, let us now examine how some of the above-described influences are manifested in the training of professional social workers. Learning objectives with respect to Group Work Methods are declared to be:

a. That the student understand the social conditions constituting the context in which group work is practiced;
b. that the student know the general theories of group work;
c. that the student know the criticisms which have been made of group work;
d. that the student be trained in the organization, development, and evaluation of groups;
e. that the student be capable of contributing to the definition of a social work with groups which is in accordance with the changes in Nicaragua's social reality; and
f. that the student [be able to] analyze groups in the light of the Nicaraguan social context.[26]

Course content dealing with group work falls into five sections. The first, dealing with the emergence and development of group work, addresses the socio-economic and political factors which produce the need for group work, and also the influences of economic, political, and ideological factors on the nature of this form of practice. The second section touches on theory related to group dynamics, drawing on theory from the field of social psychology. The following two sections deal with group work theory and practice: theories of group work methods, fields of practice in group work, discussion of the organization and development of groups, and aspects of internal and external dynamics of groups. Finally, there is attention to a critical analysis of group work. This involves an exploration of alternatives which would contribute to the transformation of Nicaragua's global social process.[27]

Significantly, materials used in teaching methods of group work are ones put together at the School itself: no textbooks currently available were considered appropriate to the Nicaraguan context. These materials consist of a collection of readings virtually entirely on the theme of the methods of popular education, or "education for critical consciousness." This emphasis implies a number of assumptions about what should be the nature of group work practice. First, it implies the giving of priority to working among the rural and urban poor in a process which leads to action for change. This is an approach which involves the developing of class consciousness and the strengthening of popular organization, placing the worker in a role of facilitating the linkages between research and organization by and for the popular classes. Most importantly, its purpose is to strengthen the ability of people to organize themselves.

In terms of methodology, the process is one which begins with the concrete experience of the participants in the group, and proceeds to reflection on that experience in order to effect positive change. This can be described as a dialectical methodology for connecting theory with practice: beginning with the concrete experiences of the participants (practice), this method "helps them develop a critical scientific understanding of those experiences (theory), and leads them to more strategic action based on the new and deeper understanding (practice)."[28] It is an ongoing collective process, with a high level of participation, in which people teach each other and learn by doing. It is *critical*, seeking the structural and historical origins of problems, and it is *systematic*, demanding rigor in both its reflective and active phases. It involves full participation of people in both action and research, and also the use of cultural art forms in drawing on the creativity and energy of the people.

To what extent are these views of the School of Social Work on what should be the nature of social work practice reflective of the thinking/ practice of social workers in general in Nicaragua? While the data available at this stage enable us only to make some guesses at the answer to this, some clues are provided in the nature of the process through which the design for this curriculum was developed. Many informants commented that the 1980 closure of the School had been a healthy thing for both the school and the profession. It is said to have stimulated a great deal of positive discussion and raising of consciousness among social workers and social work educators. Some months after the closure, a national symposium of social workers was held to examine the role of social work in the new society. It is out of this process that the conception of the new social worker and the new curriculum evolved.[29] Ties between the School and the practice community appear to be very close, with a sense of "ownership" toward the School and its program on the part of the National Association of Social Workers.[30]

CONCLUSIONS

There is a great deal of interest in Latin America and elsewhere in the kind of social work practice which is evolving in Nicaragua. What have been presented here are some preliminary indications of approaches to the practice of social work, and of group work in particular, which are emerging in this revolutionary context. It is important to emphasize that the discussion here is based only upon preliminary data and, more importantly, that it relates to developments which are *in process*. A variety of constraints, barriers, limitations, and mistakes have been, and continue to be, a part of the story of this process.

The deepening economic crisis, further exacerbated by the devastation of hurricane Joan, has presented social work practitioners and educators with overwhelming material constraints in the carrying out of their work. Also, the historical legacy of the experience of the population of hundreds of years of authoritarian rule represents a major obstacle to be overcome in the development of the popular democracy, which is seen as central to the function of social workers. To declare a participatory democracy is one thing; to realize this in the context of a people with virtually no experience of democracy of any kind is a daunting task.

Foreign observers have sometimes expressed discomfort with the openly partisan support of both the Nicaraguan Association of Social Workers (ANTS) and the national School of Social Work for the *sandinista* political project. Some of the concern with this issue undoubtedly derives from the unique and sometimes confusing mixture of socialist and liberal democracy which characterizes the *sandinista* revolution, and which itself requires further critical analysis. The question, however, may be less difficult than it first appears. There is an important distinction to be made between support of the *political project* of the *sandinistas* and identity with, or uncritical support of, the *sandinista* state and its policies and programs. That is to say, support of the *sandinista* political project is not seen as in any way precluding the important role of social workers as critics of social policy.

In accounting for the striking lack of division among Nicaraguan social workers on this point, one is likely to be referred by representatives of the profession to the traditional values of the social work profession, which are affirmed to be perfectly congruent with the political project of the *sandinistas*. On this question, a policy statement called *Peace and Human Rights in Central America*, adopted by the National Association of Social Workers Board of Directors in June 1988, observed that

> Social work is grounded in a profound belief in the essential dignity and right to self-determination of the human person . . . These basic social work values are recognized as universal; they apply to all people, everywhere. Wherever these fundamental values are challenged or violated, social workers have a professional responsibility

to respond: to call attention to such situations, to object, to educate others, and to act.

Nicaraguan social workers accordingly played very active roles in the prolonged struggle to topple the Somoza dictatorship, with important heroes and martyrs of the popular insurrection coming from among their ranks. Not surprisingly, social workers have since been consistent in their commitment to defend the revolution and its attendant gains for the popular masses.

The process of reconceptualizing and redefining the profession in Nicaragua, begun in the early 1970s, then, has advanced in the context of the influences of political and professional developments in Nicaragua and elsewhere in Latin America, and of the historical, economic, and political constraints of the Nicaraguan reality. It is a process in which errors have been made, as was illustrated by the overreaction to the excess of *tecnicismo* which produced in the 1970s a high level of theoretical development which was unaccompanied by a matching level of development in social work methods. The bringing of these elements into balance and integration is a struggle in which the Nicaraguan professionals and professional educators continue to be engaged. Among the interesting sets of contributions to this process will be those of the 1988 graduates of the first cohort of students to be admitted to the newly reopened School of Social Work.

A final comment is in order. In attempting to describe the influences and struggles involved in the emergence of new approaches to practice, we have omitted giving serious attention to an important aspect of the reality of the context of these developments: the war. If the overriding mission of Nicaraguan social workers is to enhance "the organized participation of the people in the development of the society . . . as the practice of the popular democracy,"[31] then there must be an understanding of this, too, as a barrier to the exercise of this "popular democracy."

"Wartime is obviously not the most propitious moment in which to develop popular participation and democracy."[32] However, a protracted low intensity war is a fact of the social reality in Nicaragua within which social workers must carry out their work. It is important to recognize that this condition of war is not to be seen as anomalous, but rather as *normative* in the experience of young third world revolutionary states. Thus, the creative responses of Nicaraguan social workers to the challenge of carrying out their mission under these circumstances will be instructive to their counterparts around the globe.

REFERENCE NOTES

1. Data for this analysis were collected from a number of sources, including interviews conducted on site in 1986 and 1987 with practicing social workers and social work educators, and documents and publications of the Nicaragua's national School of Social Work and the Nicaraguan Association of Social Workers. Lic. Xanthis Suárez Garcia, then president of the Asociación Nicaragüense de Trabajadores Sociales (the Nicaraguan Association of Social Workers), was of great assistance during the 1986 field trip in providing background information, and in arranging interviews and site visits. Interviews and meetings were held with social workers in various offices of the Nicaraguan Institute of Social Security and Social Welfare, the Ministry of Health, the Nicaraguan Red Cross, the Ministry of Education, the Organization of Revolutionary Disabled, and the Berta Calderón Women's Hospital, as well as with representatives of the Nicaraguan Association of Social Workers, the School of Social Work (Universidad Centroamericana), the Heros and Martyrs National Council of Professional Associations, the Luisa Amanda Espinosa Association of Nicaraguan Women, the government Women's Legal Office, the Autonomy Commission for the Atlantic Coast, the National Commission of Support for Combatants, the Nicaraguan Institute of Economic and Social Research, the National Autonomous University of Nicaragua's medical school, and other hospital, day care, primary school, juvenile, and old age services. The Escuela de Trabajo Social of the Universidad Centroamericana, located in Managua, is the nation's only school of social work. The assistance is gratefully acknowledged of Gilma Yadira Tinoco Fonseca, who was the School's Director at the time of the 1986 field trip, and of Lic. Iris Prado Hernandez, the School's current Director.

2. Thomas Walker (ed.), *Nicaragua: the First Five Years* (New York: Praeger, 1985). In summarizing the impact of the Alliance for Progress, the editor of *Inter-American Economic Affairs* observed:

> During that period the distribution of income became even more unsatisfactory as the gap between the rich and the poor widened appreciably. During most of the period a very heavy proportion of the disbursements went to military regimes which had overthrown constitutional governments, and at the end of the period, with almost half of the population under military rule, a significant portion of the aid was going *not* to assist "free men and free governments" [in Alliance rhetoric] but rather to hold in power regimes to which the people had lost their freedom.

(Simon Hansen, *Five Years of the Alliance for Progress*, Inter-American Affairs Press,1967, p. 1, quoted in Noam Chomsky, *Turning the Tide: the U.S. and Latin America*, Black Rose Books, Montréal, 1987, p. 45.)

3. "Práctica historica del trabajo social en Nicaragua," no author, *Revista de Trabajo Social*, No. 1, November 1985 (Managua: Universidad Centroamericana), p. 12. This is a scenario that had been repeated several times since the arrival of the Spaniards in 1522. With a late 19th century coffee boom, for in-

stance, had come the Pedro Joaquin Chamorro Law of 1877, which drove peasants and Indians off the land. Five thousand rural poor were killed in a rebellion against this in 1881 in the infamous *"War of Comuneros."*

4. Walker, op. cit.

5. Inter-American Development Bank, *Economic and Social Progress in Latin America: 1987 Report* (New York: IDB, 1987), pp. 350-357.

6. Walker, op. cit. p. 297. It should go without saying that this progress has been seriously impeded by the draining of funds and labor by the *contra* war.

7. E. Bradford Burns, *At War in Nicaragua: the Reagan Doctrine and the Politics of Nostalgia* (New York: Harper & Row, 1987).

8. Tom Barry and Deb Preusch, *The Central America Fact Book* (New York: Grove Press, 1986), p. 294.

9. The Council of Professionals (CONAPRO "Héroes y Mártires") of which the Nicaraguan Association of Social Workers is a member is pro-*sandinista*. A number of other professional groups, however, divided over support of the *sandinistas*, and there is another CONAPRO (Council of Professionals) made up of those not in support of the revolution.

10. María del Carmen Mendoza Rangel, *Una opción metodológica para los trabajadores sociales* (no publisher, no date).

11. Ibid. On popular education see, for example, Paolo Freire, *Education for Critical Consciousness* (New York: Continuum Publishing, 1983), *Pedagogy of the Oppressed* (New York: Continuum Press, 1970), *Pedagogy in Process* (New York: Seabury Press, 1978); Gatt-Fly, *AH-HAH! A New Approach to Popular Education* (Toronto: Between the Lines, 1983); Francisco Vio Grosso, "Popular Education: the Latin American Experience," *International Review of Education*, Vol. 30, No. 3, pp. 303-314. The interest in this model among Latin American social workers was reflected in the selection of "Social Movements, Popular Education and Social Work" as the theme of the triennial joint meeting of the Latin American Federations of Social Work/Schools of Social Work/Centre for Research in Social Work held in Medellin, Columbia in July of 1986.

12. In 1984 it was moved again to the Central American University (UCA). Documents of the Escuela de Trabajo Social, Universidad Centroamericana.

13. Reinaldo Antonio Tefel, Humberto Mendoza Lopez, and Jorge Flores Castillo, "Social Welfare," in Walker, op. cit., p. 366.

14. Unpublished documents of the Escuela de Trabajo Social, Universidad Centroamericana.

15. Ibid.

16. Ibid.; "Práctica historica del trabajo social en Nicaragua," "Reapertura de la carrera y la situación actual," no author, *Revista de Trabajo Social*, No. 1, November 1985 (Managua: Universidad Centroamericana), pp. 4-5, 10-12; interviews with Xanthis Suárez Garcia, Gilma Yadira Tinoco Fonseca, August 1986.

17. Classes had previously been offered only during the evenings, and students had been almost entirely from elite or middle-class Managua families.

18. "Modelo del profesional del Trabajo Social," Escuela de Trabajo Social, Facultad de Humanidades, Universidad Centroamericana. This and all transla-

tions mine. The School of Social Work consists of a director, four full-time professors, and two student teaching assistants. It is a member of the International Association of Schools of Social Work and the Latin American Association of Schools of Social Work (ALAETS), and has close ties with the "Mildred Abaunza" Nicaraguan Association of Social Workers. It was the recipient of academic aid from two Netherlands universities between 1982 and 1986 and currently has one Belgian and one United States cooperant associated with the School, in addition to the author.

19. Escuela de Trabajo Social, Facultad de Humanidades, Universidad Centroamericana, "Modelo del profesional del Trabajo Social."

20. Ibid.

21. Ibid.

22. The Nicaraguans reportedly received criticism for not having discarded these prerevolutionary forms at the 1986 Latin American Federation meetings. Interview with Gilma Yadira Tinoco Fonseca, August 1986.

23. Edgard Macías Gómez, *Revolución y trabajo social: Del Trabajo Social en la Revolución a la Revolución en el Trabajo Social* (Managua: Servicio Educacional Sobre la Realidad, 1981), p. 47.

24. Escuela de Trabajo Social, Facultad de Humanidades, Universidad Centroamericana, "Modelo del profesional del Trabajo Social," pp. 5-6. Emphasis mine.

25. Interview with G. Tinoco, August 1986. The research currently under way by faculty and students at the school is organized around the themes of social policy and popular participation.

26. "Metodologia del Trabajo Social II: Trabajo Social de Grupo," course outline, escuela de Trabajo Social, Universidad Centroamericana, Managua, 1987.

27. Ibid.

28. Excerpt from Deborah Brandt, *Blowing Apart the Myth: Popular Education in Nicaragua*. (1988).

29. Interviews with informants identified in fn. 1.

30. When questioned about this, both the director of the School and the president of the National Association of Social Workers (ANTS, of which some 95 percent of Nicaraguan social workers are said to be members) declared there to be a very close working relationship between the School and the Association. The president of ANTS, in fact, asserted the Association to be "mamá y papá de la escuela." Interviews with G. Tinoco and X. Suáez, August 1986.

31. Ref. p. 8 of text.

32. Peter E. Marchetti, S.J., "War, Popular Participation, and Transition to Socialism: the Case of Nicaragua," in Richard R. Fagen, Carmen Diana Deere and José Luis Coraggio (eds.), *Transition and Development: Problems of Third World Socialism* (New York: Monthly Review Press, 1986), p. 304.

Index

315